# Health Information Management Compliance

## Guidelines for Preventing Fraud and Abuse

### Fourth Edition

## Sue Bowman, RHIA, CCS

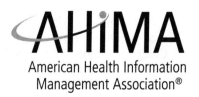

American Health Information
Management Association®

The Web sites listed in this book were current and valid as of the date of publication. However, Web page addresses and the information on them may change or disappear at any time and for any number of reasons. The user is encouraged to perform his or her own general Web searches to locate any site addresses listed here that are no longer valid. Web sites listed in this book are assumed to be preceded by http://www.

ISBN 1-58426-168-4
ISBN-13 978-1-58426-168-1
AHIMA Product No. AB102107

AHIMA Staff:
Claire E. Blondeau, MBA, Project Editor
Sue E. Bowman, RHIA, CCS-P, Director of Coding Policy and Compliance
June Bronnert, RHIA, CCS
Michelle Dougherty, RHIA, CHP
Katie Greenock, Assistant Editor
Susan M. Hull, MPH, RHIA, CCS, CCS-P
Carol Ann Quinsey, RHIA, CHPS
Rita Scichilone, MHSA, RHIA, CCS, CCS-P
Melissa Ulbricht, Editorial/Production Coordinator
Ken Zielske, Director of Publications

*AHIMA strives to recognize the value of people from every racial and ethnic background as well as all genders, age groups, and sexual orientations by building its membership and leadership resources to reflect the rich diversity of the American population. AHIMA encourages the celebration and promotion of human diversity through education, mentoring, recognition, leadership, and other programs.*

American Health Information Management Association
233 North Michigan Avenue, 21st Floor
Chicago, Illinois 60601-5800

http://www.ahima.org

# Contents

### Part I   General Compliance Guidance for All Healthcare Settings
*Sue Bowman, RHIA, CCS*

### Part II   Supplemental Compliance Guidance for Specific Practice Settings

*Susan M. Hull, MPH, RHIA, CCS, CCS-P, and*
*Sue Bowman, RHIA, CCS*

*Lynn Kuehn, RHIA, CCS-P, FAHIMA*

*Carmilla Marsh, RHIA*

# Appendices

## Resources on CD-ROM

Practice Brief: Guidelines for EHR Documentation to Prevent Fraud

Practice Brief: Delving into Computer-assisted Coding

Practice Brief: Update: Maintaining a Legally Sound Health Record—Paper and Electronic

Automated Coding Software: Development and Use to Enhance Anti-Fraud Activities

Report on the Use of Health Information Technology to Enhance and Expand Health Care Anti-Fraud Activities

## Sample Audit Tools on CD-ROM

ADL scoring review

Ambulatory coding review worksheet

Audit of therapy services

Audit summary sheet

Behavioral compliance audit worksheet

Coding audit review sheet

Coding audit summary

Coding compliance review daily worksheet: Inpatient summary

Coding compliance review: Inpatient summary

Coding compliance review: Outpatient summary

Coding and DRG variation form

Coding services review tool

Coding validation worksheet

Compliance audit

E&M audit tool 1995

E&M audit tool 1997

E&M shadow audit form

HHPPS coding audit tool

HHRG worksheet

Inpatient rebilling log

Inpatient review: Variations by coding professional

LTCH coding audit form

LTCH sample audit

MDS assessment schedule

Medicare certification-recertification requirements

# About the Editor and Authors

**Sue Bowman, RHIA, CCS,** is director of coding policy and compliance for the American Health Information Management Association (AHIMA). She holds a bachelor of science degree in medical record administration from Daemen College in Amherst, New York, and has earned the credentials of registered health information administrator (RHIA) and certified coding specialist (CCS) through the AHIMA. Prior to her current position, she held management positions in health information management (HIM) and utilization review in an acute care facility.

Sue is responsible for AHIMA's initiatives related to coding policy and compliance. She participates in the development of the *ICD-9-CM Official Guidelines for Coding and Reporting* and the content of the American Hospital Association's *Coding Clinic for ICD-9-CM*. In addition, Sue represents the AHIMA in meetings of the ICD-9-CM Coordination and Maintenance Committee and the American Medical Association's CPT Editorial Panel. She also has participated in the development of the Office of Inspector General's (OIG) compliance program guidances, including the guidance documents for hospitals, home health agencies, third-party billing companies, the hospice and nursing home industries, and physician office practices. Moreover, she has provided HIM consultative services to the OIG, the Federal Bureau of Investigation, and the Department of Justice on fraud and abuse and compliance issues. She has provided an educational program to OIG officials on health record documentation and coding practices.

Finally, Sue has written numerous articles and provided a number of media interviews on fraud and abuse, compliance, and coding issues, and has given a number of presentations on issues related to coding and compliance.

**Susan M. Hull, MPH, RHIA, CCS, CCS-P,** was a practice manager at AHIMA from 2002 to 2006. In her role as practice manager, Susan provided professional expertise to AHIMA members, the media, and outside organizations on coding practice issues and developed written products aimed at furthering the art and science of coding. Susan had more than 20 years experience in the HIM field. Before joining AHIMA in 2002, she served as Senior Executive Director for HMI Corporation where she oversaw coding reviews; chargemaster maintenance and development; and presented seminars in outpatient, inpatient, and physician documentation and coding. Prior to this, Susan worked in numerous HIM roles, including consultant, HIM department director, and HIM software developer and manager. In addition to AHIMA, Susan was actively involved as a volunteer in the HIM profession. She presented on timely HIM topics to the Health Information Management Associations of California, Tennessee, and Southern Illinois, as well as the Southern Illinois Healthcare Financial Management Association. Susan was also responsible for the development of education materials for a medical billing certificate program at Coastline Community College and Mt. San Antonio Community College in Southern California. Susan received a bachelor of arts degree and a master of public health in Health Services and Hospital Administration from the University of California, Los Angeles. Susan passed away on April 8, 2006.

**Ella James, MS, RHIT, CHPQ,** is the director of corporate health information management and health information security and the privacy officer at Center of Special Care in New Britain, Connecticut, which includes a 228-bed long-term acute care hospital and a 280-bed skilled-nursing facility. Ella is a former president of the Connecticut HIMA and has served twice on the board of directors for the organization. She is an AHIMA facilitator for long-term care. Ella also chairs the coding committee of the National Association of Long Term Hospitals (NALTH) and has presented programs on long-term acute care coding for NALTH regionally and nationally. Ella provides coding audit and educational services through NALTH for long-term acute care hospitals. She is a frequent presenter at state, regional, and national levels for several organizations, with topics including correct coding practices for long-term care coding, Center for Medicare and Medicaid Prospective Payment System for long-term acute care hospitals, and HIPAA. Ella has written and contributed to several AHIMA publications.

**Lynn Kuehn, RHIA, CCS-P, FAHIMA,** is president of Kuehn Consulting in Waukesha, Wisconsin. Previously, she was director of office operations for Children's Medical Group in Milwaukee. Additionally, she has served in HIM and coordination positions in a variety of healthcare settings. In her volunteer role, Lynn served as secretary and chair of the Ambulatory Care Section of AHIMA and the chair of several national committees. She has been a member of the AHIMA Board of Directors from 2005 to 2007. Moreover, she has presented at numerous meetings and seminars in the field of physician office management, coding, and reimbursement. Lynn has been the recipient of the AHIMA Educator-Practitioner Award and the Wisconsin HIMA Distinguished Member Award. Additionally, she has authored the AHIMA publication *CPT/HCPCS Coding and Reimbursement for Physician Services* since 2001.

**Carmilla "Kelli" Marsh, RHIA, RAC-C,** is a consultant and educator in the long-term care setting. As vice president of support services for Omnicare Pharmacies of Northern and Central Ohio, her responsibilities include providing consultation and services to numerous long-term care facilities on certification and licensure issues, quality assurance, and other related topics. She has taught numerous workshops on a variety of topics relative to long-term care. Carmilla previously served as the chairman of the long-term care section of AHIMA and received AHIMA's Volunteer Award for significant contributions in 2001. She is a member of the Ohio Nursing Facility Advisory Committee and the Indiana Casemix Advisory Committee and also serves as an instructor for the Ohio State University Administrator in Training Program for the Core of Knowledge.

**Linda Martins, RHIA,** is the operations manager for health information and reimbursement at Butler Hospital in Providence, Rhode Island, where she also serves as compliance auditor. She has 25 years of experience in behavioral healthcare including coding, compliance, and documentation. Linda is active in local and national policy issues, and has presented programs on Inpatient Psychiatric Facility Prospective Payment Systems for the National Association of Psychiatric Systems and the Rhode Island HIMA. Linda has served as education director and president of Rhode Island HIMA and was recipient of their Outstanding New Professional Award in 2001.

**Ruby Nicholson, RHIT,** has been director of quality improvement/health information at The Kent Center for Human & Organizational Development in Warwick, Rhode Island, where she has been employed for the past eighteen years. In addition to her role as director of the quality improvement and HIM departments, she is responsible for the organization's accreditation process, compliance program, and human rights office. Ruby has been involved in many state and national public policy forums. She has served as a member of AHIMA's Public Policy Task Force, past chair of AHIMA's Behavioral Health Section, and president of the Rhode Island Health Information Management Association. In 1995 and 2004, Ruby had the privilege to participate as a member of an HIM delegation to the People's Republic of China. Her enthusiasm and dedication to the HIM profession have been recognized by her peers both nationally and within her state. She was the recipient of AHIMA's Champion Award in 2000 and the Rhode Island HIMA Distinguished Member Award in 2003.

**Therese Rode, RHIT, HCS-D,** currently serves as senior coding manager for Inova VNA Home Health in Springfield, Virginia. During her 16 years of experience, she has served as a coding professional/analyst, privacy liaison, medical record manager/supervisor, and revenue cycle chart auditor in home health and acute care divisions of the Inova Health System. Prior to joining Inova VNA, Therese served in coding and medical record management positions for EHS Home Health Services (now Advocate Healthcare) in Oak Brook, Illinois. She is a member the District of Columbia Health Information Management Association and the Association of Home Care Coders.

**Patricia Trela, RHIA,** is the manager of PATrela Consulting in Quincy, Massachusetts.

# Acknowledgments

The author and publisher wish to extend their thanks to the following individuals for contributing electronic versions of audit tools:

**Prinny Rose Abraham, RHIT, CPHQ,** hiqmConsulting, Minneapolis

**Michelle Dougherty, RHIA, AHIMA,** Chicago

**Lynn Kuehn, RHIA, CCS-P, FAHIMA,** Kuehn Consulting, Waukesha, Wisconsin

**Mary Schafianski, RHIT, CCS,** St. Mary's Medical Center, Grand Rapids, MI

**Mary Stanfill, RHIA, CCS, CCS-P,** AHIMA, Chicago

**Anna Tran, RHIA,** Deloitte & Touche, Philadelphia

**Patricia Trela, RHIA,** Deloitte & Touche, Boston

The author and publisher also thank **Ida Blevins, RHIA,** for serving as a manuscript reviewer.

# Foreword

During the past several years, the need for health information management (HIM) professionals to understand and implement effective compliance programs has continued to grow.

We all strive to stay abreast of updates and changes to local, state, and national activities, in addition to the OIG model compliance program for hospitals, small group practices, and other types of healthcare organizations. It is of the utmost importance to have a resource available that is directed to the HIM professionals managing the highly complex issues surrounding compliance.

*Health Information Management Compliance: Guidelines for Preventing Fraud and Abuse* is ideal for HIM professionals working on compliance-related activities for facilities and other healthcare settings, as well as those professionals who are working to develop or revise HIM-related compliance policies. Advanced HIM students also will gain knowledge from this book that will position them for success as they enter the workforce, as it offers pertinent and up-to-date information applicable to the ever-changing health information landscape.

Health information managers should routinely validate their organization's existing compliance program. *Health Information Management Compliance* offers us the opportunity to ensure that we are aware of and are addressing the top priorities, and just as importantly, are offering solutions and tools to facilitate and implement a successful compliance program. This book offers helpful tips and tools to make this happen.

In today's fast-paced HIM world, we all constantly face new information, increased responsibilities, and rapidly changing technology. In order to sort through and adapt to it all while maintaining high levels of performance, we must capitalize on valuable resources. I hope that you will find, as I have, *Health Information Management Compliance* to be one such necessary resource.

Gail S. Garrett, RHIT
Assistant Vice President, Regulatory Compliance Support
Hospital Corporation of America

# Part I
# General Compliance Guidance for All Healthcare Settings

# Chapter 1
# Introduction

*Sue Bowman, RHIA, CCS*

The American Health Information Management Association (AHIMA) has developed this model health information management (HIM) compliance program to assist healthcare organizations[1] in formulating their own programs to ensure compliance with applicable reimbursement regulations and policies with respect to HIM.

Fraud is a significant drain on the US healthcare system. The National Health Care Anti-Fraud Association estimates that 3 percent of the nation's annual healthcare outlay—$51 billion—was lost to outright fraud in 2003. Other estimates by government and law enforcement agencies place the loss as high as 10 percent of annual expenditure, or $170 billion. Healthcare fraud is a serious and growing crime nationwide, linked directly to the nation's increasing healthcare outlay.

Fraud in healthcare is defined independently by a number of legal authorities, but all definitions share common elements:

- A false representation of fact

- A failure to disclose a fact that is material to a healthcare transaction

- Damage to another party that reasonably relies on the misrepresentation or failure to disclose

Only a small percentage of the estimated 4 billion healthcare claims submitted each year are fraudulent. Taken in total, however, the resulting cost is high, and the scope of activity is wide. Fraud takes many different forms, such as incorrect reporting of diagnoses or procedures to maximize payments, fraudulent diagnoses, and billing for services not rendered (Hanson and Cassidy 2006).

This model program provides guidance on HIM compliance with respect to fraud and abuse prevention. The publication's goal is to assist all types of healthcare organizations in formulating their own HIM compliance programs to ensure compliance with applicable

---

[1]"Organization" is used generically throughout this book to refer to all types of healthcare facilities and physician practices.

reimbursement regulations and policies with respect to HIM. The focus of this model program is primarily coding and health record documentation. The Office of Inspector General (OIG) within the Department of Health and Human Services (HHS) has noted in its Supplemental Compliance Program Guidance for Hospitals that perhaps the single biggest compliance risk area for healthcare organizations is the preparation and submission of claims or other requests for payment from federal healthcare programs (OIG 2005).

Specifically, this model program covers the HIM aspect of the key elements of a corporate compliance program (described in the section titled "Elements of an HIM Compliance Program" in chapter 2). The development of HIM policies or procedures, including those with respect to internal coding practices, documentation requirements, and medical necessity requirements, the provision of education to coding and other healthcare professionals, and auditing or monitoring methodologies are discussed extensively.

Chapter 6 describes the impact of electronic health records on HIM compliance and unique compliance challenges that have emerged in an electronic environment.

Chapters 7 through 13 provide supplemental guidance specific to settings other than acute care, short-term, or inpatient hospital services including hospital outpatient services, physician practices, long-term care, rehabilitation facilities, home health agencies, long-term care hospitals, and psychiatric facilities. Each of these settings has unique risk areas and compliance strategies because they are subject to different laws, rules, and regulations, including different Medicare reimbursement systems. Chapters 1 through 6 should be reviewed first, as **the chapters specific to certain healthcare settings provide supplemental information only and do not replace the general compliance guidance provided in the other chapters.** The general compliance guidance provided throughout the rest of the book is applicable to all healthcare settings.

The appendices provide helpful resources in the development of an HIM compliance program, including the following:

- High-risk areas for fraud and abuse enforcement related to coding and documentation issues

- Sample tools for implementation of an HIM compliance program, such as communication tools for improving physician[2] documentation

- Relevant AHIMA position statements and practice guidelines

- Suggested resources for obtaining additional information concerning Medicare reimbursement policies, correct coding practices, benchmarking, compliance program development, and fraud/abuse enforcement initiatives

An accompanying **CD-ROM** contains sample audit tools for various healthcare settings. These tools can help guide HIM professionals in the design of customized data collection

---

[2]Because healthcare professionals other than physicians may be legally permitted to order tests, provide healthcare services, or establish a diagnosis, the use of the term "physician" throughout this book is intended to include these other categories of healthcare providers. For example, the *ICD-9-CM Official Guidelines for Coding and Reporting* allows the health record documentation of nonphysician healthcare professionals, such as nurse practitioners and physician assistants, to be used for coding purposes when these healthcare providers are considered legally accountable for establishing a diagnosis within the regulations governing the provider and the facility.

tools for coding and documentation audits in their own organizations. Additional sample audit tools can be found on healthcare organizations' Web sites. For example, some quality improvement organizations'(QIOs) Web sites offer sample audit tools.

This model HIM compliance program is not intended for implementation by healthcare organizations "as is." Rather, the elements contained in this model program are intended to provide guidance to healthcare organizations as they design, implement, and refine their own HIM compliance programs. In addition, this book is not intended to cover healthcare reimbursement systems in depth but, rather, to concentrate on unique characteristics of current reimbursement systems that should be specifically addressed in compliance programs. It is also not intended to address compliance with all regulatory requirements affecting HIM practice, such as privacy. The focus of this publication is the components of an HIM compliance program designed to prevent fraud and abuse. Visit AHIMA's Web site (ahima.org) for resources pertaining to HIM practices outside the scope of this publication.

Every healthcare organization must design an HIM compliance program that meets its internal needs and addresses its specific risks. One size does not fit all. The actual content of the program depends on a number of characteristics unique to the organization, including culture, size, structure, setting type (clinic, acute care hospital, long-term care facility), and operational processes.

The OIG encourages the provider community to become involved in an extensive, good faith effort to work cooperatively on voluntary compliance to minimize errors and to prevent potential penalties for improper billings before they occur. As a result of this initiative, healthcare organizations have developed corporate compliance programs. A corporate compliance program is a systematic process aimed at ensuring that the organization and its employees and medical staff (and perhaps business partners) comply with applicable laws, regulations, and standards. This includes a comprehensive strategy to ensure the submission of consistently accurate claims to federal, state, and private payers (HCCA 2003).

An HIM compliance program is the component of a corporate compliance program that delineates policies and procedures and other requirements focused on HIM. The HIM compliance program must be developed in concert with the corporate compliance program because it must support the corporate program and have the commitment of the organization's top-level management. Because the compliance program encompasses HIM organizationwide, it is not confined to the boundaries of the HIM department.

A sincere effort by healthcare providers to comply with federal laws and regulations through an effective compliance program is a mitigating factor toward reducing a provider's liability. However, consideration of a reduction in penalties will occur only when the provider can demonstrate that an effective compliance program was in place before a criminal or civil investigation began. A compliance program will be effective in preventing and detecting regulatory violations when it has been reasonably designed, implemented, and enforced to do so. Moreover, an effective HIM compliance program is essential to the success of a corporate compliance program because the cornerstone of HIM—documentation of the provision of healthcare services—is the cornerstone of fraud investigations and the evidence of compliance. (See appendix A on pp. 261 and 262 for a description of HIM background and skills.)

The effectiveness of the HIM compliance program is measured by the success of the outcome (that is, compliance), not by the impressiveness of the processes that have been created. Additionally, the size and scope of a compliance program are not necessarily indicators of its effectiveness. An important objective is to *keep it simple.* Most organizations already have many elements of a compliance program in place. Existing policies, procedures, and standards (policies and procedures pertaining to coding, documentation practices, and health record completion requirements) need to be brought under the umbrella of the compliance program.

Each organization has an affirmative duty to ensure the accuracy of the claims it submits for reimbursement. A sound compliance program requires that reasonable measures be instituted to detect errors and potential fraud in the claims preparation process. Thus, there must be evidence of compliance through detecting, correcting, and preventing coding and billing problems and documentation deficiencies. It is important to note that providers are not subject to criminal, civil, or administrative penalties for innocent errors or negligence. The civil False Claims Act covers only offenses that are committed with actual knowledge of the falsity of the claim, reckless disregard, or deliberate ignorance of the falsity of the claim (Office of the Deputy Attorney General 1998). The Civil Monetary Penalties Law has the same standard of proof. For criminal penalties, a criminal intent to defraud must be proved beyond a reasonable doubt. Although not fraud, innocent billing errors are a significant drain on the healthcare reimbursement systems. Therefore, providers, Medicare contractors, government agencies, and consumers need to work cooperatively to reduce the overall error rate.

However, it is not enough to simply develop a compliance program. In addition to being effective, the program must have the full commitment of the organization's governing body, management, and employees. Adherence must be demonstrated at all levels of the organization. The OIG in the Department of Health and Human Services has indicated that it will consider a poor compliance program, or lack of adherence to the program, as being worse than having no program at all. Compliance controls need to be integrated into the very fabric of the healthcare organization's operations. A compliance program is never finished; rather, it is an ongoing, evolving process for continuous quality improvement.

Part I provides general compliance guidance for all healthcare settings. Part I should be read before the material related to specific healthcare settings. The setting-specific chapters in Part II provide supplemental compliance information focused on certain healthcare settings.

## References

American Health Information Management Association. ahima.org

Civil Monetary Penalties Law, 42 USC § 1320a-7a.

Hanson, S.P., and B.S. Cassidy. 2006. Fraud control: New tools, new potential. *Journal of American Health Information Management Association* 77(3):24–27,30.

Health Care Compliance Association. 2003. *Evaluating and Improving a Compliance Program: A Resource for Health Care Board Members, Health Care Executives, and Compliance Officers.* Minneapolis: HCCA.

Office of the Deputy Attorney General. 1998 (June 3). Memo: Guidance on the Use of the False Claims Act in Civil Health Matters. Available online from http://www.usdoj.gov/dag/readingroom/chcm.htm.

Office of Inspector General. 2005 (Jan. 31). *OIG Supplemental Compliance Program Guidance for Hospitals. Federal Register* 70(19):4858–76. Available online from http://a257.g.akamaitech.net/7/257/2422/01jan20051800/edocket.access.gpo.gov/2005/pdf/05-1620.pdf.

Office of Inspector General. n.d. Background on Civil Monetary Penalties. Available online from http://oig.hhs.gov/fraud/enforcement/administrative/cmp/cmp.html.

# Chapter 2
# Overview of an HIM Compliance Program

*Sue Bowman, RHIA, CCS*

The benefits of an HIM compliance are many, whereas the elements presented here are relatively simple to tailor to meet the needs of an organization. This chapter will present a description of the benefits and describe the elements that should be covered in an organization's compliance program.

## Benefits of an HIM Compliance Program

In addition to decreasing exposure to potential negligence, the benefits of establishing and adhering to an HIM compliance program will help an organization's bottom line. This section describes the specific benefits of an HIM compliance program.

The benefits include increases and improvements in the following areas:

- Internal controls

- Coding and documentation

- Education

- Communication, productivity, and efficiency

- Ethical practices

### Internal Controls

Effective internal controls ensure compliance with federal regulations, payment policies, and official coding rules and guidelines. Internal controls help shape and influence organizational norms and employee values. Internal controls constrain the system to function in a particular manner and also safeguard assets. A compliance program improves internal controls in three categories: preventive, detective, and corrective controls (LeBlanc 2006).

## Coding and Documentation

Although an organization's coding and documentation procedures may be effective, there is always room for improvement. Enacting a compliance program can improve an organization's existing procedures by:

- Identifying problematic coding and documentation practices and initiating prompt and appropriate corrective action
- Improving health record documentation
- Improving coding accuracy
- Reducing claims denial, which will improve financial performance

## Education

Even a highly educated and experienced staff requires continuous training and refresher courses. Ongoing education of staff is also supported by AHIMA's philosophy of lifelong learning as a guiding principle for professional development. The House of Delegates approved a lifelong learning resolution at AHIMA's 76th National Convention and Exhibit in 2004. The resolution is intended to affirm AHIMA members' commitment to lifelong learning and to encourage them to develop a professional development plan to prepare for the electronic health information management (e-HIM) future. "It really is important to make a statement about who we are and what we do, and a resolution is a way to do that," said [then] AHIMA president Melanie Brodnik, PhD, RHIA, during the meeting. (See figure 2.1.)

Enacting a compliance program will result in improved education for organizational staff and physicians as well as show an organization's recognition of the importance of ongoing education for HIM staff.

## Communication, Productivity, and Efficiency

Bringing HIM staff up to speed on a new compliance program will naturally result in increased interdepartmental communication by improving collaboration and cooperation among healthcare practitioners and those processing and using health information. These increased checks and balances among employees in various job roles will also increase productivity as a result of staff better understanding the intricacies of compliance, and will result in greater operational efficiency and improved financial performance. Ultimately, an organization can expect an end result of improved employee performance and morale.

## Ethical Practices

Creating a compliance program entails examining all existing procedures. This scrutiny could result in identifying previously undetected HIM practices that may be considered unethical and potentially illegal. Those who draft the compliance policy should refer to AHIMA's Code of Ethics (see appendix E).

Having a compliance policy in place reduces exposure to civil and criminal penalties and sanctions in the event of a fraud investigation. Even if wrongdoing is discovered by the government, the severity of penalties imposed will be reduced.

## Elements of an HIM Compliance Program

An effective HIM compliance program consists of the following nine elements:

1. Mission

2. Code of conduct

3. Oversight

4. Policies and procedures (discussed in chapter 3)

**Figure 2.1.   Lifelong Learning Resolution**

---

**Embracing Lifelong Learning: The Guiding Principles for Professional Development**

At the AHIMA 76th National Convention and Exhibit (Washington, DC; Ocotober 2004), the House of Delegates approved the following resolution to raise awareness and promote lifelong learning to AHIMA members:

- Whereas, the healthcare and technology environment will continually change the HIM professionals' role;

- Whereas, data show that individuals who continually advance their educational standing are rewarded with the highest compensation;

- Whereas, the most sought-after professionals are flexible and can demonstrate their knowledge and skills;

- Whereas, HIM professionals' skills and competencies are a valuable and integral part of the healthcare arena; and

- Whereas, ultimate success depends on the willingness of individual members to take responsibility for preparing for new roles by acquiring new knowledge and skills; therefore, be it

- Resolved, that AHIMA make available the new knowledge and skills that will enhance members' value in the marketplace;

- Resolved, that AHIMA members commit to mentoring and helping others to advance HIM practice; and

- Resolved, that AHIMA members make the commitment to lifelong learning and professional development so that HIM professionals continue to be vital players in ensuring quality healthcare through quality information.

---

Source: AHIMA 2004.

5.  Training and education (discussed in chapter 4)

6.  Communication

7.  Auditing and monitoring (discussed in chapter 5)

8.  Enforcement

9.  Problem resolution and corrective action

## Mission

An HIM mission statement should be written and consistent with the healthcare organization's mission statement. Although its exact wording should be unique for each organization, just as each healthcare organization's mission statement is slightly different, certain key points should be addressed, including the following:

- HIM staff are committed to ethical and legal business practices.

- HIM staff are committed to making every effort to comply with federal and state statutes and regulations, private payer policies, official coding rules and guidelines, and the accepted standards governing the practice of health information management, including appropriate clinical documentation practices.

- HIM professionals value health information of the highest quality, as evidenced by its integrity, accuracy, consistency, reliability, and validity.

- HIM professionals demonstrate behavior that reflects integrity, supports objectivity, and fosters trust in professional activities.

- HIM professionals refuse to participate in illegal or unethical acts and to conceal the illegal, incompetent, or unethical acts of others.

- HIM professionals believe that collaboration and cooperation among healthcare practitioners and those processing and using health information are essential to ensure high-quality health information and accurate claims submission.

- HIM professionals respect the confidentiality of individually identifiable health information.

- HIM professionals are committed to developing internal policies and procedures that are consistent with reimbursement regulations and policies, official coding rules and guidelines, and prohibit coding practices that inappropriately maximize reimbursement.

It is very important that the organization expressly prohibits maximization and affirms this prohibition in the mission statement, code of conduct, and policies and procedures. **Maximization** involves manipulation of the sequence of codes or adding codes that are not substantiated by the health record documentation. However, **optimization** is acceptable and even encouraged. Optimization involves sequencing and selecting the codes such that the organization receives the optimal reimbursement to which it is entitled, while adhering to all of the applicable rules and guidelines pertaining to proper coding and documentation.

## ② Code of Conduct

Along with an HIM mission statement, the healthcare organization should develop an HIM code of conduct. The AHIMA recommends that its Standards of Ethical Coding be used as the basis for the organization's HIM code of conduct. (See appendix E.) Every employee, in addition to contracted consultants and independent contractors (such as outsourced coding staff), involved in the coding function should be asked, initially at the time of employment and annually thereafter, to sign and date a statement affixed to a copy of the code of conduct. (See figure 2.2.) The signed copy of the code of conduct should be kept in the employee's personnel file.

An organization also may choose to specifically include adherence to federal and state regulations, payer reimbursement policies, and the organization's own policies and procedures in the code of conduct. The code of conduct should be reviewed annually, perhaps at the time of the annual performance evaluation.

## ③ Oversight

The AHIMA recommends that an HIM professional with demonstrated honesty and integrity and a strong background in coding be charged with responsibility for overseeing the HIM compliance program. Depending on the size of the organization, this responsibility may be the individual's sole duty or added to other responsibilities. This position is referred to as the HIM compliance specialist throughout this document for illustration purposes. However, the specific title of this position may vary from organization to organization. (Appendix C contains a sample job description for the position of HIM compliance specialist.)

Depending on the organization's size and structure, this position might be either part of the HIM department or external to the HIM department. Locating this position outside the HIM department allows more objectivity in the responsibilities of this position because

**Figure 2.2.   Example of a statement regarding the code of conduct**

I have read and understand these Standards of Ethical Coding and agree to abide by them at all times. If at any time I believe I have reason to suspect that one of these standards has been violated, either by an internal or external entity, I will report this incident according to the organization's internal reporting policy.

_____        _____
              Employee Signature                                    Date

the individual will not report to the HIM director, thereby avoiding any potential conflicts of interest. It might make the most sense for the HIM compliance specialist to report to the corporate compliance officer. However, in smaller organizations it may not be feasible for this position to be outside the HIM department. The HIM compliance specialist should be accountable to the corporate compliance officer and should sit on the organization's compliance committee.

For multifacility systems or integrated delivery networks, one individual should oversee HIM compliance systemwide and one individual should oversee compliance activities at each healthcare organization within the system. The corporate individual should work closely with his or her counterparts at the individual organizations to ensure a consistent, cohesive process for implementation of, and adherence to, the corporate compliance program. Depending on the size of the organization, the person responsible for oversight of the HIM compliance program may or may not have individuals reporting to him or her.

Both the individual responsible for oversight of the HIM compliance program and the HIM director should serve on the organization's compliance committee or task force. An organization may choose to establish a coding compliance committee that is separate from (but reports to), or is a subcommittee of, the corporate compliance committee. The coding compliance committee should include representatives from pertinent departments such as registration, billing, utilization management, and quality management, as well as coding professionals and physicians. This committee should:

- Monitor the effectiveness of the coding compliance program
- Oversee development of policies and procedures related to coding
- Review results of auditing and monitoring of coding practices
- Assist with development of audit protocols
- Develop educational programs on coding and documentation issues
- Oversee corrective actions that are within the scope of the committee (such as changes to coding policies and procedures)

In a multifacility organization, a systemwide committee can be used to develop policies and procedures, evaluate system problems, and establish benchmarks for use by facilities within the system.

 **Communication**

An established mechanism for employees to report perceived compliance violations must be in place. Organizations must be able to demonstrate that all reports of perceived violations are promptly investigated and that, when necessary, appropriate corrective action is taken. The organization's lines of communication and reporting protocol for compliance-related issues should be clearly communicated to all employees. For example, the organization may wish to stipulate the types of issues to be reported to the employee's supervisor rather than directly to the HIM compliance specialist or corporate compliance officer.

However, employees should be encouraged to report any issue to the HIM compliance specialist or corporate compliance officer that they either do not feel comfortable reporting to a supervisor or do not believe the supervisor has adequately investigated and addressed. Although every effort should be made to educate employees on what a compliance-related issue is and the purpose of the organization's compliance reporting protocol, employees should not be reprimanded when they use the wrong reporting channel (for example, calling the corporate compliance officer with a human resources–related issue). Employees who believe they have been reprimanded for using the compliance-reporting protocol (regardless of the reason) will be less likely to report issues in the future, including true compliance issues.

An established mechanism should be in place for employees, physicians, and contractors to receive clarification on a policy or procedure, an element of the compliance program, or an answer to a billing or coding question. The defined process should specify a designated resource person to contact. Employee inquiries and the responses to them should be documented, dated, and maintained by the HIM compliance specialist or corporate compliance officer. Depending on the nature of the inquiry, it may be appropriate to share the clarification with other staff members. If several employees require clarification on the same issue, it may be necessary to revise the written policies and procedures to alleviate confusion.

Policies and procedures should address how a significant change in a regulation or guideline will be expeditiously communicated to all affected staff. Changes that significantly affect reimbursement may not be able to wait until the next scheduled coding professionals' meeting (unless the implementation date of the change is well after the meeting date). Communication strategies for sharing and disseminating information should be created, such as educational programs, newsletters, committee meetings, and administrative memos. A formalized tracking system can be developed to monitor the sharing of the Hospital Payment Monitoring Program (HPMP) with all staff. For example, schedule face-to-face meetings about HPMP issues to foster interaction among key staff members.

All reporting mechanisms should take into consideration employees who work evenings or weekends when a supervisor, HIM compliance specialist, and corporate compliance officer may not be available. Moreover, a centralized source and systematic process for distributing information on healthcare statutes and regulations should be in place. It is imperative that coding staff be informed of all local, state, and federal regulations governing the coding of health data. A mechanism should also be in place to ensure that all affected staff are informed of payment policies, regulatory changes, new guidelines, and other important information. Therefore, when a provider bulletin or other transmittal communicating information about new or revised regulations or payment policy is received in one department, there also must be a process for its timely distribution outside that department. Communication to affected staff on updated regulations, standards, policies, or procedures should occur as soon as possible after the updated information becomes available and certainly before the effective date of the change. When a memo advising staff of a policy, procedure, or regulatory change is disseminated, the staff members should be asked to sign it, thereby acknowledging their receipt of the information. The memo, along with the staff signatures (and the date read by the staff), should be kept on file.

It is often difficult, if not downright impossible, for all of the affected staff to read all of the new or revised material pertaining to coding and billing requirements. One solution would be to designate certain staff members as responsible for reading particular types of material and updating the other staff. This task could be accomplished on a rotating basis to give everyone an opportunity to serve in this capacity.

All documents containing regulatory information affecting coding should be maintained with the coding policies and procedures. Additionally, an established mechanism should be in place for communicating effectively with physicians on coding and documentation issues. If the organization has evening, weekend, part-time, or as-needed staff, it also should consider ways to expeditiously communicate important regulatory information to these staff members.

A positive, collaborative working relationship between the HIM and billing departments is essential to an effective coding compliance program. Constant interaction and exchange of information between these departments will help to ensure the submission of accurate claims.

The Centers for Medicare and Medicaid Services (CMS) acknowledge that the Medicare provider communities have been affected by the number, frequency, and complexity of Medicare changes and that these changes are not always relayed to providers in an easy, timely, and consistent manner. In order to improve their process for communicating changes in Medicare rules to providers, CMS implemented an initiative called Consistency in Medicare Contractor Outreach Material (CMCOM). This initiative is designed to provide more timely information on Medicare changes. The product of this effort is a series of articles titled "Medlearn Matters: Information for Medicare Providers," which are prepared by actual clinicians and medical coding/billing experts. The articles are tailored, in content and language, to the specific provider types who are affected by the Medicare changes. The Medicare contractors are still responsible for local provider education, but the "Medlearn Matters" articles will support their efforts to communicate the content of change requests (CRs) in a way that focuses the information toward providers. The articles appear on the Medlearn Web site: www.cms.hhs.gov/medlearn/.

It is difficult to stay abreast of all of the new and updated regulatory information that comes out on a daily basis. However, the Internet has made it much easier to stay current. Organizations should consider subscribing to one of the free software programs that can monitor Web sites of interest and provide automatic notification of any changes or updates. This automatic notification eliminates the need to continually check the sites. Many government agencies also offer an e-mail notification service that announces the release of new regulations, policies, or instructions. It also is helpful to stay in touch with colleagues. The AHIMA's Communities of Practice are an excellent way for AHIMA members to stay in touch with colleagues and get up-to-the-minute information concerning regulatory or legislative changes.

## Enforcement

Because noncompliance is a significant organizational risk, enforcement of adherence to the organization's compliance program is mandatory. Appropriate and consistent disciplinary mechanisms should be instituted for employees or physicians who violate the organization's standards of conduct, policies and procedures, or federal or state laws, or have otherwise engaged in wrongdoing. Any noncompliant behavior, including an employee's failure to detect a violation that is attributable to his or her negligence or reckless conduct, should result in disciplinary action.

After a violation is detected, the organization must take all reasonable steps to respond appropriately to the offense and take action to prevent similar offenses in the future, including any necessary modifications to the compliance program. In addition to being appropriate to the circumstances, responses to detected violations should be consistent. In other words, all levels of employees should be subject to the same disciplinary action for the commission of similar offenses. Disciplinary action should be fair and equitable. The organization's managerial staff, compliance officer, and human resources department should work together to develop disciplinary policies that are in accordance with the Health and Human Services Office of Inspector General's (OIG) expectations (as described in the OIG compliance program guidances). The human resources department's policies pertaining to disciplinary action, including requirements for documentation of disciplinary actions taken, should be consistent with the compliance program, and these policies should be communicated and followed.

The various levels of disciplinary action (up to and including termination) that may be imposed on executives, managers, employees, physicians, and independent contractors for failure to comply with standards, policies, statutes, and regulations should be clearly spelled out and communicated to all involved. The individual responsible for carrying out each level of disciplinary action also should be determined (such as a supervisor, a human resources representative, or a member of administration).

For new employees being hired to fill positions that carry discretionary authority to make decisions involving compliance with the law (including coding professionals and the HIM compliance specialist), a reasonable and prudent background investigation should be conducted. The investigation should include a careful check of references.

Managers, supervisors, medical staff, and others in a supervisory capacity should be held accountable for failing to comply with, or encouraging or directing employees to violate, regulatory requirements. The applicable standards, procedures, and laws should be followed by everyone. The appropriate manager or supervisor should be disciplined for failing to adequately instruct his or her subordinates or to detect noncompliance with applicable policies and regulations. When it has been determined that reasonable diligence on his or her part would have led to the discovery of a problem, a manager is obligated to provide the organization an opportunity to correct it. Adherence to the provisions of the compliance program also should be a factor in every employee's annual performance evaluation. Contractual agreements, with either individuals or companies, should stipulate that the contracted entity's failure to comply with the organization's standards of conduct, policies and procedures, and federal and state laws and regulations is cause for immediate termination of the contract.

## Problem Resolution and Corrective Action

The healthcare organization must be able to demonstrate that reasonable steps have been taken to achieve compliance with policies, standards, and regulatory requirements and that all reports of perceived violations disclosed by employees or others are investigated and appropriate actions taken. Reasonable steps must be taken to resolve any identified problems and ensure that similar problems do not recur. When a potential problem or unusual trend is identified, through either the review process or some other mechanism (such as employee identification or external agency notification), a facility should conduct an internal investigation to determine its cause, scope, and consequences. The HIM compliance specialist should be involved in all internal investigations of coding issues or other HIM concerns and determination of subsequent corrective action. It is important to remember that many compliance issues are not simple and straightforward, but rather, they may be linked to complex processes in multiple departments. Therefore, they may require significant time and resources to investigate, ascertain whether a problem really exists, and determine the best corrective action plan. When multiple potential compliance issues have been identified, it may be necessary to prioritize the investigations. Issues with the greatest potential for involving criminal violations or significant overpayments should be tackled first.

Organizations should consider developing a set of warning indicators that trigger further review to determine if a problem exists. Triggers might include the following:

- Significant changes in the number and/or types of claim rejections and denials

- Correspondence from payers challenging the medical necessity or validity of claims

- Illogical patterns or unusual changes in the pattern of Healthcare Common Procedure Coding System (HCPCS) (Current Procedural Terminology [CPT] or HCPCS level II) or International Classification of Diseases, Ninth Edition, Clinical Modification (ICD-9-CM) code utilization

When a trend is evident, it should be determined whether the trend is related to clinical factors, data management, or coding practices and if the issue is isolated, limited to a given time period, or an ongoing problem. Unusual trends are not necessarily representative of problems that need to be corrected. For example, the case-mix index can be affected by changes in physicians' admitting patterns, new services being provided, and changes in overall admission patterns.

If the trend appears to be coding related, all pertinent policies and procedures, regulations, and official coding guidelines should be reviewed to determine whether the coding practice is improper. The review may reveal that a trend can be explained by a change in a code or coding guideline. If the review is inconclusive as to whether the coding practice in question is improper, an official source should be contacted for further information. For example, contact a Cooperating Party organization if it is an ICD-9-CM–related issue or the American Medical Association (AMA) if it is a CPT-related issue. The coding errors may be related to poor documentation or the coding process (for example, coding without all necessary documentation available). The organization should consider whether encoder software logic or information system planning is a factor in the identified errors. Staff should be interviewed to determine how the practice might have started. For example, a new coding professional or supervisor, consultant, or instructor may have initiated the practice or implemented a new software program for claims processing.

A statistically valid sample of cases should be reviewed to determine whether the problem is isolated (that is, having occurred during a set time period) or widespread and ongoing. Use of the OIG's free statistical sampling software, RAT-STATS should be considered (OIG n.d.). All the facts are needed to develop a reasonable explanation regarding the practice's development and to determine the best course of action to correct the situation. Information can be obtained by interviewing staff and/or researching the issue. Possible factors such as initiation of a new service provided by the organization, addition of a specialist to the medical staff, loss of a specialist on the medical staff, a new or revised code, a diagnosis-related group (DRG) revision, or a new or revised coding guideline should be considered. The coding staff may have attended a seminar around the time the change in coding practice occurred or a consultant may have conducted a coding review. Perhaps a change in patient mix has occurred or a procedure that was usually performed on an inpatient basis has shifted to the outpatient setting, or vice versa.

Changes in reimbursement methodology also may be a relevant factor. For example, implementation of a new prospective payment system is likely to result in changes in utilization and coding and billing patterns. After implementation of the outpatient prospective payment system (PPS), procedures previously performed as an outpatient may have shifted to the inpatient setting because they are part of the CMS's "inpatient only" list. CPT codes previously reported separately may be bundled now as part of the National Correct Coding Initiative (NCCI) edits. Significant volume decreases in high-volume, low-weight DRGs can result in an increase in the organization's overall case-mix index. Changes in the case-mix index may have occurred because a physician with several patients in a high-volume, low-weight DRG left the medical staff, or perhaps utilization review has successfully encouraged physicians to use observation services for some of the patients assigned to a specific DRG. If the frequency of assignment of the critical care codes has increased significantly, perhaps the physicians received education on the proper use of these codes and now do a better job of documenting time spent rendering critical care. Perhaps the number of critical care beds has increased or the physician's practice has shifted such that he or she has more critical care patients. Or perhaps an individual coding professional misunderstands the proper use of the critical care codes and he or she is assigning a critical care code whenever a patient occupies an intensive care unit (ICU) or critical care unit (CCU) bed.

If a reasonable explanation for the pattern or aberration is found, the reason should be documented along with the evidence and official resources to support it so that it can be readily produced in the event of a fraud investigation. When a legitimate explanation for the deviation is found, and no improper activity is indicated, no corrective action may be necessary.

When an internal investigation has concluded that a problem exists, corrective action should be promptly initiated to ensure that the identified problem does not recur. Internal organizational policy should dictate the point at which the corporate compliance officer is to become involved. Internal policy also should stipulate the appropriate course of action regarding various types of violations. The specific action that should be taken depends on the circumstances of the situation. In some instances, this action might consist of simply generating a repayment to the affected payer with an appropriate explanation. In certain situations, consultation with a coding or billing expert may be helpful in order to determine the best course of action.

Typical corrective actions for resolving problems identified during a coding audit include:

- Revisions to policies and procedures

- Development of additional policies and procedures

- Process improvements

- Further education of coding professionals, physicians, and/or other organizational staff, depending on the nature of the identified problem

- Revision or addition of routine monitoring activities

- Additions, deletions, or revisions to systems edits (for example, encoder, billing system)

- Documentation improvement strategies (for example, a clinical documentation improvement program might be implemented as a strategy for addressing problems with the completeness or quality of health record documentation)

- Disciplinary action

Education may consist of targeted education for a coding professional or physician, or education on a particular diagnosis, procedure, or coding rule or guideline. All of a coding professional's work or a physician's documentation may need to be reviewed until the problem has been resolved. The particular problem area may need to be monitored on an ongoing basis, such as reviewing 100 percent of the records with a certain diagnosis code. An internal coding policy may need to be revised or developed to prevent recurrence of the problem. The type and urgency of corrective action depends on the severity of the problem, including the impact on reimbursement and the prevalence of the problem. Although any corrective action taken as the result of an internal investigation will necessarily vary depending on the organization and the specific situation, every organization should strive for some consistency by using sound practices and disciplinary protocols.

When a problem related to coding errors has been identified, the organization must determine whether overpayments resulted from claims submitted with the errors. Whenever an overpayment is identified, regardless of whether it is the result of an honest error or potential fraud, it should be reported to a manager or the corporate compliance officer, according to the organization's reporting policy. Organizations should develop refund and disclosure policies to ensure that any detected violations are handled consistently.

Types of errors and violations should be categorized according to severity, and the appropriate actions to take regarding each category should be clearly delineated in the organization's policies and procedures. For example, a clear, consistent policy should be in place outlining the circumstances for which a simple refund of an overpayment will be made to the payer versus reporting the incident to the federal government.

The corrective action plan should include time frames for implementation of each action item and time frames for follow-up audits to ensure that the corrective action has been successful and the problem resolved. The organization should develop a checklist for all identified errors and deficiencies that need to be addressed. Each deficiency should have a follow-up plan associated with it and be backed up by documentation that the plan has been completed and there is evidence that an acceptable level of improvement has been made. Improvement can be evidenced through testing, ongoing monitoring between audits, and follow-up auditing. If a follow-up audit shows little or no improvement, modifications to the corrective action plan may be required.

If the results of an investigation reveal evidence of misconduct that may violate criminal, civil, or administrative law, the issue should be promptly reported to a government authority within a reasonable period of time (not more than 60 days after determining there is credible evidence of a violation). The OIG has indicated that instances of noncompliance must be determined on a case-by-case basis and that the existence or amount of a monetary loss to a healthcare program is not the sole determinant of whether the conduct should be investigated and reported to government authorities. In fact, in some instances in which there is no monetary loss to a healthcare program, corrective action and reporting to government authorities is still necessary to protect the integrity of the applicable healthcare program and its beneficiaries. The OIG believes that some violations may be so serious that they warrant immediate notification to government authorities, prior to, or simultaneous with, commencing an internal investigation, such as the following instances:

- Clear violations of criminal law

- Conduct that has a significant adverse effect on the quality of care

- Evidence of a systemic failure to comply with applicable laws, an existing corporate integrity agreement, or other standards of conduct, regardless of the financial impact on the healthcare program

Regardless of the organization's specific policy on self-reporting to the government, any identified overpayments (from any payer) should be refunded promptly to the applicable payer. Failure to repay overpayments within a reasonable period of time could be interpreted as an intentional attempt to conceal the overpayment, thereby establishing an independent basis for a criminal violation with respect to the organization, as well as any individuals who may have been involved.

After an internal investigation has confirmed the existence of a problem, the HIM compliance specialist, in conjunction with HIM staff, should review the circumstances related to the issue and make every effort to identify and investigate similar or related areas. For example, if an internal investigation uncovers the overcoding of complications or comorbidities in one pair of DRGs, it would be logical to look at other complication/comorbidity (CC)/non-CC DRG pairs to see whether overcoding occurred elsewhere.

All aspects of the internal investigation should be documented. Records of the investigation should contain the following elements:

- Documentation of the alleged violation
- A description of the investigative process
- Copies of notes from interviews with staff, physicians, and/or external entities
- Copies of key documents such as a pertinent coding guideline or a *Coding Clinic for ICD-9-CM* reference
- A log of the people interviewed and the documents reviewed
- The results of the investigation (for example, any disciplinary action taken and/or corrective action implemented)

Records of the investigation should be maintained by the corporate compliance officer. The HIM compliance specialist, under the direction of the corporate compliance officer, should take appropriate steps at the initiation of an internal investigation to prevent the destruction or loss of documents or other evidence relevant to the investigation.

## References

American Health Information Management Association. 2004. Code of Ethics. Available online from ahima.org.

American Health Information Management Association. 2004. Lifelong Learning Resolution. Available online from http://campus.ahima.org/.

Centers for Medicare and Medicaid Services. n.d. Medlearn. Available online from http://www.cms.hhs.gov/MLNGenInfo/.

LeBlanc, M.M. 2006. Work design and performance improvement. Chapter 23 in LaTour, K., and S. Eichenwald *Health Information Management: Concepts, Principles, and Practice,* 2nd ed. Chicago: AHIMA.

Office of Inspector General. 2001 (June). Special Advisory Bulletin: Practices of business consultants. Available online from http://oig.hhs.gov/fraud/docs/alertsandbulletins/consultants.pdf.

Office of Inspector General. 1998 (Feb. 23). OIG Compliance Program Guidance for Hospitals. *Federal Register* 63(35):8987–98. Available online from http://oig.hhs.gov/authorities/docs/cpghosp.pdf.

Office of Inspector General. n.d. Office of Audit Services, RAT-STATS program. Available online from http://www.oig.hhs.gov/organization/OAS/ratstat.html.

## Additional References

Hammen, C. 2001. Choosing consultants without compromising compliance. *Journal of American Health Information Management Association* 72(9):26, 28, 30.

Russo, R. 1998. Seven Steps to HIM Compliance. Marblehead, MA: Opus Communications.

Scichilone, R. 2002. Best practices for medical necessity validation. *Journal of American Health Information Management Association* 73(2):48, 50.

# Chapter 3
# Policies and Procedures

*Sue Bowman, RHIA, CCS*

Clear written policies and procedures that are communicated to all employees are important to ensure the effectiveness of a compliance program. Written standards and procedures reduce the prospect of erroneous claims and fraudulent activity by identifying risk areas and establishing tighter internal controls, while also helping to identify any aberrant billing patterns. Comprehensive policies and procedures on coding, documentation requirements (including retention), payer regulations and policies, and contractual arrangements for coding consulting and outsourcing services should be developed. Coding policies and procedures serve as guidelines for coding and billing functions and provide documentation of the organization's intent to correctly report services provided. Policies should include requirements for accurate, complete, and timely documentation and coding practices as well as incorporate the laws and regulations governing coding and billing. Complying with these policies is key to preventing coding errors or delayed reimbursement. In addition to the statutes, regulations, and guidelines of federal and state health insurance programs, the policies and requirements of private health plans and managed care organizations should be addressed. Consistent with the prohibition against maximization, the policies and procedures should stipulate that no financial incentive will be provided for upcoding (that is, maximization). It should be clear that this policy applies to staff and external consultants.

All HIM policies and procedures should be approved according to the organization's policy on review and approval of departmental policies and procedures. An up-to-date, user-friendly index for the HIM policies and procedures should be maintained so that specific information can be readily located. In addition, policies and procedures should be kept in a location that is easily accessible to all HIM staff. Ideally, policies and procedures should be maintained on-line, such as on an organization's intranet. On-line availability ensures easy, simultaneous access and facilitates updating the policies and procedures. Policies and procedures should be revised promptly in response to code revisions, regulatory changes, or other new or revised requirements impacting policies and procedures.

In addition to the organization's own policies and procedures, the HIM department should maintain up-to-date resources related to pertinent government regulations and payer policies, including:

- Medicare manuals

- Other pertinent manuals addressing government requirements such as those dealing with the Minimum Data Set (MDS) and Outcome and Assessment Information Set (OASIS) completion and submission for long-term care facilities and home health agencies, respectively

- Medicare transmittals (change requests)

- Medicare contractor, private payer, and quality improvement organization (QIO) newsletters and bulletins

- National coverage determinations (NCDs) and local coverage determinations (LCDs)

Key coding references are addressed in more detail in the upcoming section on internal coding practices, starting on page 24. Additionally, AHIMA publications on coding and professional practice standards are excellent resources. Bookmarking useful Web sites in an Internet browser also facilitates ready access to a variety of excellent resources. The organization's HIM compliance program document should specify where information on regulatory or payer-specific requirements can be located.

Laws, regulations, and guidelines are constantly changing, and regular review of the coding policies and procedures is necessary to ensure compliance with the current requirements. Policies and procedures should be updated as changes occur, affected staff should be notified of the changes, and a complete review of the policies and procedures should be conducted annually. Routine monitoring of compliance to policies and procedures should be conducted.

## Risk Assessment

Written policies and procedures should take into consideration the regulatory exposure for each function or department. Organizations should conduct an assessment of the particular risk areas to which they are vulnerable in order to identify potential problems, develop policies and procedures to address these problems, and prioritize focus areas for educational programs and auditing and monitoring activities. Assessing the level of risk with respect to nationally recognized high-risk areas is a good place to start. Nationally recognized high-risk areas include those identified by the following:

*External (National)*

- The Health and Human Services (HHS) Office of Inspector General (OIG) in its annual work plans, inspection reports, fraud alerts, compliance program guidances, and semiannual reports

- The Centers for Medicare and Medicaid Services (CMS) in its transmittals

- Private payers in their memoranda, newsletters, and other communications with providers

- Healthcare experts in journals, newsletters, and other publications

Common risk areas associated with claim submission include:

- Incorrect coding

- Upcoding or undercoding

- Unbundling of services

- Billing for uncovered or medically unnecessary services

- Billing for services not provided

- Duplicate billing

- Lack of health record documentation to support the reported diagnosis and procedure codes

- Reporting incorrect discharge status code

Incorrect coding, including upcoding and undercoding, can lead to inappropriate diagnosis-related group (DRG) assignment—a major compliance risk in healthcare settings subject to a Medicare Prospective Payment System (PPS) based on DRGs. Undercoding will result in receipt of payment that is less than what would have been appropriate. Although underpayment does not represent a loss to the Medicare program, it is still considered a Medicare payment error. Upcoding results in the hospital receiving a payment that is more than would have been appropriate and is also considered a Medicare payment error. In addition, this type of billing constitutes fraud, and a related conviction can result in significant fines, penalties, and other adverse actions. Regardless of whether incorrect DRG assignment results in an underpayment or overpayment, mistakes in this area are a serious matter. Both of these types of errors indicate that the organization's processes lack the necessary controls to ensure correct payment and that claims are being submitted that contain erroneous information.

High-risk areas applicable to certain healthcare settings are described in Part II, chapters 7–13. (See appendix B for a list of high-risk areas related to HIM practice, including a list of high-risk DRGs in the hospital inpatient setting.) Although these lists of risk areas are not exhaustive or static, they serve as a good starting point for an internal review of the organization's potential vulnerabilities. As new risk areas are identified by government agencies and payers, they should be incorporated into the HIM compliance program. Areas of risk that are unique to an organization also should be assessed, through auditing and monitoring interviews of staff, a review of claims denials and rejections, and a review of systems and processes. Identified areas of risk should be incorporated into the organization's policies and procedures, training and educational programs, and auditing and monitoring activities.

HIM policies and procedures should explicitly address weak areas identified through a risk assessment so that appropriate measures can be implemented to resolve problems or improve system weaknesses. For example, a clinic may discover that a certain procedure is being reported incorrectly because separate codes are being assigned for its individual components (that is, the procedure has been unbundled). A hospital might discover that certain diagnoses are being reported as complications or comorbidities with unusually high frequency. Perhaps the coding accuracy is much higher for inpatient claims than for outpatient claims. Further analysis of problem areas might reveal that the problems are caused by missing physician orders, outdated codes on the chargemaster, poor documentation, inadequate understanding of the procedure performed, or misunderstanding of the appropriate use of the affected codes or modifiers. After the problems are identified, their causes can be determined, and appropriate corrective actions instituted to prevent their recurrence.

The HIM department also needs to work together with the billing and ancillary departments to verify that appropriate charges, codes, and edits are in place and that denials are reviewed and, when appropriate, appealed. Ongoing review, update, and maintenance of the chargemaster are required to verify that all billable services are captured.

The HIM and billing departments should collaborate on establishing the systems edits needed to identify errors prior to claim submission.

Claim denial history and claims that have resulted in repeated overpayment should be examined, causes identified, and the most frequent sources of these denials and overpayments corrected.

Utilization of external data sources for benchmark comparison purposes is a good way to identify potential risk areas associated with current organizational coding practices. For instance, Medicare provider analysis and review (MEDPAR) data from the CMS can be used to compare the distribution of DRGs for Medicare discharges. MEDPAR data are also available for skilled nursing facilities. The CMS has a number of data files available on its Web site, including the MEDPAR data files. (See appendix F for a list of sources of comparative data and appendix B for a list of identified high-risk areas.)

## Internal Coding Practices

Current written policies and procedures related to the coding of health data must be maintained. Coding policies establish the organization's guidelines to be followed in the coding process. If all of the organization's coding professionals follow the same set of clear, well-written guidelines, the organization will be more likely to achieve a higher level of coding consistency. Written policies and procedures pertaining to proper coding should reflect current regulatory requirements, including the following:

- The official coding guidelines promulgated by the Cooperating Parties (CMS, National Center for Health Statistics, American Hospital Association [AHA], and AHIMA)

- Current Procedural Terminology (CPT) rules promulgated by the American Medical Association (AMA)

- Uniform Hospital Discharge Data Set requirements (for inpatient hospital-izations)

- Requirements for uniform claims reporting established by the National Uniform Billing Committee and National Uniform Claims Committee

- Requirements for completion of patient assessment instruments (such as the PAI for rehabilitation facilities or OASIS for home health agencies)

- Individual payer policies

## Coding Resources

Policies and procedures should identify the coding resources that are available to the coding staff. Inappropriate or outdated coding resources pose a compliance risk, as their use can lead to incorrect coding and billing. Essential coding resources include the following:

- Up-to-date International Classification of Diseases, Ninth Revision, Clinical Modification (ICD-9-CM); CPT; and Healthcare Common Procedure Coding System (HCPCS) Level II codebooks

- *ICD-9-CM: Official Guidelines for Coding and Reporting*

- Medical dictionary

- Anatomy/physiology textbook

- *Physicians' Desk Reference*

- Current subscription to AHA's *Coding Clinic for ICD-9-CM*

- Current subscription to AHA's *Coding Clinic for HCPCS*[1]

- Current subscription to AMA's *CPT Assistant*

- Current version of the National Correct Coding Initiative (NCCI) manual

- Payer-specific coverage policies (for example, LCDs and NCDs)

- Payer bulletins and memoranda that contain instructions or policies affecting the coding process

This list covers only the minimum requirements. Each organization should identify any additional coding resources that need to be available to the coding staff.

These resources should be maintained in a location that is readily accessible to the coding staff. They should be kept in close proximity to the coding professionals' work-stations and not in a private office (such as a supervisor's office) that sometimes may be inaccessible. Ideally, if possible, resources should be made available electronically so they are literally at one's fingertips when they are needed. The HIM compliance special-ist should periodically (at least annually) check to ensure the availability and timeliness

---

[1]*Coding Clinic for HCPCS* provides authoritative advice on the proper use of Level I HCPCS (CPT codes) for hospital providers and certain Level II HCPCS codes for hospitals, physicians, and other health professionals. The Editorial Advisory Board for *Coding Clinic* publications includes AHA, AHIMA, CMS, and other stake-holders from the healthcare industry.

of the coding resources described in the policies and procedures. Using inappropriate or outdated coding resources places the organization at high risk for patterns of coding errors. In addition, the compliance program's effectiveness might be questioned if the organization was not relying on official or up-to-date coding resources (for example, allowing a subscription to *Coding Clinic for ICD-9-CM* to lapse). Even if an encoder is used, it remains important to provide access to current ICD-9-CM and CPT codebooks because there may be times when coding personnel need to verify the appropriateness of an encoder code selection or edit. **Encoders** are computer software programs that assist coding professionals in assigning appropriate codes.

The only official sources of coding advice and guidelines are the AHA for ICD-9-CM and the AMA for CPT. Although the healthcare organization may choose to subscribe to other vendors' coding publications for educational purposes, these are not considered official sources of coding advice and should not be relied on for verification of coding accuracy in the event of an audit or investigation.

## Coding Process

Policies and procedures should describe the necessary steps the coding professional should take during the course of reviewing a health record. Direction also should be provided on the proper steps to take in those situations when an official source does not provide guidance (for example, when neither the codebook nor *Coding Clinic for ICD-9-CM* provides direction on the most appropriate ICD-9-CM code for a stated diagnosis or procedure).

To ensure consistency, coding policies and procedures should identify the optional codes the organization wishes to collect (such as morphology codes or procedure codes that are not required for reporting purposes). The organization's use of E codes should be described.

The OIG's Supplemental Compliance Program Guidance for Hospitals[2] states that underlying assumptions used in connection with claims submission should be reasoned, consistent, and appropriately documented, and hospitals should retain all relevant records reflecting their efforts to comply with federal healthcare program requirements.

An advantage of electronic health records (EHRs) is that submitted codes can be closely linked to the relevant documentation and audit trails track any changes to the codes or documentation, along with the date of the change and the identity of the person who made the change. The use of computer-assisted coding software offers the advantage of an electronic coding audit trail, which allows reconstruction of the reason a particular code was selected. (See chapter 6 and the CD-ROM for more information on computer-assisted coding.) The

---

[2]The Supplemental Compliance Program Guidance for Hospitals builds on the OIG's original compliance program guidance for hospitals issued in 1998. Collectively, the two documents offer a set of guidelines that hospitals should consider when developing and implementing a new compliance program or evaluating an existing one. For those hospitals with existing compliance programs, the Supplemental Compliance Program Guidance for Hospitals may serve as a benchmark or comparison against which to measure ongoing efforts and as a roadmap for updating or refining their compliance plans. It includes a section on expanded risk that highlights areas of significant risk for hospitals and offers guidance designed to help them identify potential problems. In addition, the Supplemental Compliance Program Guidance for Hospitals sets forth practical questions that hospitals can use to gauge the effectiveness of their compliance programs. Although these questions were drafted with hospitals in mind, many of them can also be used to gauge the effectiveness of compliance programs in other industry sectors.

use of EHR documentation facilitates the coding process and improves coding accuracy and productivity by allowing the coding professional to route records to supervisors for coding questions, to physicians for coding query, or to auditors for prebill review.

### Facility-specific Coding Guidelines

Facility-specific coding guidelines should be developed for situations that are not addressed by the official coding rules and guidelines. Facility-specific coding guidelines must be documented in the coding policies and procedures and must be applied consistently to all records coded.

*Facility-specific coding guidelines must not conflict with official rules and guidelines.* When official advice addressing the situation has been received, the organization-specific guideline is invalidated and should not be used again. Facility-specific coding guidelines should not be developed to replace the physician documentation needed to support code assignment. For example, an internal facility guideline should not interpret abnormal findings to replace physician documentation or physician query. The guideline may provide assistance in determining when a physician query is appropriate, but it may not interpret abnormal test results.

HIM professionals can work together with their medical staff to develop coding guidelines that promote complete documentation needed for consistent code assignment. Specific and detailed coding guidelines that cover the reporting of typical services provided by the organization are tools for data consistency and reliability by ensuring that all coding staff interpret clinical documentation and apply coding principles in the same manner. These guidelines can reveal to the coding professionals the circumstances in which they should query physicians for clarification of documentation. The coding guidelines should be specific to the settings to which they apply.

An example of a situation that might warrant a facility-specific guideline is an unusual diagnosis or a new procedure for which there is no official instruction regarding the appropriate code assignment. In this situation, the issue must be researched to ensure that the diagnosis or procedure has not been addressed previously by an official source of coding advice. If the diagnosis or procedure has not been previously addressed, the issue should be submitted, along with appropriate health record documentation, to the proper source for determination of an official answer (for example, the AHA's Central Office on ICD-9-CM is the official source of advice for ICD-9-CM coding issues). Publication of an official answer will ensure consistency in coding because all healthcare providers will be using the same code when they encounter a particular diagnosis or procedure. While waiting for an official answer, the coding professional may:

- Consult the attending physician for direction on the most appropriate code
- Solicit buy-in on this code selection by other physicians on the medical staff who are likely to encounter the same diagnosis or procedure
- Develop a facility-specific guideline for application of this code whenever this diagnosis or procedure is encountered

Another example of a situation when facility-specific guidelines are appropriate is in the development of clinical criteria, through collaboration of coding staff and physicians, for determining the circumstances when querying the physician is appropriate. (See appendix D for a practice brief on developing a physician query process). The appropriate medical staff committee should give final approval of any facility-specific coding guidelines that involve clinical criteria to ensure appropriateness and physician consensus.

If the facility-specific guidelines are maintained electronically, they should be searchable by key terms. Placing guidelines on a facility intranet or internal computer network is an efficient way to ensure their accessibility and consistent use and also enables timely and efficient updating and distribution. If the computer network permits access to the Internet, live links can be incorporated to Web sites containing regulatory requirements related to documentation, claims submission, and code assignment.

### Clarification of Coding Advice

When ambiguity or conflicting advice regarding a coding or reimbursement issue exists, official sources should be contacted for clarification and all responses documented. All supporting and relevant data relating to the coding, documentation, or billing issue should be retrieved. A summary document outlining all sources contacted, responses, and clarification and instructions obtained should be prepared. Depending on the nature of the issue, it may be appropriate to do one of the following:

- Research the *Federal Register,* Medicare contractor bulletins, and CMS transmittals

- Visit a government, Medicare contractor, or private payer Web site

- Contact a professional association such as the AHIMA, AHA, AMA, Healthcare Financial Management Association (HFMA), or Medical Group Management Association (MGMA)

## Coding Accuracy Standards

Healthcare organizations should establish their own acceptable coding accuracy standards. These standards should be based on each organization's unique characteristics and realistic expectations with consideration given to standards that are reasonable and yet minimize the risk of erroneous claims submission.

## Claims Denials and Rejections

An organizational policy and procedure should be developed for processing claims denials and rejections. Every healthcare organization should be reviewing information about claims denials and implementing prevention strategies. All rejected or denied claims pertaining to a diagnostic or procedure coding issue must be returned to the coding staff for review and, if necessary, code correction. If the claim pertains to the chargemaster, it should be forwarded to the affected ancillary department for review and resolution.

The business office generally receives claim denials and rejection, but may not share those involving coding issues with the HIM department. As a result, coding personnel may not be aware that code assignments have caused claim denials or delays. Reducing claims denials and rejections requires a collaborative, multidisciplinary approach. Staff from the appropriate departments should work together in identifying rejections and denials, tracking denial trends, and taking corrective action. Organizational policy should emphasize that diagnosis and procedure codes, including modifiers, should never be changed by billing personnel without the consensus of the department that assigned the original codes. If there is disagreement between the coding and the billing staff, the issue should be referred to the coding supervisor. If necessary, the coding supervisor should forward it to the HIM compliance specialist or, if this position does not exist, to the corporate compliance officer.

When an error in code assignment or a discrepancy between the code(s) reported by the coding staff and the code(s) submitted on the claim is discovered after claim submission, the organization should implement its established process for updating and correcting the information system and amending or correcting the claim. Denials are often related to the ongoing battle of obtaining appropriate documentation. Ways to reduce denials may include physician education, improved processes for charge capture, or more frequent review and updates of the chargemaster.

The number of denials and value by category should be reported to the organization's compliance committee. A denial management team should oversee prospective prevention and claims recovery. An effective claims-monitoring process should result in an efficient claims submission process and a reduction in revenue losses resulting from medical necessity denials, as well as mitigation of the risk of denial patterns triggering a fraud investigation.

## Requests to Change Codes

A policy and procedure should be established for handling patient and physician requests to inappropriately change codes to those for which the patient's insurance will provide reimbursement. The policies and procedures should stipulate that codes will not be assigned, modified, or excluded solely for the purpose of maximizing reimbursement. Codes should not be changed or amended at the request of the physician, patient, or member of the patient's family in order to have the service covered by the patient's health insurance. If the initial code assignment did not accurately reflect the service provided or the reason for the service, the code(s) may be revised based on supporting documentation (any verbal information provided by the physician that justifies reporting a revised or additional code must be incorporated into the health record documentation and signed by the physician). Disputes with physicians or patients regarding coding issues should be handled by the coding manager and appropriately logged for review. Requests to change codes should be monitored for patterns. If a pattern of requests coming from the same physician practice is identified, the reasons these requests are occurring should be investigated and corrective action taken to reduce the incidence of requests. Appropriate corrective action might consist of providing education to the physician and staff on medical necessity requirements and the importance of providing accurate diagnostic information regarding the reason a service was ordered.

## Disputes with Physicians

Appropriate methods for resolving coding or documentation disputes with physicians also should be described in the organization's HIM policies and procedures. For example, the issue might be referred to a physician liaison or a medical staff committee for resolution.

If the final outcome is such that the organization faces a compliance risk (for example, the attending physician absolutely refuses to allow a code to be reported in compliance with an official coding guideline), detailed documentation of the issue, including all steps taken to attempt to resolve it, should be maintained.

## Physician Query Process

Organizations should use physician queries as a communication or educational tool in working with physicians to enhance health record documentation. However, a physician query should not be used as a substitute for appropriate health record documentation. CMS has stipulated that a query form is only acceptable to the extent that it provides clarification and is consistent with other health record documentation. CMS requires that QIOs disregard query forms that are leading in nature or that introduce new information.

Codes should be based on physician documentation. Physician documentation is the cornerstone of accurate coding. Documentation is not limited to the face sheet, discharge summary, progress notes, history and physical, or other report designed to capture diagnostic information. Ensuring the accuracy of coded data is a shared responsibility between coding professionals and physicians. Accurate diagnostic and procedural coded data originate from collaboration between physicians, who have a clinical background, and coding professionals, who have an understanding of classification systems. Compliance issues often arise when physicians lack time or sufficient understanding of the methodology behind coding and how documentation (or lack thereof) affects coding, billing, and the integrity of the health record. In other instances, compliance issues arise because coding professionals, who should never make clinical judgments in the absence of proper documentation, are hesitant to approach physicians when documentation is ambiguous or needs clarification. Sometimes organizational processes or culture can inhibit direct interactions with physicians to amend ambiguous or inadequate documentation.

If evidence of a diagnosis exists in the health record and the coding professional is uncertain whether it is a valid diagnosis because the documentation is incomplete, unclear, or contradictory, it is the coding professional's responsibility to query the attending physician to determine if the diagnosis should be coded and reported. For example, if a laboratory or radiology finding supports the selection of a more specific diagnosis than the physician has documented, then the physician should be queried to clarify the diagnosis. An inpatient guideline from the *ICD-9-CM Official Guidelines for Coding and Reporting* states: "Abnormal findings (laboratory, x-ray, pathologic, and other diagnostic results) are not coded and reported unless the physician indicates their clinical significance. If the findings are outside the normal range and the physician has ordered other tests to evaluate the condition or prescribed treatment, it is appropriate to ask whether the diagnosis should be added."

It is important to keep in mind that the purpose of a physician query is clarification of health record documentation. The physician should not be queried when there is no clinical information in the record to indicate the possible presence of the condition being queried. For example, to query the physician about gram-negative pneumonia on every pneumonia case, regardless of whether there is any clinical indication that the pneumonia might be gram-negative, is inappropriate and would be considered "leading" the physician. Some of the examples of situations when physician queries are appropriate that have been published in *Coding Clinic for ICD-9-CM* include clarification of:

- Whether a condition that developed after surgery is a complication of the procedure
- The relationship between diabetes mellitus and other documented conditions, such as peripheral vascular disease
- Whether a patient with sepsis and hypotension has septic shock
- Whether urosepsis represents a urinary tract infection or sepsis
- The type of heart failure
- Whether a "history of" represents a current condition or past medical history
- Which diagnosis represents the reason for admission
- The stage of chronic kidney disease
- The clinical significance of abnormal findings

As stated in AHIMA's practice brief titled "Developing a Physician Query Process:"

The query forms should not:

- "Lead" the physician
- Sound presumptive, directing, prodding, probing, or as though the physician is being led to make an assumption
- Ask questions that can be responded to in a "yes" or "no" fashion
- Indicate the financial impact of the response to the query
- Be designed so that all that is required is a physician signature" (Prophet 2001).

Some of the QIOs have sample query forms or examples of appropriate queries on their Web sites. See figure 3.1 for several examples of appropriate queries from one QIO.

Policies regarding the circumstances when physicians will be queried should be designed to promote complete and accurate coding and complete documentation. The process of querying physicians is an effective and necessary mechanism for improving the quality of coding and health record documentation and capturing complete clinical data. Query forms must be used as a communication tool meant to improve the accuracy of code assignments and the quality of physician documentation, not to inappropriately maximize reimbursement. It would be inappropriate to implement a policy requiring that the physician be queried only when reimbursement is affected because such a policy would skew national healthcare data and could lead to charges of upcoding.

Each healthcare organization should develop a process for obtaining physician clarification. For example, the policies and procedures might include a statement authorizing the coding professionals to contact a physician directly regarding a record that is being coded. Such a statement will clarify that communication with physicians is not restricted to supervisory personnel. Coding professionals must have access to—and be empowered to—query physicians when necessary.

**Figure 3.1.    Standard wording for a nonleading physician query**

This document was developed in collaboration with representatives from PPS hospitals in Maine, New Hampshire and Vermont and is intended to serve as a guideline to assist in composing non-leading physician queries. It does not represent required wording for queries. Coding professionals should use their professional judgment and hospital policies/procedures when assessing clinical documentation and in querying physicians for code assignment.

**EXAMPLE #1**

This wording would be appropriate to obtain correlation between diagnoses or between a diagnosis and results such as cultures.

- Diabetes and possible manifestations/complications
- Infections and organisms in lab work
- Anemia and blood loss
- Determining drug/medical/surgical complications

> **A cause and effect relationship between diagnoses may not be assumed and coded unless documented as such by the attending physician.**
>
> **The patient presented with** *insert clinical indicators/reference supporting medical record documentation.*
>
> **Please document the relationship, if any, between** *insert diagnoses.*

**EXAMPLE #2**

This wording would be appropriate to obtain clarification of urosepsis.

> **"Urosepsis" is a non-specific term, which requires further physician clarification to ensure accurate coding. From a coding perspective, urosepsis may mean that sepsis is localized to the urinary tract OR it may mean that the urinary infection has become generalized septicemia.**
>
> **Please document the diagnosis that best represents your intended meaning of the term "urosepsis."**

**EXAMPLE #3**

This wording would be appropriate to obtain documentation of the significance of abnormal findings for the possible addition of a diagnosis.

> **Codes may not be assigned based on abnormal results from diagnostic studies without physician documentation of the significance of the findings.**
>
> **The** *insert diagnostic study* **demonstrates** *insert abnormal findings.*
>
> **Please document the significance, if any, of these abnormal findings.**

**EXAMPLE #4**

This wording would be appropriate to obtain additional documentation of diagnoses that are being treated, but which are not clearly documented.

> **All diagnoses that affect the management of the patient should be documented and coded.**
>
> **The patient is receiving** *insert treatment.*
>
> **Please document the diagnosis(es) that requires this treatment.**

**Figure 3.1.** *(Continued)*

**EXAMPLE #5**

This wording would be appropriate to help determine the principal diagnosis.

> **The patient's principal diagnosis has not been clearly identified and cannot be selected without further clarification.**
> **The patient presented with** *insert presenting symptoms/admitting diagnosis.*
> **Please document which diagnosis, after study, accounted for the patient's presenting symptoms and was the reason for this inpatient admission.**

**EXAMPLE #6**

This wording would be appropriate to obtain additional specificity.

> **The documented diagnosis** *insert diagnosis* **lacks the required specificity to ensure accurate coding.**
> **Please provide documentation regarding** *insert issues (such as site, chronicity, etc.).*

**EXAMPLE #7**

This wording would be appropriate to resolve conflicting documentation.

> **The medical record documentation is conflicting.** *Insert references to conflicting information.*
> **Please provide clarification as to the most appropriate diagnosis.**

**EXAMPLE #8**

This wording would be appropriate to obtain clarification of illegible documentation.

> **We are unable to read** *insert references to illegible entry.* **Please print the entry so that we may complete the coding of this record.**

**EXAMPLE #9**

This wording would be appropriate to obtain clarification of an abbreviation that is unknown or that may have more than one definition.

> **The abbreviation** *insert abbreviation* **[is not familiar] OR [has more than one meaning].**
> **Please write out the definition of this abbreviation.**

**EXAMPLE #10**

This wording would be appropriate to obtain a more definitive diagnosis if the documented diagnosis is a symptom.

> **Symptoms should not be coded when the underlying cause is known.**
> **If known, please document the underlying diagnosis causing the patient's** *insert symptom(s).*

**EXAMPLE #11**

This wording would be appropriate when there is indication of a diagnosis that has not been documented by the physician.

> **The patient presented with** *insert clinical indications,* **which may indicate** *insert diagnosis.*
> **Please document the diagnosis if you feel that it accurately reflects the patient's condition—OR—**
> **If it does not accurately reflect the patient's condition, document a more appropriate diagnosis.**

Source: This material was prepared in April 2002 by the Northeast Health Care Quality Foundation under a contract with the Centers for Medicare and Medicaid Services (CMS). The contents presented do not necessarily reflect CMS policy.

In an EHR environment, the physician query process will be automated—through e-mail communication or flagged documentation in the EHR itself. As with paper-based records, it is still important to establish a written policy regarding whether or not the physician query (for example, e-mail communication, question inserted in comment field) will be maintained as part of the permanent health record. Any amendments made to the EHR documentation as a result of the physician query should follow the guidelines outlined in chapter 6, Impact of Electronic Health Records on HIM Compliance.

A physician query is not necessary if a physician (including consulting physicians) involved in the care and treatment of the patient has documented a diagnosis and there is no conflicting documentation from another physician. If there is conflicting documentation from different physicians, clarification should be obtained from the attending physician, who is ultimately responsible for the final diagnosis.

Patterns of incorrect physician documentation (for example, use of the term *urosepsis* without indicating whether the patient has a urinary tract infection or septicemia)—whether for an individual physician or all physicians—should be addressed in physician educational programs and monitored to determine the severity of the problem. If no improvement is noted after a predetermined time period, corrective action should be initiated.

The healthcare organization may wish to designate a physician to provide guidance to the coding staff on clinical issues and to serve as a liaison to the medical staff. Appendix C offers sample communication tools for improving physician documentation.

See Appendix D for a Practice Brief titled "Developing a Physician Query Process," which provides additional guidance on the appropriate use of physician queries.

## Payment Policies

Organizations should document their efforts to comply with applicable statutes, regulations, and federal healthcare program requirements. When advice is requested from a government agency (including a Medicare contractor) charged with administering a federal healthcare program, a record of the request and any written or oral response must be documented and retained. A log of oral inquiries between the organization and third parties (government and private entities) will help document the organization's compliance efforts. These records could become relevant in a subsequent investigation to the issue of whether the organization's reliance on this advice was reasonable and whether it exercised due diligence in developing procedures and practices to implement the advice.

Payment policies affecting code assignment should be incorporated into coding policies and procedures. A copy of the provider bulletin or any other official memorandum addressing payment policy should be filed with the policies and procedures so that the organization will be able to produce documentation supporting the coding practice. Should the payer provide advice or direction on a particular policy verbally, the organization should request that information in writing. If the organization's encoder allows customized edits, payer-specific edits for the code(s) affected by a payer policy should be created.

With respect to Medicare, information concerning specific payment policies should be available from the Medicare contractor under the Freedom of Information Act. Information concerning Medicare NCDs and LCDs is available on the Internet. (See appendix F for the specific Web site.) If attempts to obtain the information in writing are unsuccessful, the conversation with the payer should be documented, including the date(s), the name(s) of the individuals involved in the conversation(s), and the provider organization's interpretation of the payer's advice. A copy should be faxed to the payer along with a request that the payer representative sign the document and fax it back. Finally, a copy of the confirmation that the fax was successfully delivered should be kept on file. Another method is to send a letter to the payer via certified mail and request a reply if the payer does not concur with the summary of the conversation. Even if the payer fails to provide its advice in writing, sign the summary of the discussion, or reply to the certified letter, the provider organization will still have evidence that a summary of the conversation was provided to the payer. This documentation should be kept in the policy and procedure manual.

Payment policies sometimes appear to conflict with official coding rules, conventions, and guidelines. Under the Health Insurance Portability and Accountability Act (HIPAA), regulations pertaining to electronic transactions and code sets (discussed in more detail in the next section), payers are required to accept valid codes and modifiers and to adhere to the *ICD-9-CM Official Guidelines for Coding and Reporting.* However, HIPAA does not require adherence to coding rules and guidelines for other code sets. If a payer has a policy that conflicts with official coding rules or guidelines, every effort should be made to resolve the issue directly with the payer. First, whether the issue is related to coding or coverage should be determined. For example, the denial may be referred to the HIM department with a message from the business office that the claim was denied because code V72.5, Radiology examination, was an unacceptable diagnosis. Many insurance policies do not include coverage for routine services (such as annual physical examinations and screening tests), and this code is assigned when the patient has no signs or symptoms. Therefore, the denial may really be related to noncoverage of the service provided rather than to the accuracy of the reported code.

If it is determined that the problem is not related to a coverage issue and does involve a conflict between a payer requirement and the official coding rules or guidelines, the payer should be contacted and an attempt made to explain the problem. For example, a letter could be sent to the payer (if the payer is Medicare, a letter could be sent to the fiscal intermediary or carrier) pointing out the conflict and the problems it could cause with data consistency and comparability. The applicable coding rule or guideline should be included. (AHIMA's *Payer's Guide to Healthcare Diagnostic and Procedural Data Quality,* available at www.ahima.org, may be used as a tool to support the organization's position and the underlying rationale.) If the payer involved is Medicare and no satisfactory resolution is achieved with the Medicare contractor, the appropriate CMS regional office should be contacted. An organization's business office or Medicare contractor can provide contact information for the CMS regional office with jurisdiction in a particular area.

If the conflict involves a HIPAA violation (such as nonacceptance of a valid code or violation of an ICD-9-CM coding guideline), the payer should be informed that it is a HIPAA violation and of the consequences (that is, civil monetary penalties) of noncompliance with HIPAA.

If the payer refuses to change its policy, an attempt should be made to obtain its policy in writing. If the payer refuses to provide the policy in writing, all conversations with the payer should be documented, including dates, names of individuals involved, and substance of the discussion. Furthermore, the payment policy should be confirmed by a representative of the payer's management. A file should be kept of all documentation on communications with the payer regarding this issue. If the issue involves a HIPAA violation and the payer refuses to change its policy to comply with HIPAA, the organization's recourse is to follow the HIPAA enforcement protocol, which involves reporting the violation to the CMS Office of HIPAA Standards. This office handles all violations of the HIPAA standards for electronic transactions and code sets committed by any covered entity.

If the issue seems to be a misinterpretation of CMS Medicare policy by a Medicare contractor, the organization should work with the contractor to resolve the issue. If necessary, the CMS regional office may need to become involved. The organization also may wish to solicit assistance from its state hospital association or component state association of AHIMA. If the issue appears to be relatively broad in scope (that is, involving multiple Medicare contractors or payers), soliciting AHIMA's assistance to resolve the issue at a national level should be considered. If satisfactory resolution of a HIPAA violation involving a medical coding issue is not obtained from the Office of HIPAA Standards, AHIMA may be able to offer assistance in resolving the matter.

## Use of Encoding Software

The organization's policies and procedures should address the use of encoders or other computer software (see chapter 6 for information on computer-assisted coding technology). Following are four basic rules to follow when writing such a policy:

1. The organization should not rely solely on encoding software for code assignment. The encoder may not include all of the information found in the codebooks. To verify codes, notes, cross-references, and other conventions and instructions, up-to-date ICD-9-CM and CPT codebooks should be readily available.

2. If the encoder permits customized edits, they should be used for coding rules or guidelines that are difficult to remember. For payment policies affecting code assignment, payer-specific edits might be incorporated in the encoder to help coding professionals remember the policy.

3. Coding staff should familiarize themselves with the ICD-9-CM and CPT code revisions so that they are able to identify errors in encoder software. (Keep in mind that changes to both code sets become effective twice a year—CPT on July 1 and January 1, and ICD-9-CM on April 1 and October 1.

4. Coding staff should be educated to detect errors in logic or in encoding software. Procedures for addressing perceived errors in logic or inappropriate edits in encoder, billing, or other types of software should be developed. Suggested steps to take when a possible error is identified include the following:

   • Coding staff should immediately report the issue to the coding manager, and it should be reported to the vendor promptly.

- If the software error is an unequivocal conflict with official coding rules and guidelines, immediate corrective action should be implemented. Coding staff should be informed of erroneous instruction and directed to disregard software instruction; if software permits customized edits, an edit should be developed to remind coding staff of the error and the appropriate code assignment.

- Follow-up with the vendor should be done on a regular basis until the issue has been resolved satisfactorily.

- All communication with the vendor should be documented, including organizational inquiries and vendor responses.

- All software errors should be documented, including the date the error was detected and how it was handled, and the date it was resolved. This documentation should be kept with the coding policies and procedures.

- If the error resulted in an overpayment by a payer, every reasonable effort should be made to identify overpaid claims and return the overpayment to the payer (with a letter of explanation).

- Software logic or edit errors affecting reimbursement should be reported to the HIM compliance specialist, who should report it to the corporate compliance officer.

## Documentation Requirements

Policies and procedures should address appropriate documentation requirements. The OIG's Supplemental Program Guidance for Hospitals states that all claims and requests for reimbursement from federal healthcare programs, and all supporting documentation, must be complete and accurate and reflect reasonable and necessary services ordered by an appropriately licensed medical professional who is a participating provider in the healthcare program from which the individual or entity is seeking reimbursement.

Documentation of all physician and other professional services should be proper (that is, according to regulatory standards and generally accepted documentation practices), complete, and timely to ensure that only accurate and properly documented services are billed. A number of regulatory standards and requirements address complete and accurate documentation. For example, medical staff standards of The Joint Commission include a standard pertaining to medical staff participation in the measurement, assessment, and improvement of patient care processes, including those related to accurate, timely, and legible completion of patients' health records. The management of information and performance improvement standards also contains a standard pertaining to ensuring accurate, timely, and complete health record documentation. The principles and standards for complete and accurate documentation are equally applicable to paper-based and electronic health records, although the processes may be different. Just as with paper-based records, clinicians using electronic documentation are responsible for the completeness and accuracy of their entries.

Claims should be submitted only when appropriate documentation supporting them is present in the health record and available for audit and review. Processes for ensuring that health record documentation is adequate and appropriate to support the coded diagnoses and procedures need to be in place. Given the compliance risks associated with the wrong discharge status being reported on inpatient claims, it is also important for the documentation to clearly indicate the discharge disposition of the patient.

Figure 3.2 lists the types of questions one should ask when evaluating the appropriateness of documentation.

The level of care to be provided should be clearly documented in the initial orders. For example, simply documenting "admit" is confusing because it is not clear if the patient is to be admitted as an inpatient, for outpatient surgery, or to outpatient observation. The order for level of care should be explicitly documented, such as "admit as inpatient," "admit to outpatient surgery," or "admit to observation." If the admission order is unclear, the physician should be asked to clarify the intended level of care and this clarification should be documented in the health record.

Health record documentation for any physician involved in the care and treatment of the patient, including documentation by consulting physicians, is appropriate for the basis of code assignment. It is also permissible to use the health record documentation for nonphysician healthcare providers, such as nurse practitioners and physician assistants, as the basis for code assignment, if they are considered legally accountable for establishing a diagnosis within the regulations governing the provider and the facility.

Health records should be organized and legible so that they can be coded accurately and audited readily. Documentation that should be available at the time of coding should be specifically described in the organization's policies and procedures. In an electronic environment, it is still necessary to have written policies and procedures defining when the record is complete for coding purposes. Accurate documentation is particularly important in an electronic environment because health record documentation may be maintained in multiple information systems, making it more difficult to determine when the documentation necessary for coding purposes has been completed. In a hybrid environment (mix of paper-based and electronic documentation), the format (paper or electronic) in which the reports will be made available to the coding staff should also be defined. If coding staff will be viewing health records online, they must be granted access to all clinical reports for any record they are responsible for coding.

No federal requirement exists on the specific health record documents that must be present when the health record is coded. However, the OIG's *Compliance Program Guidance for Hospitals* states that "the documentation necessary for accurate code assignment should be available to coding staff" (OIG 1998, 8991). Therefore, if an organization chooses to exclude certain reports from having to be available at the time of coding, and it is ultimately determined that one of these reports contains information affecting code assignment and that this information is not present elsewhere in the health record, this may be viewed as evidence of noncompliance. Examples of necessary but excluded reports are the discharge summary, certain consultation reports, the operative report, or complete office note documentation.

**Figure 3.2.  Questions to ask when evaluating documentation**

- Is the chief complaint and/or reason for the patient encounter or hospitalization documented?

- Do the initial orders for patient care reflect the level of care to be provided?

- Is there an appropriate history and physical examination?

- Are all services that were provided documented?

- Does documentation clearly explain why support services, procedures, and supplies were provided?

- Is assessment of the patient's condition included in the documentation?

- Does documentation include information on the patient's progress and treatment outcome?

- Is there a documented treatment plan?

- Does the plan for care include, as appropriate, treatments and medications (including frequency and dosage), any referrals and consultations, patient and family education, and follow-up instructions?

- Are changes to the treatment plan, including rationale, documented?

- Is there documentation of the medical rationale for services rendered?

- Does documentation support standards for medical necessity?

- Are abnormal test results addressed in the physician documentation? If abnormal test results are returned after discharge, are they documented in an addendum, along with the action taken?

- Are relevant health risk factors identified?

- Does documentation support intensity of patient evaluation and/or treatment, including thought processes and complexity of decision making?

- Are significant changes in the patient's condition and action taken documented?

- Is the status of unresolved problems documented?

- Is planned follow-up care documented?

- Is the hospital discharge status, including transfers to another hospital or to postacute care, clearly documented? Are any plans for home health services clearly documented?

- Does documentation support the level of care provided?

- Does documentation meet the criteria for the evaluation and management code billed?

- Does the documentation for the patient encounter include an assessment, clinical impression, or diagnosis?

- Are all diagnoses and procedures documented as specifically as possible?

- Are all complications and comorbidities documented?

- Do clinical reports include all elements required by regulatory and accreditation agencies?

- Are health record entries appropriately dated and authenticated?

- Is the documentation legible?

Coding without complete documentation or using preliminary information must be avoided. It is highly recommended that organizational policy prohibit coding records in the absence of final, physician-generated documentation or any other documentation the coding staff deems critical for proper coding. Coding from incomplete or preliminary documentation, and submitting these codes on the claim, can result in discrepancies between the final, completed health record and the reimbursement claim. When final reports do not match the submitted claim, the organization must rebill. Rebilling results in unnecessary additional work and may result in billing errors, because there is a risk that the discrepancy between the final record documentation and the codes reported on the claim will not be caught.

**In order to avoid re-reviewing the record and possibly having to rebill the claim, it is highly recommended that records not be coded until all physician-generated reports, including the discharge summary, are available.** HIM policies/procedures should identify any additional types of reports that should be present prior to coding. It is important to remember that there may be alternate methods of accessing the necessary information, such as in a hybrid environment (whereby there is a mix of both paper and electronic documentation). The coding staff should be involved in developing policies/procedures that define when a record is "complete for coding purposes" to ensure that documentation necessary for complete and accurate coding is available at the time of coding. (Of course, concurrent coding, in which codes are assigned and updated throughout the hospitalization but are not finalized and submitted on a claim until a final review of the completed record has been performed after discharge, is acceptable because the "preliminary" codes are not submitted to the payer.)

Standards for the timely completion of health records stipulated in the medical staff bylaws or policies should be adhered to. In addition to addressing requirements from regulatory agencies (for example, JCAHO), the healthcare organization's standards for health record completion should take into consideration the documentation necessary for coding. Health record completion standards should reasonably ensure that unnecessary delays in the coding process are not inadvertently built into the record completion process. Ideally, services should be documented at the time the service is provided or as soon afterward as is practical. Because physician documentation is critical to accurate and compliant coding, it is essential that documentation be completed in a timely manner and that adherence to the organization's policies for record completion be strictly enforced, whether the documentation is in a paper or electronic format. Violations should be taken seriously and disciplinary action should be taken against physicians who fail to comply with the organization's record completion policies. Full support from senior management and the Board of Directors is essential for enforcement of these policies. Given the importance of complete and accurate documentation, it is recommended that the medical staff leadership agree on minimum documentation standards necessary to retain medical staff privileges.

In addition to considering the timely completion of report dictation by clinicians, the timeliness of the transcription and filing of dictated reports should be addressed.

## Medical Necessity

Medicare, as well as most other payers, will not pay for any items or services it does not consider to be reasonable and necessary for the diagnosis or treatment of illness or injury

Non covered vs. Covered
medically    unnecessary
necessary                    Policies and Procedures        41

or to improve the functioning of a malformed body member. The first step in determining medical necessity is to determine whether the payer considers the services as covered or noncovered. Services that are classified as noncovered by a payer are never reimbursed by that payer, regardless of the diagnosis or the circumstance.

Covered services can be judged to be either medically necessary or unnecessary. NCDs and LCDs help providers avoid billing Medicare for items and services that are not covered or are coded incorrectly. CMS establishes NCDs to specify the circumstances under which Medicare covers specific medical items, services, treatments, procedures, or technologies. The Social Security Act defines an NCD as:

> . . . a determination by the Secretary with respect to whether or not a particular item or service is covered nationally by Medicare, but does not include a determination of what code, if any, is assigned to a particular item or service covered under this title or a determination with respect to the amount of payment made for a particular item or service so covered (CMS 2003).

NCDs are published in the *Medicare National Coverage Determinations Manual,* and they become effective as of the date listed in the transmittal that announces the manual's revision. If an NCD does not specifically exclude an indication or circumstance, or if the item or service is not mentioned at all in an NCD or in a Medicare manual, it is up to the individual Medicare contractors to make the coverage decision.

National coverage determinations apply nationwide and are binding on all Medicare contractors, QIOs, health maintenance organizations, competitive medical plans, and healthcare prepayment plans for purposes of Medicare coverage.

In the absence of a specific NCD, coverage decisions are made at the discretion of the Medicare contractors. LCDs are determinations by a Medicare contractor with respect to whether a particular item or service is covered in accordance with the "reasonable and necessary" provisions of the Social Security Act on an intermediary- or carrier-wide basis. LCDs are formal statements developed by Medicare contractors to outline coverage criteria, define medical necessity, and provide references upon which a policy is based.

According to the *Medicare Program Integrity Manual,* Medicare contractors must develop medical review policies for services that have one or more of the following characteristics:

- They are being furnished to an extent that raises questions of abuse or overutilization.

- They appear to have been furnished under conditions inconsistent with standards of practice or accepted technology.

- They appear not to be medically reasonable and necessary.

Private payers also develop specific coverage policies and may use differing definitions of medical necessity.

Because medical necessity is determined by the ICD-9-CM diagnosis code(s) describing the patient's symptom(s) or condition(s) necessitating the service, accurate code assignment is critical. Because of the need to establish medical necessity prior to rendering care, this coding may be performed by individuals who have not received adequate coding education and training, resulting in inaccurate (or incorrect) code assignments. Also, missing, incomplete, or unclear documentation from the physician ordering the service can lead to coding inaccuracies.

Submitting claims for services that the provider should know will not be paid by Medicare can subject the provider to civil monetary penalties or fines. When a provider sees that a service is not medically necessary, as evidenced by a denied claim, the provider's persistent submission of claims for these services is considered "reckless disregard."

## Documentation to Support Medical Necessity

The Balanced Budget Act of 1997 requires physicians and qualified nonphysician practitioners (NPP) to provide diagnostic information when ordering services furnished by another entity when the Medicare contractor has a local coverage policy requiring such diagnostic information from the entity performing the service. This diagnostic information must be provided at the time the item or service is ordered. It is highly recommended that organizations require physicians and nonphysician practices to provide diagnostic information each time they order items or services. This policy promotes consistent documentation practices, lessens confusion as to when diagnostic information is necessary, and ensures that the documentation needed to support medical necessity is readily available. The ordering physician or nonphysician practitioner should provide this information in narrative form, and the trained HIM coding staff at the organization performing the diagnostic test(s) should translate it to ICD-9-CM code(s). A complete order is one that is dated, includes the test(s) being ordered and the reasons (diagnoses or symptoms) for each test, and is signed by the physician.

If tests are ordered electronically, the diagnosis field should be a mandatory field. If hard-copy requisition forms are used, the field for the diagnosis should be prominent and the form should contain a reminder about the necessity to document the reason for the test on the form. The entity performing the service must maintain the documentation that it receives from the ordering physician or qualified NPP. The ordering physician or qualified NPP must maintain documentation of medical necessity in the patient's health record. Upon request by CMS, the provider performing the test and submitting the claim for the service must be able to provide documentation of the order for the service billed (including sufficient information to enable CMS to identify and contact the ordering physician or NPP), documentation showing accurate processing of the order and submission of the claim, and diagnostic or other medical information supplied by the ordering physician or NPP.

Medicare regulations require that all diagnostic tests, including x-ray tests and laboratory tests, must be ordered by the physician who is treating the patient for a specific medical problem and who uses the results in the management of the patient's specific medical problem. CMS has indicated that this requirement does not necessarily mean that there must be a physician's signature on the test requisition. However, documentation that the physician or NPP ordered the test must be available upon CMS's request. According to CMS, although the signature of a physician on the requisition is one way of documenting that the treating physician has ordered the test, it is not the only permissible way of documenting that the treating physician ordered the test. For example, the treating physician may document the ordering of specific tests in the patient's health record. The *Medicare Carrier Manual* defines an order for a diagnostic test as a communication from the treating physician or NPP requesting that a diagnostic test be performed on a patient. In CMS Program Memorandum AB-01-144 (2001), CMS has indicated that an order may include the following forms of communication:

- A written document signed by the treating physician/practitioner that is hand-delivered, mailed, or faxed to the testing facility

- A telephone call by the treating physician or NPP or his or her office to the testing facility

- An electronic mail message by the treating physician or NPP or his or her office to the testing facility

The use of order forms or test requisition forms that only list the payable ICD-9-CM codes for a given test is not recommended, because this practice can result in charges of "code jamming."

For orders communicated via telephone, CMS requires both the treating physician or NPP and the testing facility to document the telephone call in their respective copies of the patient's health record. Organizations' medical staff rules and regulations should address the policy and procedure for processing telephone orders and indicate who is authorized to receive them.

In the event that there is no diagnosis on the physician's order, efforts should be made to obtain diagnostic information from the ordering physician's office prior to performing the service. Many facilities have established a policy that when an order is incomplete or does not meet medical necessity criteria, the patient is instructed to call the physician's office to obtain more information. In other instances, the coding or registration staff is responsible for contacting the physician's office. When the physician's office must be contacted for diagnostic information pertaining to an ordered service, either before or after the service is rendered, this information should be obtained only from the physician or a designated member of his or her office staff. When diagnostic information is obtained from a physician or his or her staff after receipt of the specimen and request for services, it should be documented by the HIM staff, including the diagnosis supporting the diagnostic test, the date the information was obtained, and the name of the individual providing the information. This information should be maintained in the patient's health record. The organization's policies and procedures should stipulate the specific location in the health record where this information should be maintained.

In the event that the ordering physician or NPP has not supplied diagnostic information related to a test that has been ordered and is unavailable, CMS allows organizations to obtain diagnostic information directly from the patient as to the reason a test is being performed (per Program Memorandum AB-01-144). However, this practice is not recommended. Patients may not accurately describe the reason for the test or may describe the reason in nonmedical terms, which then must be translated into clinical terms by staff, and their description of the reason for the test may not be supported by health record documentation. When no diagnostic information is provided by the ordering physician or NPP and that person is unavailable, it may be preferable to issue an advance beneficiary notice (ABN), which is discussed in more detail in the next section, than to rely on diagnostic information provided by the patient. Prior to submitting the claim, the ordering physician or NPP should be contacted for diagnostic information.

Documentation supporting medical necessity of the service rendered should be maintained in the patient's health record (at the organization performing the diagnostic tests) and should be legible. The provider performing the service may request additional diagnostic and other medical information to document that the services performed are medically necessary. However, habitually contacting physicians for more information because the physician's order or test requisition lacked diagnostic information or the provided diagnostic information did not support medical necessity of the ordered services is not the ideal practice and is potentially risky from a compliance perspective. Contacting physicians for additional documentation or modified orders after the service has been rendered or after the service has been denied as medically unnecessary is particularly risky. This practice places the organization in a position of appearing to "doctor" the documentation. If not handled correctly and objectively, these actions could be perceived as "prompting" the physician.

Instances when diagnostic information supporting tests must be obtained after the fact should be the exception rather than the norm. Physicians should be expected to provide the necessary diagnostic information at the time the service is ordered. The HIM department should monitor physician compliance to identify patterns. When a pattern of noncompliance by a particular physician is identified, appropriate corrective action should be taken. This action might include targeted education, refusal to perform tests in the future until diagnostic information has been obtained, or initiating penalties for repeated noncompliance. Patterns that should be closely monitored include lack of provision of any diagnostic information on the test requisition, provision of unacceptable diagnostic information (such as a rule-out diagnosis without specification of the patient's symptoms), provision of diagnoses that do not meet Medicare's definition of medical necessity (as defined in NCDs and LCDs), and no issuance of an ABN. When there is a recurring pattern of noncompliance, organizational policy should delineate appropriate disciplinary action.

Ideally, periodic random reviews of physicians' office records for situations in which diagnostic information was provided verbally to coding staff should be conducted to ascertain that the information provided is documented appropriately. However, physicians' practices that are not owned by the healthcare organization are not required to permit the organization access to their records. These reviews can only be conducted if the physicians grant their consent. When patterns of problems are identified, education should be provided to the physicians whose office documentation is found to be inadequate.

If a provider believes that an ICD-9-CM code has been inadvertently omitted from a payer's coverage policy, or an appropriate diagnosis is not included in the indications for the item or service, the issue should be brought to the attention of the payer, along with documentation to support the inclusion of the code or diagnosis. Medicare contractors are required to solicit public comments on their draft local coverage policies. They generally accomplish this by posting their draft LCDs on the Internet (draft LCDs are available online from cms.hhs.gov/coverage), publishing them in bulletins, and holding advisory committee meetings that are open to the public. It is important for HIM professionals to review these draft policies and ensure that the listed ICD-9-CM codes are complete and accurate and consistent with coding rules and guidelines. HIM professionals also are encouraged to actively seek ongoing involvement in the development of LCDs through volunteering to serve on the local Medicare contractor's advisory committee or attending all advisory committee meetings. Any identified errors in the listed codes or missing codes should be brought to the attention of the payer. These actions ensure that providers receive the appropriate reimbursement for the item or service without being required to violate coding rules and guidelines. The importance of ensuring that coverage policies are consistent with ICD-9-CM coding rules and guidelines in light of the HIPAA requirement for adherence to the *ICD-9-CM Official Guidelines for Coding and Reporting* should be stressed to payers. During the process of reviewing draft coverage policies, input from physicians also should be sought to ensure that the clinical indications for the item or service are complete and accurate. It is also important for the narrative indications stated in a coverage policy to be consistent with the ICD-9-CM codes that support medical necessity.

Because private payers' coverage policies can differ from Medicare's, it is important to also communicate with other payers regarding their process for developing coverage policies pertaining to medical necessity and to take advantage of opportunities to provide public input on these policies.

### Advance Beneficiary Notices

If the healthcare provider has reason to believe that Medicare will deny an item or service because Medicare's coverage criteria have not been met, an advance beneficiary notice (ABN) should be issued to the Medicare patient or his or her legal representative before performing the test. An example of such an instance is when the physician (or other ordering provider) has provided a reason for ordering a diagnostic test or therapy services for a Medicare beneficiary, but it does not meet Medicare's medical necessity standards. The ABN relieves the provider of the item or service of liability because the notice is proof of the beneficiary's prior knowledge of the likelihood of noncoverage. It also allows the provider to collect payment for the item or service from the patient if Medicare denies the claim.

Items or services that are statutorily excluded from Medicare coverage do not require an ABN, such as routine physicals or cosmetic surgery.

CMS created a program called the Beneficiary Notices Initiative (BNI). The purpose of this program is to wed consumer rights and protections with effective beneficiary communication so that beneficiaries are given the opportunity to exercise their rights and protections in a well-informed and timely manner. As part of this program, CMS developed standardized ABN forms that contain model language.

The purpose of the ABN is to inform Medicare beneficiaries, before they receive specified items or services, that Medicare certainly or probably will not pay for them on that particular occasion. The ABN also allows beneficiaries to make informed consumer decisions whether or not to receive the items or services for which they may have to pay out-of-pocket or through other insurance coverage. In addition, the ABN allows beneficiaries to better participate in their own healthcare treatment decisions by making informed consumer decisions. If the provider, practitioner, or supplier expects payment for the items or services to be denied by Medicare, the provider, practitioner, or supplier must advise the beneficiary before items or services are furnished that, in his or her opinion, the beneficiary will be personally and fully responsible for payment. To be "personally and fully responsible for payment" means that the beneficiary will be liable to make payment out-of-pocket, through other insurance coverage (for example, employer group health plan coverage), or through Medicaid or other federal or nonfederal payment source.

An ABN must be signed by the patient after the service is ordered and before it has been performed. Each ABN should meet the following requirements:

- Be expressed in writing in lay language

- Identify the specific items or services for which payment will be or is likely to be denied

- State the specific reason why the physician or other provider believes the service will be or is likely to be denied

- Be delivered to the patient (or the patient's authorized representative) before the indicated items or services are furnished

- Be signed by the patient (when another person signs for the patient, that person's name and relationship to the patient should be documented) acknowledging that the required information was provided and that the patient assumes responsibility for paying for the service

The beneficiary cannot refuse to sign a properly executed ABN and still demand the item or service. If a beneficiary refuses to sign a properly executed ABN, the provider should consider not furnishing the item or service. Additionally, the provider may annotate the ABN, and have the annotation witnessed, indicating the circumstances and persons involved. In this instance, the claim for services can be submitted with an indication that an ABN was given.

An ABN is not acceptable evidence if the following occurs:

- The notice is unreadable, illegible, or otherwise incomprehensible

- The patient (or authorized representative) is incapable of understanding the notice because of the particular circumstances (even if others may understand)

- The notice is given during an emergency, or the beneficiary is under great duress

- The patient (or authorized representative) is, in any way, coerced or misled by the notifier, by the contents of the notice, and/or by the manner of delivery of the notice

A telephone notice to a beneficiary or authorized representative is not sufficient evidence of proper notice for limiting any potential liability, unless the content of the telephone contact can be verified and is not disputed by the beneficiary. If a telephone notice was followed up immediately with a mailed notice or a personal visit at which time written notice was delivered in person and the beneficiary signed the written notice accepting responsibility for payment, the contractor will accept the time of the telephone notice as the time of ABN delivery.

An ABN will not be considered acceptable if the patient is asked to sign a blank form. An ABN should never be issued routinely without regard to a particular need, as the ABN must state the specific reason the physician or other provider anticipates that the particular service will not be reimbursed. Each time diagnostic information is missing on the test requisition, an ABN should not be routinely issued to the patient in lieu of contacting the ordering physician for a diagnosis. This practice could be construed as routine issuance of ABNs, which is prohibited by Medicare. "Routine issuance" means giving ABNs to beneficiaries when there is no specific, identifiable reason to believe Medicare will not pay. If the Medicare contractor identifies a pattern of routine notices in situations in which such notices clearly are not effective, he or she will write to the provider and remind the provider of these standards. In general, routinely given ABNs are defective notices and will not protect the notifier from liability. There are a few exceptional circumstances when ABNs may "routinely" be issued, such as for services that are always denied for medical necessity or for services for which Medicare has established a statutory or regulatory frequency limitation on coverage.

For any ABN process to be successful, a policy must be established and enforced. The components of an effective policy include the following:

- A determination of who will obtain the ABN (Physician's office? Registration department at site where test is to be performed? Ancillary department where test is to be performed?)

- A determination of what constitutes a valid order

- Action that will be taken when a valid order is not received

- Action that will be taken when a patient arrives with an invalid order

- Action that will be taken when a patient's specimen arrives with an invalid order or no order

- Action that will be taken when the patient refuses to sign the ABN

- Type of monitoring that will occur to gauge the effectiveness of the ABN policy and assignment of responsibility for this monitoring

An ideal approach to handling ABNs is an online application for entering diagnoses and symptoms to ascertain the necessity of an ABN, and the ability to generate an ABN automatically.

Ideally, the physician's office should issue the ABN. The ABN is supposed to provide sufficient information to the patient in advance of the service so that the patient can make an informed decision whether to bear the financial responsibility for the service without "undue pressure." Physicians are in the best position to explain their rationale for ordering the test. Staff at the facility where the test is to be performed will not be in a position to explain to the patient a physician's rationale for ordering the test. The LCDs of the local Medicare contractor should be made available to physicians so that they are able to determine when an ABN needs to be issued. If the physician is charged with responsibility for issuing the ABN, his or her knowledge of Medicare's medical necessity standards is continuously reinforced, and the physician is more likely to keep these standards in mind when ordering diagnostic tests.

If the physician is responsible for issuing the ABN, a copy of the notice should be attached to the test requisition or order form and sent to the organization providing and billing for the item or service. This action ensures the organization that the ABN has been issued and meets Medicare requirements.

Given the complexity of obtaining ABNs, providers may be tempted to simply not obtain them. However, providers who do this may be considered to be providing inappropriate incentives for patients by providing "free" care, leading to allegations of antikickback violations. Because a provider cannot bill the patient without an ABN, failure to obtain ABNs can give the appearance that the provider is attempting to use improper inducements to attract Medicare patients. CMS encourages Medicare contractors to identify providers who do not submit ABNs and investigate them under antikickback statutes. Also, denials resulting from lack of medical necessity are not considered "bad debt" because the services were never billed to the proper payer, which is the Medicare beneficiary or his or her secondary insurance. The only way to stay in compliance is through front-end medical necessity determinations and issuance of the ABN as appropriate. Review of claims and supporting health record documentation prior to submission of the claim serves as a good final check to ensure compliance with Medicare policies, but it is too late at that point to obtain an ABN. However, this final review before the claim is submitted can ensure that the diagnosis documented as the reason for the service is accurately reflected on the claim. Although the ABN may be issued by either the organization providing the item or service or the physician ordering it, the organization must produce a copy of the ABN upon Medicare's request. Also, the organization that billed for the item or service will not be protected from liability if at least one of the following situations is true:

- The provider of the item or service believes the physician issued an ABN, but in actuality the physician did not.

- The ABN issued by the physician is unacceptable to Medicare (for example, it does not contain all of the information required by Medicare or was not issued before the service was provided).

- The physician's office cannot locate the ABN (and the provider of the item or service does not have a copy).

The financial liability protection offered by the issuance of an ABN cannot be afforded to providers when a finding of fraud or abuse has been made with respect to the provider's billing practices or in other situations in which the provider furnishes and claims payment for services that are so patently unnecessary that all providers could reasonably be expected to know they are not covered. For example, this would include services that are inconsistent with accepted sound medical practice and are clearly not within the concept of reasonable and necessary as defined by law or regulation. ABNs cannot be used to avoid bundling rules determined by the National Correct Coding Initiative edits.

### Medical Necessity Screening Software

Some facilities use screening software to check for medical necessity. Medical necessity software applications supply information to providers regarding whether a particular service (represented as a CPT code) will be covered by Medicare based on the ICD-9-CM diagnosis codes identified in the applicable medical coverage policy. Most coverage policies contain examples of covered and noncovered ICD-9-CM codes, but in many situations a service would meet medical necessity criteria based on the narrative indications for the test described in the coverage policy that are not explicitly identified by the ICD-9-CM diagnosis codes listed in the policy. Furthermore, some services have such a wide variety of conditions that all possible codes are not listed. These services would be denied under certain circumstances, which may or may not be clearly indicated in the policy (Scichilone 2002, 48). Also, coverage policies may be revised, but the software may not be immediately updated.

This software should be used with caution. It is inappropriate to rely solely on software applications to provide the appropriate information to substantiate medical necessity for items and services ordered. Software programs only create an efficient way to manage coverage policies; they cannot substitute for familiarity with the entire coverage policy and review of the health record documentation to validate medical necessity (Scichilone 2002, 48). Medical necessity screening software is best used after a coding expert has coded the diagnostic information provided by the ordering physician or practitioner. For example, is the software going to be able to recognize that a diagnosis of "history of venous thrombosis" means a past history, not a current condition? Will it know what to do with a "rule-out" diagnosis?

The risk of reliance on screening software has some pitfalls that should be recognized before investment. When the software to screen for medical necessity is used **prior to the service,** the following can occur:

- ABNs may be issued by the hospital when the service does not appear to be medically necessary, though the documentation in the record kept by the ordering physician supports coverage. Medicare beneficiaries may end up believing they must pay out-of-pocket for services that should be covered when a claim is filed. Also, it is possible that a covered diagnosis code may be assigned by the hospital coding staff based on information confirmed by a physician following the test results, when prior to the test, the clinician did not have enough information to report a diagnosis on the covered list. Medicare would pay for the service claimed and there would be no need to bill the patient, even though the patient was told up front that Medicare might not pay for the service.

- When the software rejects the service as not medically necessary, the patient has to decide whether to pay for the test or ask the provider to submit a claim for the purpose of obtaining a denial. Faced with these choices, a patient may elect not to receive a service their physician believes is needed. This situation can become complicated when it occurs in a hospital; the physician is usually not available to speak with the patient and explain why the service was ordered. If the hospital indicates that it will go back to the physician for a "better" diagnosis, questions may be raised about the ethics of the coding process.

- Valuable time and resources are wasted selecting an "acceptable" diagnosis from the physician to progress with the service rejected by the screening software, even though the diagnosis provided would be appropriate and necessary for the condition, despite not being listed in the coverage policy table.

When the software is used on the back end of the process, **before a claim is filed,** the following can occur:

- Some providers using screening software might elect not to file a claim for a questionable or noncovered service and will write off the costs rather than submit a claim to the payer. If this is a routine practice, there are instances when hospitals are losing money that they deserve and are not taking advantage of the appeal process to [effect] coverage changes. These providers are also increasing the risk of providing inappropriate incentives for patient services by waiving patient coinsurance and deductibles and providing free care. For questionable services involving medical necessity, a claim must be filed to determine coverage requirements for the patient. As described in the Medicare Hospital Manual, there are only a few circumstances when a provider should not submit a claim to Medicare.

- The "back door" approach [ensures] that patients receive the services the physician ordered without delay or questions but increases compliance risks by encouraging the search for a "payable code." In the case of Medicare, this can also cause the hospital to lose money by providing services that will be denied because they are not covered and then cannot be billed to the patient because no ABN was completed at the time of service.

- When a service is rejected with the code provided, the hospital may try to find a covered code using inappropriate methods such as assumptive coding, creation of leading inquiries to physicians, or using a source document for a code not appropriate for that encounter (such as documentation from a previous encounter). All of these practices are ethically questionable and increase the likelihood of false claims allegations against the hospital. Software tools should never be used as a reason to change or manipulate a patient's diagnosis for claims reporting without full knowledge and consent of the physician and assurance that clinical documentation supports the actual condition reported (Scichilone 2002, 48,50).

Organizations should research medical necessity screening software carefully and seek feedback from other organizations using the same software prior to purchase. The software can serve as a useful tool but should not completely replace human review. Educated and ethical coding practices should continue to form the cornerstone of the billing process.

## Managing Medical Necessity Requirements

Following are some tips for achieving compliance with payers' medical necessity requirements:

- **Report the patient's actual condition** that reflects the reason for the test. If a hospital allows ordering physicians to submit the diagnosis codes rather than the narrative description of the reason for service, there is a risk that the code is not fully accurate when compared to the source document. Further, the narrative description enables the technician carrying out [the test] to understand the indications for the service and not have to translate the numeric code back to clinical information.

- **Use a requisition form** that documents the reason for the service and enforces its use. Then, a coding professional specifically trained in coding conventions and reimbursement requirements can translate the information into ICD-9-CM codes used on the claim form.

- **Make sure** clinical documentation forms or formats **prompt** the users to fully document medical necessity for services ordered.

- When ABNs are required, they are best **administered by the ordering physician** so that the patient is fully informed of the implications of payment or declining the service. This is much harder to accomplish at the hospital. Software assistance is most useful at this stage to educate physicians concerning Medicare coverage requirements and policies.

- Audit claims with medical necessity denials and **look for patterns** by actual service or by ordering physician. When trends are identified, targeted education can help improve documentation or communication of the reason for services to minimize denials and rejections for covered services. This education can ensure that noncovered services are identified in time to get the required notices given and allow the patient to make a fully informed choice.

- **Use software as a tool** for managing coverage requirements and providing readily available education. Avoid reliance on any product that suggests codes when the conditions cannot be fully supported in documentation. Also, confirm that the product is using the correct set of guidelines. For hospitals, those are the policies that apply to institutions submitting claims to fiscal intermediaries (FIs). There are currently differences by locality and also between FIs and carriers for the same service, so make sure the tool being used applies the correct set of guidelines to the reported services.

- **Ask** the software vendor to illustrate how the software will help the facility manage those services where discrete code sets are not available or all-inclusive and the policy relies on text descriptions rather than ICD-9-CM code lists.

- **Be confident** that when accurate clinical data is translated into the appropriate clinical codes, the correct coverage decision will result with or without software assistance. When it does not, be sure to exercise the right to appeal (Scichilone 2002, 50).

The healthcare organization's compliance program should include processes for ensuring that medical necessity criteria are checked prior to performing the test and that the test was ordered by a physician or other appropriately licensed individual. If feasible, assigning a coding professional to the registration area helps to ensure the accuracy of the process for verifying that medical necessity requirements have been met. In addition to the importance of correct assignment of the diagnosis codes, it is also important to identify the correct procedure code so that the applicable NCD, LCD, or private payer coverage policy will be used for determining medical necessity. Of course, it is probably unrealistic for an organization to be able to staff the registration area with coding personnel 24 hours a day, but certainly providing coding staff during the time when most of the diagnostic outpatient services are being performed would address many of the medical necessity issues.

The best approach to ensure compliance with medical necessity requirements is complete and accurate diagnostic information provided by the ordering physician or practitioner at the time a test is ordered. The key to achieving this is thorough, ongoing education of the medical staff on medical necessity requirements and the importance of providing complete, accurate diagnoses describing the reason(s) test(s) are being ordered, supported by the documentation in their office health records. The organization performing the diagnostic tests should regularly educate physicians on the medical necessity definitions and rules of the various payers it does business with. Physicians should be educated on the reasons they are required to provide diagnostic information when ordering tests. Examples include the following:

- The Medicare requirement that services are reasonable and necessary for diagnosis and treatment

- The development of NCDs/LCDs containing diagnoses that support Medicare's definition of medical necessity

- The development of coverage policies pertaining to private payers' definitions of medical necessity

- The likelihood that the provider furnishing the test will not be reimbursed unless a diagnosis supporting the medical necessity of the test is submitted on the claim or an ABN has been issued to the patient

- The possibility that the Medicare contractor will request a copy of the physician's office record if insufficient or nonsupportive diagnostic information is submitted on the claim

Educational programs should emphasize that the diagnostic information provided on the requisition must accurately reflect the patient's condition and be supported by documentation in the physician's office record. It is *never* appropriate to simply select a payable diagnosis in order to ensure that the test will be reimbursed by Medicare.

It is unethical and fraudulent to report a diagnosis code on the claim that is not supported by health record documentation simply because it is "payable." If the service does not meet the payer's medical necessity standards, the patient should be informed of the likelihood of the service being denied prior to furnishing the service, and, in the case of Medicare, an ABN should be issued. The patient should be allowed the option of choosing to forego the test. If the patient decides not to have the test, the ordering physician or practitioner should be notified.

In all healthcare settings, the applicable medical necessity requirements should be reviewed and appropriate processes put in place to ensure compliance. For example, in the home health setting, the plan of care must be certified by a physician who is a doctor of medicine, osteopathy, or podiatric medicine. Periodic clinical reviews, both prior and subsequent to billing for services, should be conducted to verify that patients are receiving only medically necessary services. Home health agencies should examine the frequency and duration of the services they perform to determine, in consultation with a physician, whether the patient's medical condition justifies the number of visits provided and billed. Policies and procedures should be implemented to verify that beneficiaries have actually received the appropriate level and number of services billed. The importance of accurately documenting the services performed and billed should be stressed to caregivers. Confirmation that services were provided as claimed could be obtained by periodically contacting (via e-mail, telephone, or in person) a random sample of patients and interviewing the clinical staff involved. Home health agencies need to establish processes to ensure that physician orders are received and properly documented prior to billing for services. A leading reason for home health claims denials is failure to obtain physician orders in a timely manner.

## Other Policy/Procedure Issues

Facilities also should create policies or procedures for issues including consultant arrangements, record retention, confidentiality, compliance in relation to an employee's performance review, and HIPAA.

### Arrangements with Consultants

Although a coding consultant can help to identify and resolve errors and improve coding accuracy, reliance on improper advice from a consultant substantially increases an organization's risk of sanctions and/or fines. Therefore, it is imperative for an organization to select a consultant carefully. The OIG released a Special Advisory Bulletin in June 2001 regarding certain consulting practices. The bulletin addressed the following questionable practices that have been identified in healthcare consulting:

- **[Making] Illegal or misleading representations:** Some consultants have made claims that they have "special" relationships with the CMS or the OIG, including statements that they are "endorsed" by one of these agencies. Neither of these agencies endorses consulting companies.

- **[Making] Promises and guarantees:** Consultants may make financial promises or guarantees that cannot be met. Such guarantees may include a promise that consulting services will result in a certain dollar or percentage increase in reimbursement. The practices used to keep these promises may be fraudulent.

- **Encouraging abusive practices:** Healthcare consulting companies may educate providers to use inappropriate codes to increase reimbursement or to misinterpret coding rules and regulations to maximize reimbursement. The provider may not question the vendor and, in fact, trust the information provided as part of the vendor education.

- **Discouraging compliance efforts:** Certain consultants discourage certain compliance efforts, such as coding compliance reviews. Compliance reviews are a recommended component of the OIG's Compliance Guidance. Should problems remain undetected, the provider may be at risk for potential fraud and abuse violations (Hammen 2001, 26).

According to the OIG advisory bulletin, the consultant's role is as follows (OIG 2001, 2):

Responsible consultants play an integral role in developing and maintaining practices that enhance a client's business objectives, as well as in improving the overall integrity of the health care system. [The OIG] believes that most consultants, like most providers, are honest, and that the vast majority of relationships between providers and consultants are legitimate business activities. Unfortunately, a small minority of unscrupulous consultants engage in improper practices or encourage abuse of the Medicare and Medicaid programs. Depending on the circumstances, these practices may expose both the consultants and their clients to potential legal liability. Hiring a consultant does not relieve a provider of responsibility for ensuring the integrity of its dealings with the Federal health care programs.

In June 2001, the General Accounting Office (GAO) issued a report that discussed instances of inappropriate or fraudulent advice given by a consulting company (GAO 2001). This advice could result in violations of both civil and criminal statutes. During the course of the education, advice was provided regarding the following:

- Avoidance of reporting and refunding overpayments

- Creation of documentation to support higher-level evaluation and management (E/M) code assignments when a lower level code is appropriate

- Limitation of services to Medicaid patients to avoid the lower payments usually associated with Medicaid

The GAO suggested to the OIG that workshops and seminars should be monitored to identify advice that could result in improper or excessive claims for reimbursement.

Healthcare providers need to be vigilant and exercise prudence when selecting and relying on consultants (Hammen 2001, 26).

Criteria to assist providers in selecting external coding consulting companies is detailed in figure 3.3.

**Figure 3.3.   Consulting vendor criteria**

- **Follows the cooperating parties' official guidelines for coding and reporting.** Under the HIPAA regulations for electronic transactions and code sets, all providers and payers must adhere to the cooperating parties' *ICD-9-CM Official Guidelines for Coding and Reporting.* The cooperating parties are AHIMA, AHA, CMS, and the National Center for Health Statistics. It may be worthwhile to review the vendor's internal coding guidelines to ensure consistency with the official coding guidelines. Additionally, if a physician coding quality review is conducted, the vendor should be well versed in the application of E/M documentation guidelines that have been approved by CMS in assigning the appropriate level of CPT evaluation and management codes.

- **Reports overcoding, undercoding, and coding quality errors that do not affect reimbursement.** The primary goals should be to assess and improve coding accuracy. High-quality coded data depend on complete and accurate coding that reflects the documented diagnoses and procedures. The provider can then be assured that the billing is accurate and that its healthcare statistics will provide an accurate view of the case mix for determining future services, managed care contracting, and profiling.

- **Charges fixed fees instead of contingency fees.** The OIG compliance program guidance advises that compensation for billing consultants should not provide any financial incentive to improperly upcode claims. By charging the healthcare provider a fixed fee for coding quality reviews rather than a percentage of the money "found," the incentive for upcoding is eliminated.

- **Employs only AHIMA-credentialed coding staff and is willing to provide proof of the credential status of each employee providing services.** Attainment of an AHIMA credential indicates that the individual has met AHIMA competencies for the particular credential and participates in ongoing continuing education.

- **Justifies recommendations for changes to coding or DRG assignment through the use of appropriate references.** Appropriate references would include the use of the official coding guidelines, E/M documentation guidelines, *Coding Clinic for ICD-9-CM,* or *CPT Assistant.* If the consultant cannot justify a recommended change, the healthcare provider may want to contact an official source (the Central Office on ICD-9-CM for ICD-9-CM questions or the American Medical Association for CPT questions) prior to agreeing with the consultant's recommendation.

- **Educates consulting staff on consistent application of official coding guidelines.** The vendor should be able to produce documentation indicating the provision of at least annual or semiannual educational programs for its consulting staff. This may represent an educational session developed and presented by the company itself or sending the consulting staff to external programs.

- **Assesses its own compliance and provides you a copy of its program.** If a coding compliance vendor does not have a compliance program in place, how can it assist you in ensuring your compliance? Their program should be verified for consistency with your organization's compliance program. The coding philosophy of the selected vendor should reflect your organization's philosophy in ensuring complete and accurate coding. In any case, the firm's representative should be asked to sign an agreement that any personnel assigned to the healthcare organization will abide by the elements of its compliance program.

- **Monitors the quality of work performed by its consulting staff and institutes corrective action to address unacceptable levels of coding accuracy.** The vendor should be able to provide assurance that its work meets certain quality standards.

*(Continued on next page)*

**Figure 3.3.**    *(Continued)*

- **Educates provider staff as a component of its services.** A good external coding quality review should include education related to findings of upcoding, undercoding, and data quality as a component of its services. Education should be provided for both the coding staff and the physicians in order to address findings related to coding quality and documentation. Technical or clinical education related to trends identified during the audit process should be included in the educational component.

- **Possesses a clean record.** In keeping with the regulations for providers in the Balanced Budget Act of 1997, vendors who have been convicted of fraudulent practices should be avoided. It is in the best interest of the healthcare provider to ensure that they are receiving high-quality, ethical services.

- **Provides services under attorney-client privilege.** When an attorney representing a provider requests auditing services under attorney-client privilege, the vendor will work with and report only to the attorney. There will be no communication between the vendor and the healthcare provider. This protects the results of the coding compliance audit from future "discovery."

- **Possesses credible client references.** Do not settle for a prepared list of references—this list will only give you the names of individuals with whom the vendor wants you to speak. Request a list of and contact the five clients most recently served by the vendor. Ensure that they were satisfied with the coding philosophy of the vendor, the fees, and the quality of service.

Adapted from Hammen 2001, 26, 28, 30.

Before signing a contract for coding consulting services, the qualifications of the firm providing the services should be evaluated carefully. The following questions offer some guidance:

- What is the background of the firm's management staff?

- What experience and qualifications do its personnel have?

- What are the firm's continuing education requirements for its staff?

- What mechanisms does the firm have in place to monitor the quality of its work? How is quality measured? What are its accuracy standards?

- Does the firm have a corporate compliance program? If so, is it consistent with the healthcare organization's compliance program?

- How is the firm reimbursed for services (flat fee, hourly rate, per record rate, contingency based)?

The references and specific qualifications of the individuals responsible for conducting the work at the healthcare organization should be checked thoroughly. Do they possess an HIM credential? Does their experience match the type of work they will be doing? For example, does the person performing DRG validation have inpatient coding experience in a PPS hospital, or does the individual reviewing a physician's E/M services have experience with this type of coding? Organizations should contact the most recent clients served by the consultant to determine the quality of the work performed and the level of satisfaction with the services provided.

The organization's policies and procedures should stipulate that it has the right to refuse to implement a consultant's recommendation when it can demonstrate that the consultant's advice conflicts with official coding guidelines or regulatory requirements. For every recommendation accepted that is contingent on additional physician documentation, the physician should incorporate the documentation in the health record before submitting the claim containing the revised codes (or, if it is a retrospective review, before resubmitting a claim or submitting a higher-weighted DRG adjustment request).

A healthcare provider can protect itself from investigation by ensuring that the coding consulting company selected provides high-quality, ethical services and adheres to all applicable federal and state laws and regulations. As the OIG notes in the conclusion of its advisory bulletin, "if a consultant's advice seems to be too good to be true, it probably is" (OIG 2001, 2).

## Retention of Records

Written policies and procedures should be established to address the creation, distribution, retention, storage, retrieval, and destruction of all types of documents. Types of documents include health records, claims documents, and compliance documents. Health records and claims documentation should be retained according to applicable federal and state law and regulations.

All organizations should develop and implement a system for maintaining all records necessary to demonstrate the integrity of the compliance process and confirm the effectiveness of the program. Documents include the following types:

- Employee certifications relating to the code of conduct, training, and other compliance initiatives
- Copies of compliance training materials
- Results of auditing/monitoring activities, including corrective action plans and follow-up
- Reports of investigations
- Outcomes
- Disciplinary actions taken
- Relevant correspondence with CMS, Medicare contractors, private health insurers, and state survey and certification agencies

The organization's legal counsel should be consulted regarding the retention of compliance records (such as employee training documentation, reports from the hotline, results of internal investigations, and results of auditing and monitoring). These records must be maintained for a sufficient length of time to ensure their availability to prove compliance with laws and regulations, if needed.

Health records must be secured against loss, destruction, unauthorized access, unauthorized reproduction, corruption, and damage. All health record documentation should be secured in a safe place and access should be limited to avoid accidental or intentional fabrication, alteration, or destruction of records.

Policies and procedures should be developed to ensure the integrity of the information maintained by the organization and to ensure that records can be easily located and accessed within a well-organized filing or alternative retrieval system. There should be a backup system to ensure the integrity of data, and policies should provide for regular system backup to ensure that no information is lost.

When seeking advice from a representative of a federal healthcare program or other payer, a record of the request and any written or oral response (or nonresponse) should be retained in order to support any actions taken or policies and/or procedures developed as a result of the advice received.

## Confidentiality

Policies and procedures ensuring the confidentiality and privacy of financial, medical, personnel, and other sensitive information should be developed, implemented, audited, and enforced. Policies and procedures should address both electronic and hard-copy documents. Policies and procedures related to privacy of medical information should be developed and/or updated to ensure compliance with the HIPAA privacy regulations.

## Compliance as an Element of Performance Review

Organizational policy should stipulate that the promotion of, and adherence to, the elements of the compliance program is a factor in the performance review of managers and supervisors. Managers and supervisors of the coding process have a duty to discuss compliance policies, official coding guidelines, and regulatory requirements affecting the coding process with all coding staff. If the organization outsources part or all of the coding function, managers and supervisors should ensure that the outsourced staff members are made aware of these requirements.

Managers and supervisors should inform coding staff that strict compliance with these policies and requirements is a condition of employment. With outsourced staff, the company employing the coding professionals should be informed that compliance by its personnel is a condition of the contractual arrangement and that violations will be cause for termination of the contract. Managers and supervisors also should explain to their personnel the consequences (that is, disciplinary action) of violating policies and regulatory requirements. Fulfillment of these managerial responsibilities should be a factor in managers' and supervisors' performance evaluations.

## Health Insurance Portability and Accountability Act

An organization's HIM compliance program should address compliance with all of the regulations promulgated under HIPAA.

## Standards for Electronic Transactions and Code Sets

HIPAA requires the adoption of standards for code sets for data elements that are part of all healthcare transactions. The regulation pertaining to electronic transactions and code sets promulgated under HIPAA named the following standard code sets:

- ICD-9-CM volumes 1 and 2 are to be used in all healthcare settings to report diseases, injuries, impairments, and other health problems and their manifestations.

- ICD-9-CM volume 3 is to be used for acute care hospital inpatient services to report procedures or other actions taken to prevent, diagnose, treat, and manage diseases, injuries, and impairments.

- A combination of CPT and HCPCS is to be used to report physician and other healthcare services.

- HCPCS is to be used for all other substances, equipment, supplies, or other items used in healthcare services.

- Current Dental Terminology (CDT) is to be used for dental services.

- HCPCS is to be used for drugs and biologics by entities other than retail pharmacies (retail pharmacies are to use the National Drug Codes).

It is not HIPAA compliant for organizations to report codes on a claim that are from a code set that is not the HIPAA standard for that healthcare service, even if the HIPAA-compliant codes also are reported. For example, prior to HIPAA implementation, some hospitals reported ICD-9-CM volume 3 codes as well as CPT codes for outpatient claims in order to have comparable procedural data across the inpatient and outpatient settings. Although hospitals may continue to collect ICD-9-CM volume 3 codes for outpatient services for internal purposes, they no longer may report them on outpatient claims.

The standard code sets include both the codes and modifiers, if the code set contains modifiers. Although HIPAA does not require payers to reimburse for all valid codes within the standard code sets, payers are required to accept all valid codes within a standard code set. The version of the code set that is valid at the time healthcare services are furnished must be used by both providers and payers.

For ICD-9-CM, HIPAA requires both providers and payers to adhere to the *ICD-9-CM Official Guidelines for Coding and Reporting*. Operational guidelines and instructions are not included as part of the other standard code sets.

## Privacy and Compliance—Dual Role?

The final regulation for the standards for privacy of individually identifiable health information promulgated under HIPAA requires covered entities to designate a privacy official who is responsible for the development and implementation of policies and procedures relative to privacy.

Because the primary responsibilities for both the privacy official and the individual responsible for HIM compliance involve oversight of regulatory compliance related to

HIM, some organizations may decide to charge one individual with both sets of responsibilities. However, depending on the organization's size and structure, this may not be feasible. Also, because of the differences in skill sets related to privacy and coding expertise, the individual most qualified for the HIM compliance specialist position may not be the individual most qualified to serve as the privacy official. It is imperative that the individual or individuals charged with oversight for compliance with reimbursement regulations and policies and for compliance with the privacy regulations not be overburdened with myriad responsibilities and have sufficient resources to be effective. Even if an organization decides that the responsibilities are too great for a single individual to assume, it may choose to link these roles through a reporting relationship (for example, both positions might report to the same individual or department). Certain functions of both roles also may be consolidated appropriately. For example, it may be appropriate to develop training programs that address both privacy issues and compliance with reimbursement regulations.

## References

AHIMA's Coding Policy and Strategy Committee. 2001. Payer's Guide to Healthcare Diagnostic and Procedural Data Quality. Available online from ahima.org.

Centers for Medicare and Medicaid Services. 2003 (Nov. 7). Medicare Program: Review of national coverage determinations and local coverage determinations, Final Rule. 42 CFR Parts 400, 405, and 426. *Federal Register* 68(216): 63692–731. Available online from www.access.gpo.gov/su_docs/fedreg/a031107c.html.

Centers for Medicare and Medicaid Services. 2001 (Sept. 26). Program Memorandum, Intermediaries/Carriers: ICD-9-CM coding for diagnostic tests. Transmittal AB-01-144. Available online from http://www.cms.hhs.gov/Transmittals/downloads/AB01144.pdf.

General Accounting Office. 2001 (June). Health Care: Consultants' billing advice may lead to improperly paid insurance claims. GAO-01-818. Available online from www.gao.gov/new.items/d01818.pdf.

Hammen, C. 2001. Choosing consultants without compromising compliance. *Journal of American Health Information Management Association* 72(9):26, 28, 30.

Office of Inspector General. 2001 (June). Special Advisory Bulletin: Practices of business consultants. Available at http://oig.hhs.gov/fraud/docs/alertsandbulletins/consultants.pdf.

Office of Inspector General. 1998 (February 23). OIG Compliance Program Guidance for Hospitals. *Federal Register* 63(35): 8987–98. Available online from http://oig.hhs.gov/authorities/docs/cpghosp.pdf.

Prophet, S. 2001 (October). Practice brief: Developing a physician query process. *Journal of American Health Information Management Association* 72(9):88I–M.

Scichilone, R. 2002. Best practices for medical necessity validation. *Journal of American Health Information Management Association* 73(2):48, 50.

# Chapter 4
# Training and Education

*Sue Bowman, RHIA, CCS*

The proper education and training of managers, supervisors, employees, physicians, and independent contractors and the continuous retraining of current personnel at every level are important elements of any effective compliance program. Participation in training programs should be made a condition of continued employment, and failure to comply should result in disciplinary action, including possible termination. Moreover, participation in training programs should be a factor in performance evaluations.

Policies and procedures should stipulate the credentials, education, and training of the staff responsible for coding. This includes the following:

- Credentials, education, and experience required for initial hire
- Initial orientation and training
- Ongoing education update to address code revisions and changes to coding rules/ guidelines, regulations, and reimbursement policies
- Initial and ongoing compliance education

## Qualifications for Coding Positions

Organizational policies must stipulate that coding staff meet established qualifications and stay up to date on coding regulations and practice. It is highly recommended that anyone being considered for a coding position receive formal coding education prior to assuming the position. Every healthcare organization should maintain job descriptions that outline each position's necessary qualifications and responsibilities. Positions with responsibility for coding, even if coding is only a small portion of the individual's job, should be filled with individuals who have the appropriate educational background and training. Using unqualified staff could pose compliance risks for an organization.

Qualifications for coding include formal training in the following areas:

- Anatomy and physiology
- Medical terminology

- Pathology and disease processes

- Pharmacology

- Health record format and content

- Reimbursement methodologies

- Conventions, rules, and guidelines for current classification systems (for example, ICD-9-CM and CPT)

Coding supervisory personnel should possess skills and knowledge in the following areas (Texas Medical Foundation Health Quality Institute, 8):

- Possession of HIM credential

- Coding expertise and experience (including knowledge of ICD-9-CM and CPT coding systems and coding guidelines)

- Familiarity with fraud and abuse regulations

- Chargemaster experience

- Ability to compare medical record documentation to the bill

- Understanding of the relationship between coding and billing

- Knowledge of payers' rules (private as well as government programs)

- Familiarity with the payer and the way in which claims are processed

- Communication skills

- Human relations skills

- Management skills

- Versatility (broad scope of knowledge, including ambulatory and inpatient coding and billing rules)

Coding education can be obtained from a range of sources and through various means. AHIMA offers Internet-based basic, intermediate, and advanced coding education. Many community colleges offer coding certificate programs and/or Health Information Administration (HIA) or Health Information Technology (HIT) programs that incorporate coding courses. AHIMA accredits HIA and HIT programs, signifying that the program has met established program standards and curriculum requirements. In addition, AHIMA approves coding certificate programs. The goal of program approval is for programs to meet certain criteria regarding curriculum structure and program assessment. Enrollment in an AHIMA-approved program ensures that students receive the fundamental knowledge to meet basic coding competency standards. To receive approval from AHIMA, coding certificate programs must meet established qualifications and educational standards, which can be accessed on AHIMA's Web site.

AHIMA-accredited HIA and HIT programs and AHIMA-approved coding certificate programs are listed on AHIMA's Web site. A copy of AHIMA's Coding Program Curriculum Guide also can be downloaded from AHIMA's Web site or can be obtained by contacting AHIMA. If candidates for coding positions have received their formal coding education from a coding certificate program that has not sought approval from AHIMA, or if a current HIM staff member is considering enrollment in a nonapproved program, the program's curriculum and structure should be compared against the requirements outlined in AHIMA's Coding Program Curriculum Guide to ensure that the program meets AHIMA's standards for high-quality coding education.

A job candidate's coding skills may be assessed in a number of ways, and the organization may choose to adopt one or a combination of approaches. For example, a coding assessment may be developed and administered. If this is the approach chosen, the test should meet Equal Employment Opportunity Commission (EEOC) guidelines. Working with the organization's human resources department will help ensure compliance with EEOC guidelines (EEOC n.d.). The organization must be able to demonstrate that the test reflects performance required on the job. The test must fairly reflect the type of coding required for the job and the typical types of cases coded in the healthcare organization. For example, an inpatient coding test should not be given to someone applying for an outpatient coding job. The coding test and the required passing score should be the same for all candidates for a particular position.

Successful attainment of a national coding certification is another way to determine coding competency. In addition to the general HIM credentials—registered health information technician (RHIT) and registered health information administrator (RHIA)—the AHIMA also offers several specialized coding certifications: certified coding associate (CCA), certified coding specialist (CCS), and certified coding specialist–physician-based (CCS-P). The RHIA, RHIT, and CCA credentials all denote entry-level competency. The RHIA and RHIT credentials denote entry-level competency in multiple aspects of health information practice, including coding, whereas the CCA credential denotes entry-level competency in coding alone. The CCS and CCS-P credentials signify mastery-level coding proficiency gained through experience or additional education beyond basic competency. The coding certification obtained should match the skills sought or required for the position in question. For example, possession of AHIMA's CCS-P credential does not demonstrate competency as an inpatient coding professional. The CCA credential may be appropriate for registration personnel or other access positions where a basic level of coding knowledge is important. Additional information about AHIMA's coding certifications can be found on AHIMA's Web site.

Extensive coding experience, with excellent references verifying coding expertise, may be considered sufficient evidence of an individual's coding qualifications. However, the individual's coding experience must match the type of coding required by the position for which he or she is applying. If the individual's past coding experience is only in ambulatory care and he or she is applying for an inpatient coding position, it may be necessary to administer a coding skill assessment test or to look to coding certification as a way to verify his or her inpatient coding skills. AHIMA's Internet-based Coding Assessment and Training Solutions program offers tools for assessing coding skills and identifying specific areas requiring improvement. (See AHIMA's Web site for information about this program.)

If the healthcare organization is considering hiring a graduate of a coding certificate program and that person does not possess other qualifications (such as nationally recognized coding credentials or extensive experience), the organization should check to see if the program has been approved by AHIMA (approved programs are listed on AHIMA's Web site). If it has not been approved by AHIMA, the program's curriculum and structure should be benchmarked against AHIMA's Coding Program Curriculum Guide to ensure the program meets AHIMA's standards for quality coding education. Organizations may want to consider only accepting graduates from coding programs that have been approved by AHIMA.

Successful completion of an HIM educational or coding certificate program does not, in itself, establish the advanced-level coding competency necessary for many coding positions in a complex regulatory environment. Completion of an HIM or coding program, and successful attainment of the RHIA, RHIT, or CCA credential, signifies only that an individual has met entry-level skill requirements. In the absence of requisite coding experience, the work of these entry-level professionals should be closely monitored until they have demonstrated that they are able to consistently meet the organization's quality standards.

## Continuing Education and Ongoing Training

All employees of the HIM department should receive annual training on the basic features of the compliance program so that they understand what compliance is, its importance, their role in maintaining compliance through application of standards, and their obligation to report any potential violations according to the organization's policy. Additionally, employees should be educated on the various mechanisms available to them for reporting potential violations. The organization's disciplinary policy for various types of violations should be included in the educational program that all employees attend. All HIM staff involved in coding should receive extensive ongoing coding education.

All newly hired coding professionals should receive extensive training on the organization's HIM compliance program. Key components of the program, such as the code of conduct, should be communicated to newly hired employees prior to beginning their job responsibilities. New coding staff should receive extensive training in the organization's coding policies and procedures. Random reviews of their coding should be conducted to ensure comprehension of, and adherence to, the organization's compliance program and policies and procedures. The coding reviews of newly hired employees with advanced-level competency (that is, extensive qualifications and/or experience) may be less intensive than that of entry-level personnel, but more intensive than that of seasoned departmental staff. For example, because attainment of AHIMA's CCS and CCS-P credentials signifies mastery-level coding proficiency, an organization may decide that newly hired staff with these credentials require less rigorous monitoring. Such a decision would be based on the past experience of the individuals holding these credentials.

All entry-level coding professionals should be closely monitored and supervised until their ability to code accurately (in a variety of situations), to make appropriate decisions (for example, determining when physician clarification is needed), and to apply multiple-payer regulations and policies have been ensured (the time frame will vary according to individual skills and learning curves). Current coding staff can serve as mentors and trainers for new coding professionals.

Employees, physicians, and independent contractors should be required to have a minimum number of educational hours per year with the number of required hours varying for different categories of individuals. For example, coding staff should be required to have a higher number of educational hours than file clerks or record-processing staff. Education can consist of the following:

- In-house programs by internal staff or consultants
- Seminars at an outside organization, including both face-to-face seminars and those using technological media such as audio conferencing, satellite conferencing, or Internet-based training
- Self-study instruction such as correspondence courses, videotapes, audiotapes, and software programs
- Self-assessment programs, such as taking continuing education quizzes after reading journal articles

The use of a variety of training methods is preferred to meet all learning styles. Staff should take advantage of free or low-cost training whenever possible. For example, most Medicare contractors provide training. Inexpensive educational opportunities are also available from state medical societies as well as professional associations, such as AHIMA or Medical Group Management Association (MGMA).

Computer-based training can be particularly advantageous because it improves the quality and consistency of the training (both the content and the delivery are more consistent), enhances the ability to target training, lowers training costs over the long term, and generally incorporates mechanisms to administer and measure the effectiveness of training efforts. Computer-based training is self-paced, more conducive to individual schedules, quickly updated in comparison to other types of training programs, and immediately accessed. AHIMA offers Internet-based training to enhance coding skills and other HIM skill areas. (More information is available on AHIMA's Web site.)

Regular meetings of the coding staff should be conducted to discuss difficult cases, individual questions, new or revised guidelines or regulations, and new diseases being treated or new technologies being used. Meeting frequency depends on the size of the organization and the number of coding professionals. Focused coding training programs should be developed in response to areas of deficiency identified during monitoring or auditing and as new regulatory or guideline changes occur (such as ICD-9-CM, CPT, and HCPCS revisions). Education on identified coding errors should always be provided to the coding staff, regardless of whether the errors caused accuracy rates to fall below the standard.

The coding staff should receive training not only on the coding process, but also on interpretation of physician documentation and techniques for communicating with physicians (for example, how to query the physician for clarification regarding a documentation or coding issue). They should also receive education on the health record documentation that must be present to code, how to deal with inadequate or ambiguous health record documentation, and the difference between optimization and maximization. Education should also be provided whenever the organization has started treating new medical conditions or using new medical technology. Techniques for effectively communicating with physicians and how to interpret documentation should be included in the topics for educational programs. An effective training method might be to ask the coding staff to research coding issues and discuss their findings at a future meeting. Participation in coding roundtables and AHIMA's Communities of Practice (CoPs) present economical opportunities to network with peers and discuss coding issues.

Physicians, physician extenders, nurses, and other medical professionals should be educated regarding health record documentation requirements (for paper-based records or electronic health records, depending on the type of record system being used) and the critical role they play in supporting accurate coding with clear and specific documentation. Clinicians should also be educated on the physician query process so that they understand the purpose of a physician query, under what circumstances a query will be used, and their role in the process.

*job categories* {

HIM coding staff, physicians, other healthcare professionals, and appropriate billing and ancillary department staff (such as utilization review personnel and those individuals involved in chargemaster maintenance) should receive training on the HIM compliance program on an annual basis. The training should include, as appropriate for the target audience, acceptable documentation practices (including the prohibition against altering health records); accurate coding practices; and regulatory requirements pertaining to coding, billing, and documentation. Education on regulatory or reimbursement requirements should be provided to the appropriate personnel sufficiently in advance of the effective date of the requirement to ensure that everyone is well-prepared to comply on the effective date. For example, pay-for-performance initiatives that may affect coding practices and required reporting of whether or not diagnoses were present on admission will necessitate education of affected staff.

*topics* {

Educational sessions held during orientation and routinely for all individuals with health record documentation privileges should emphasize the organization's policies and rationale for record documentation requirements. These sessions also should explain the consequences of poor documentation, provide tools and tips for documentation improvement, and address ongoing review practices for monitoring compliance. Documentation improvement can be achieved through education of healthcare professionals with health record documentation privileges; systems and record design to facilitate a complete, accurate, timely, and legible health record; and medical staff and administrative support of efforts to improve record documentation.

Part of the compliance program education should stress that manipulation, fabrication, alteration, or omission of information in an effort to falsely support medical necessity or affect health plan coverage is a compliance violation. Staff and clinicians should be encouraged to suggest ways to improve coding accuracy and documentation practices such as by the use of additional resources or revised processes. Healthcare professionals need to understand the effect documentation has on the clinical, operational, and financial aspects of healthcare delivery. (See appendix C for a list of suggested educational topics for non-HIM personnel.)

Various disciplines within the healthcare organization can participate in educating each other. For example, HIM staff can educate ancillary departments on the importance of documentation to support medical necessity of ordered tests and the need for annual updating of the chargemaster. HIM staff also can educate physicians and other departments' staff on coding, reimbursement, and documentation requirements as well as fraud and abuse issues. Physicians can educate coding personnel on new surgical or diagnostic procedures and techniques and various clinical disease processes. Coding staff should prepare questions related to the clinical topic in advance, which will help the presenter know what to cover and will improve both the coding professionals' and clinicians' understanding of the relationship between documentation and coding. Physicians' office staff should be invited to attend hospital in-house training programs. These opportunities for office and hospital staff to learn from each other will foster communication and collaboration.

The medical staff should receive education on documentation requirements and the relationship of documentation to coding. When documentation deficiencies are identified, focused training programs should be provided and may consist of one-on-one training. Examples of documentation issues that may need to be addressed in training programs for physicians include the following:

- Inconsistent health record documentation

- Incomplete progress notes

- Undocumented care

- Test results that are not being addressed in the physician documentation

- Historical diagnoses that are being documented as current diagnoses

- Long-standing, chronic conditions that are not being documented at all

- Lack of documentation of postoperative complications

- Illegibility

- Documentation that is not being completed in a timely fashion

It is best to use actual examples of documentation issues during the educational programs to demonstrate how poor documentation results in inaccurate coding and reimbursement. Physician educational programs held for short periods of time (for example, 30 to 45 minutes) tend to fit better into physicians' daily schedules. Planning programs focused exclusively on compliance issues are also better than discussing these issues in a meeting with a larger agenda. Sandwiching presentations in this way may cause compliance issues to be overshadowed. In-house newsletters serve as an excellent method in which to augment and reinforce the material presented during educational programs. Attendance should be mandatory for all employees, including physicians, and disciplinary action should be taken for lack of participation. Because physicians are best influenced by peers, seeking an advocate on the medical staff who helps to promote the importance of complete and accurate documentation can bridge the gap between ethical coding practices and clinical documentation. Penalties such as fines and imprisonment should be avoided as a way to motivate physicians. Instead, an organization should stress that improved efficiency and better patient care can result from effective documentation practices.

The compliance officer should be involved in the design of educational programs for physicians. This involvement will ensure that the programs are designed appropriately such that there is no appearance of inducing referrals through the provision of free services to the physicians. Also, documentation improvement programs for physicians must have the support of senior management. The administration must understand that proper documentation is crucial to patient care, risk management, and billing. Medical staff bylaws should reflect timely and proper medical record completion so that senior management can work with physician leadership for a common understanding of required standards and the process for handling failure to meet standards.

Allied health personnel (including therapists, pharmacists, and nurses) can educate coding staff on clinical issues pertaining to their respective disciplines. HIM staff can educate billing staff on the coding process. In turn, billing staff can educate HIM staff on the billing process and guidelines, including claims rejections and appeals. The healthcare organization might consider conducting periodic joint education programs for coding and billing staff. Such programs could address the relationship between coding and billing, the coding systems and reporting guidelines, how to communicate with payers, the importance of coding when claims are denied or delayed, and discussion of the organization's risk areas. The importance of involving coding staff in the resolution of claims denials related to coding issues and the potentially serious consequences of codes being changed on a claim without involvement of the coding staff also can be addressed.

Proactive cooperation and collaboration can prevent many inappropriate practices and inaccurate claims submissions from occurring. Registration personnel should be properly trained on the compliance impact of diagnostic and other clinical information that they obtain during the registration process. All of the employees involved in the reimbursement process, including registrars, coding professionals, schedulers, physicians, accounting personnel, case management staff, utilization review staff, quality assurance staff, ancillary clinical departments (such as laboratory, radiology), and data-entry clerks should be brought together. Staff can gain exposure to other, related functions that make up the big picture through e-mail newsletters and small interdepartmental group discussions and interactions.

Training (especially training on new or significantly modified regulations, guidelines, or codes) should be personal and interactive. Through discussion of new requirements and the use of case scenarios to show their proper application, a thorough understanding of the requirements can be demonstrated. Interactive discussions of the latest issues of *Coding Clinic for ICD-9-CM* and *CPT Assistant* can help to ensure comprehension of the content of these publications. If the healthcare organization has evening, weekend, part-time, or as-needed (also known as *pro re nata* [prn]) staff, it should consider ways to include these individuals in its training programs. Organizations need to consider educational topics unique to their business areas and ensure that they are included in educational programs. For example, skilled nursing facilities should provide focused training on Minimum Data Set completion and proper health record documentation to support the MDS.

All independent contractors and other external agents involved in the coding or reimbursement processes (such as consultants or contracted coding or billing services) should receive training on the organization's HIM compliance program. In addition, they should be asked to sign an agreement to abide by the organization's program as part of the terms of their contract.

If the organization has both contract and employed coding professionals, the contract coding professionals should be required to have at least as much training and experience as the employed coding professionals. In addition to receiving training on the organization's coding policies and procedures, the contract coding professionals' work should be reviewed for accuracy and the contract coding professionals should be expected to maintain the same accuracy standards as the employed coding professionals.

The individual responsible for overseeing the HIM compliance program should maintain attendance rosters for all training programs, as well as copies of agendas and handouts. Sign-in sheets, rather than pretyped rosters, should be used to verify attendance, and attendees should be asked to sign in at the conclusion of the program. In addition, on either the sign-in sheet or a separate document, employees should be asked to sign an acknowledgment of their comprehension of the material presented during the program. For attendance at seminars outside the organization, participants should be asked to provide a copy of the continuing education certificate (or other document verifying attendance), agenda, and handouts. These records should be made available to the corporate compliance officer upon request.

It is important to assess the effectiveness of training, such as the level of comprehension of the material presented and the effectiveness of the delivery and media used. The effectiveness of educational programs depends on establishing well-defined objectives for the program, creating a test instrument based on these objectives, and providing follow-up and appropriate corrective actions to address unacceptable test results. An objective should be developed for each specific competency that is expected to be gleaned from the program. Designing test questions around each objective will ensure that the organization is following through on the intended purpose of the program. Documentation of all test results should be maintained. Documentation of employees who have achieved acceptable scores on the test provides the organization with proof that the employee received the education and understood and internalized the concepts.

Continuous and immediate follow-up should be provided to those employees with unacceptable test scores. This follow-up should consist of retraining and retesting. Failure to obtain an acceptable score on a preestablished number of retests should result in disciplinary action. In its program guidances, the OIG states that one way to assess the knowledge, awareness, and perceptions of an organization's employees is through the use of a validated survey instrument. This can be accomplished through employee questionnaires, interviews, or focus groups. If the survey process indicates that participants did not get the intended message, the approach to training should be modified until the expected results are achieved. Program evaluations also are useful feedback tools. Because different people learn best in different ways, the best approach is to vary the manner of delivery to sustain people's interest and also ensure they get the message.

Organizational policies should require that coding staff meet the organization's established qualifications, continually improve their skills, and keep up-to-date on pertinent regulations and coding practice standards. Job descriptions and educational requirements should be regularly reviewed and updated.

# Insufficient Coding Skills as a Compliance Risk

Lack of sufficient coding skills to ensure accurate ICD-9-CM coding is a compliance risk in all healthcare settings. Personnel responsible for assignment of the ICD-9-CM codes should have the following:

- A knowledge of anatomy and physiology, disease processes, pharmacology, and medical terminology

- An understanding of the content of the health record and knowledge of documentation requirements

- A knowledge of, and an ability to apply, coding rules and conventions, the *ICD-9-CM Official Guidelines for Coding and Reporting,* and reimbursement policies and regulations

- Ongoing continuing education in coding to keep skills up to date

It may be necessary to require coding personnel to complete a formal coding program and/or to obtain coding certification.

## References

Equal Employment Opportunity Commission. n.d. Federal equal employment opportunity (EEO) laws. Available online from http://www.eeoc.gov/abouteeo/overview_laws.html.

Texas Medical Foundation Health Quality Institute. 2005 (December). Hospital Payment Monitoring Program Compliance Workbook. Available online from http://www.tmf.org/hpmp/tools/workbook/index.htm.

## Additional Resources

American Health Information Management Association. 2006 (May 30). AHIMA's Coding Program Curriculum Guide. Available online from http://www.ahima.org/academics/documents/CEPAManualMay2006.doc.

American Health Information Management Association. n.d. Approved coding education programs. Available online from http://www.ahima.org/careers/college_search/search.asp.

American Health Information Management Association. n.d. Certification standards. Available online from http://www.ahima.org/certification/.

American Health Information Management Association. n.d. AHIMA's Internet-based Coding Assessment and Training Solutions. Distance education course catalog available online from http://campus.ahima.org/campus/catalog/catalog_all.htm.

Medical Group Management Association. n.d. Education/events. Available online from http://www.mgma.com/education/index.cfm.

# Chapter 5
# Auditing and Monitoring

*Sue Bowman, RHIA, CCS*

An ongoing evaluation process is important to a successful compliance program. The process evaluates whether the standards, policies, and procedures are current and accurate, as well as whether there is compliance with them and appropriate submission of claims. If the standards, policies, or procedures are found to be ineffective or outdated, they require immediate updates. The auditing and monitoring of operations are key to ensuring compliance and adherence to government regulations, official coding rules and guidelines, and the healthcare organization's standards, policies, and procedures.

*Monitoring* is the ongoing internal review of operations conducted by an organization on a regular basis. *Auditing* is an infrequent, retrospective review usually conducted by an outside firm to ensure objectivity. Auditing is a more structured, formal reporting process than monitoring and is performed less frequently than monitoring. Auditing also tends to be focused on larger populations (Russo 1998).

An effective monitoring program allows an organization to detect and correct problems early, which minimizes the risk of civil financial penalties and administrative sanctions. Auditing and monitoring also identify areas of potential risk that may require closer attention and areas on which to focus additional education. Routine reviews help to ensure that errors and patterns of errors are identified and corrected early, before becoming major problems.

Internal organizational policy should identify the types of audits, reviews, and internal investigations, if any, that will be conducted under the direction of legal counsel so that attorney–client privilege regarding audit results is preserved, when appropriate.

## Auditing and Monitoring of Coding and Documentation

Coding accuracy should be monitored through periodic reviews and regular monitoring. Periodically, a random sample of health records should be recoded to ensure that the coding was performed properly and the code assignments accurately reflect the services provided, as documented in the health records. Coding accuracy encompasses assignment of proper codes, appropriate code sequencing, and identification of all reportable diagnoses and procedures. Reviews of coding accuracy should include an assessment of the health record documentation to ensure that it is clear, complete, and accurately reflects the codes assigned. The scope of the review, frequency of reviews, and size of the sample depend on the size of the organization, available resources, the number of coding professionals, prior history of noncompliance, the organization's particular risk factors, case complexity, and results of initial assessments. Chart-to-bill audits should be performed periodically to assess not only the accuracy of coding and the quality of health record documentation, but also the adequacy of charge capture at the department level.

Monitoring also should include the types of coding that are not typically performed by coding staff, such as the CPT codes listed in the chargemaster. Depending on the findings, subsequent reviews can be narrower in focus. A higher sample of cases in the organization's top diagnosis-related groups (DRGs), ambulatory payment classifications (APCs), diagnoses, procedures, and/or clinical services should be reviewed. (See figure 5.1.) For DRG reviews, cases may be selected in a number of ways.

In addition to evaluating coding accuracy, auditing and monitoring should include ongoing reviews of the quality of health record documentation. Aspects that should be addressed, regardless of the setting, include the following:

- Consistency in documentation among various reports and disciplines

- Contradiction in documentation without a clear reason for the differences (either between or within a discipline)

- Documentation that is missing key elements

**Figure 5.1.   Examples of various case selections**

- Simple random sample
- Medical DRGs by high dollar and high volume
- Surgical DRGs by high dollar and high volume
- Medical DRGs without comorbid conditions or complications
- Surgical DRGs without comorbid conditions or complications
- Major diagnostic category by high dollar and high volume
- Most common diagnosis codes
- Most common procedure codes (ICD-9-CM or CPT)
- Significant procedure APCs by high dollar and high volume
- Unlisted CPT codes
- "Separate procedure" CPT codes reported in conjunction with related CPT codes
- Unusual modifier usage patterns (for example, high volume of CPT codes reported with modifier 59 or modifier 25)
- Not elsewhere classified (NEC) and not otherwise specified (NOS) codes
- Highest-level evaluation and management (E/M) codes
- Consultation E/M codes
- Critical Care E/M codes
- Chargemaster review by service
- Superbill, encounter form, and charge sheet review by specialty

- Documentation that reflects the application of appropriate standards, regulations, clinical protocols, and reimbursement requirements

The organization's internal coding practices should be evaluated to ensure that they are consistent with coding rules and guidelines. If organization-specific coding guidelines have been developed, they should be evaluated to ensure that they are not in conflict with official coding guidelines or recently implemented directives. Staff compliance with coding policies and procedures should be reviewed continuously. All systems and software applications that use diagnosis and procedure codes should be identified and the code tables reviewed to ensure the codes are accurate and up to date.

In addition to coding evaluations, health information management (HIM) departments need to review the accuracy of other data elements that they share responsibility for and that affect reimbursement or clinical data management (for example, data entry of discharge status, patient's age, admission and discharge dates, clinical performance indicators, and outcomes).

## Audit Design

A formalized audit process for compliance should be established by developing audit protocols. (See figure 5.2.) These should include policies and procedures for an audit process, periodic reporting, and corrective measures for identified problems. The first step when designing an audit is to clearly define the purpose and goal of the audit.

The audit plan should include the following:

- Established frequency for performing the audit

- Established period covered by each audit

- The review population (for example, selected services, physicians, or patient types)

- Explanation of how the sample size will be determined, which will depend on the type of audit being conducted

- Description of established sample design

**Figure 5.2.   Factors to consider when designing an auditing/monitoring program**

- Objectives of the review
- Frequency of the review
- Time period to be covered
- Record selection process (review population)
- Sample size and design
- Indicators
- Whether the review will be retrospective or prospective
- Data analysis techniques to be used
- Qualifications of personnel performing review
- How results will be used to improve operations
- Report formats for tracking and analyzing audit results

- Description of the indicators and indicator specifications
- Time frame for conducting the audit
- Comparative data or benchmarks used
- Description of planned analysis techniques

Data elements for consistent data retrieval need to be identified. The value of the data element must be weighed against the time required to abstract the data.

The audit process should be approached methodically with an organized plan that begins with a review of the areas of highest vulnerability (for example, DRGs targeted by the Office of Inspector General (OIG) or statistical variations from national norms). The following questions need to be addressed:

- What will be audited?
- Who will perform the audit?
- When and how often will the audit occur?
- What type of format will be used?

The population to be reviewed might be inpatients, outpatients, ambulatory surgery patients, clinic patients, or emergency department patients. The population might consist of a subset of one of these categories, such as Medicare inpatients only or Medicare inpatients with a diagnosis of pneumonia.

The scope of the review, frequency of reviews, and sample size depend on the size of the organization, available resources, number of coding professionals, prior identification of noncompliance, and the organization's known risk factors.

Indicators need to be defined. The indicators will vary depending on the type of audit. For example, indicators used in coding audits are different from those used in claims audits. Types of indicators for a coding audit include the coding error rate, selection of principal diagnosis, accuracy of DRG assignment, and selection of discharge status. Indicators for claims audits might encompass the most frequently billed APCs and DRGs, average length of stay for each DRG, or number of short-stay admissions. The indicators can be further stratified or broken into smaller groups, if appropriate.

Indicators that measure performance in areas being scrutinized by the federal government should be developed (for example, high-risk DRGs). By analyzing multiple indicators, areas for further review can be prioritized. When the indicators have been determined, the specifications for each indicator should be described. Specifications are instructions regarding what data elements are required and where each data element can be located (that is, the database where the data element can be found). An explicit description of the indicators allows consistent replication of the indicators so that results from audits performed at different times, or by different individuals or entities, can be compared. Indicators with smaller denominators (fewer than 30) will yield results that are less stable, meaning they are more subject to random fluctuation. A high percentage in one year could be followed by a very low percentage in the following year. Indicators with denominators greater than 30 are more stable from year to year, and they represent a facility's more commonly rendered services.

Regarding sample design, in most instances a simple random sample is sufficient. However, if a systemic problem is identified, a determination of how far back the errors have been occurring will need to be made and a statistically significant sampling of claims will need to be re-audited in order to extrapolate the error rate against the entire population of claims involved. Whether a disclosure to the Medicare contractor or a self-disclosure to the OIG is warranted, the audit sampling will need to be determined more carefully. For self-disclosure, the OIG recommends the use of its Office of Audit Services Statistical Sampling Software (known as RAT-STATS), which is currently available free of charge through the OIG website (OIG n.d.). The use of statistical sampling (such as the OIG's RAT-STATS program) can also help to serve as an early detection system of risk and vulnerabilities. In conjunction with investigation of identified problems and initiation of appropriate corrective action, statistical sampling can improve the effectiveness of the compliance program. Statistically valid sampling helps to limit the cost of labor resources necessary to carry out proactive auditing and monitoring.

Use of an audit tool provides consistency in data collection and facilitates collection of required data. A few sample audit tools can be found on the CD accompanying this book. Audit tools also can be found through an Internet search. Many of the quality improvement organizations (QIOs) provide sample audit tools. Audit tools are included in the Appendices of the HPMP Compliance Handbook (Texas Medical Foundation Health Quality Institute 2005). Because many organizations are willing to share audit tools they have developed, networking is an excellent way to obtain useful audit tools that have already been developed. Participation on the AHIMA Communities of Practice (CoPs) is a great way for organizations to share audit tools they have developed.

## Sample Size and Selection

It is important that a large enough sample size be audited for the results to be statistically valid and reliable. It is also important to keep in mind that large samples do not necessarily provide more reliable results. Sampling should include the following:

- Records representative of current areas of investigative focus

- Records representative of internally identified problem areas

- Random sampling of records to determine overall accuracy

- A sample of cases in any area that shows a significant variation from benchmarks

The sample selection should include different coding professionals; various service types; various clinician types; various patient encounter types; high, medium, and low charges; diagnoses and procedures; and a variety of payment groups (for example, DRGs, APCs).

Samples should be consistent and measurable. Consistency ensures that audit results can be compared, and measurability ensures that the sample is statistically significant and reliable. The steps taken for sample selection should be documented. Also important is documentation of the specific population, any population exclusions, sample selection techniques, and the formula used for determining the sample size. Sample selection methods should be replicable so that results from reviews conducted at different times can be compared. If results indicate an increase in errors, corrective steps should be taken immediately.

There are two types of samples: statistically significant and probe. A statistically significant random sample is representative of the entire population; probe or focused samples are not. Probe samples provide a way to quickly determine if potential problems exist. Any errors identified by either a statistically significant or a probe sample must have claims resubmitted with repayment, if necessary.

## Audit Process

Initially, a baseline audit should be conducted, consisting of a fairly large sample, representative of all coding professionals, physicians, and all types of cases treated at the organization. The phrase "all types of cases" means all specialties, medical and surgical cases, and the various healthcare settings under the organization's ownership, including the following:

- Inpatient
- Outpatient surgery
- Observation
- Emergency department
- Clinic
- Physicians' offices
- Ancillary facilities
- Home health
- Subacute care
- Long-term care
- Rehabilitation
- Psychiatric facilities

A baseline audit enables providers to judge, over time, their progress in reducing or eliminating potential areas of vulnerability. Every organization needs to know its own data (that is, characteristic patterns, patient mix, and ICD-9-CM/CPT code and DRG distributions) in order to be able to recognize deviations. For this reason, the OIG recommends that organizations take a snapshot of their operations from a compliance perspective. This snapshot becomes the baseline against which variations are identified and progress in resolving problem areas is monitored. A baseline audit examines the claim development and submission process from registration through claim submission and payment and identifies elements within this process that may contribute to noncompliance or that may need to be the focus of process improvement. This audit will establish a consistent methodology for selecting and examining records. The resulting methodology will then serve as a basis for future monitoring. The OIG suggests that baseline levels for coding practices include the frequency and percentile levels of various diagnosis codes and complications or comorbidities.

When the baseline audit has been completed, follow-up reviews involving a smaller sample of cases should be conducted periodically, according to the organization's schedule. For high-risk, low-volume services, 100 percent of the records should be evaluated. These subsequent reviews should be conducted at regular intervals (that is, quarterly, semiannually, and annually) to compare current performance (for example, accuracy of coding or another HIM function) with the baseline and any previous evaluations that have been performed subsequent to the baseline. More frequent monitoring may be performed in areas that have been identified as requiring improvement. The results should be used to monitor the effectiveness of corrective action plans implemented to resolve problems identified during previous audits, which helps to demonstrate the effectiveness of the compliance program as a whole. Audits performed subsequent to the baseline audit should seek to determine if improvements have occurred in problem areas and if any deviations from the initial baseline level have occurred in areas without problems.

In order to compare the results of subsequent reviews or audits to the baseline audit, a process needs to be developed for the collection and analysis of results over time. Whenever possible, reports of auditing and monitoring activities should be maintained electronically to facilitate comparisons of results over time and to identify trends.

Organizations should conduct trend analysis or longitudinal studies that uncover deviations in specific areas over a given period of time. Comparisons should be made of year-to-year activity or one six-month time period to another. Patterns and potential problem areas often can be identified by reviewing reports (monthly, quarterly, and/or annually) of diagnosis and procedure codes and DRG frequency. Reading such reports should prompt questions such as, "Are there changes in the outpatient case-mix distribution or coding patterns since the implementation of the outpatient prospective payment system (PPS)?"

Reports providing data on the organization's code or reimbursement category (such as DRG or APC, respectively) frequency and distribution must be designed carefully to ensure that equal comparisons are being made. (See figure 5.3.)

**Figure 5.3.  Basic formulas for DRG monitors**

- Facility's CC%:

$$\frac{\# \text{ discharges in DRGs with CC}}{\# \text{ discharges in DRGs with CC} + \# \text{ discharges in DRGs without CC}} \times 100$$

- Facility's DRG Y% of DRGs Y/Z:

$$\frac{\# \text{ discharges in DRG Y}}{\# \text{ discharges in DRG Y} + \# \text{ discharges in DRG Z}} \times 100$$

- Facility's DRG A/B% of DRGs A/B/C/D:

$$\frac{\# \text{ discharges in DRG A} + \# \text{ discharges in DRG B}}{(\# \text{ discharges in DRG A} + \# \text{ discharges in DRG B}) + (\# \text{ discharges in DRG C} + \# \text{ discharges in DRG D})} \times 100$$

When reviewing records, organizations should ensure that the regulatory requirements and payment policies in effect during the applicable time period (as opposed to the regulatory requirements and payment policies in effect at the time the review is performed) are used. This includes identifying the code set version in use during the time period being reviewed.

The organization's encoder should not be used to recode records. Problems caused by encoder logic or edits will be missed if the same encoder used to code the records also is used to audit coding accuracy.

Criteria should be established for the types of occurrences that will count as errors. (See figure 5.4.) Coding errors generally can be categorized as clerical, judgmental, and systemic. Clerical errors are generally random in nature and occur infrequently. Judgmental errors can be minimized through clear, comprehensive policies and procedures and education. Systemic errors are particularly high risk for potentially triggering a fraud investigation because they involve patterns of errors. Common coding errors include the following:

- Selecting an incorrect principal diagnosis

- Selecting an incorrect code

- Failing to include or incorrectly including a fifth digit on a diagnosis code

- Coding diagnoses or procedures that are not supported by health record documentation

- Failing to code all diagnoses or procedures that are supported by health record documentation

- Failing to clarify conflicting or ambiguous documentation

- Entering data erroneously into the abstracting or billing system

Common causes of coding errors include the following:

- Missing, inadequate, or conflicting documentation

- Failure to review entire health record

- Insufficient coding education

**Figure 5.4.   Questions to consider when establishing error criteria**

- Will error rates be calculated and reported as percentages, raw numbers, or proportions?
- Will they include the number of records coded incorrectly or the number of incorrect codes?
- What is meant by an incorrect code (transposition of numbers, missing fourth or fifth digits, wrong code selected)?
- How will the selection of principal diagnosis or other sequencing occurrences be evaluated?
- Will miscoding, incomplete identification of all secondary diagnoses, and incomplete identification of all procedures be calculated differently in the error rate?
- Will errors affecting DRG assignment be treated differently from those that do not?

- Lack of coding knowledge or skills

- Lack of understanding of disease process or procedure

- Misinterpretation of coding rules or guidelines

- Incorrect coding advice

- Lack of or outdated coding resources, codebooks, and/or encoding software

- Failure to stay informed of coding rules and guidelines, reimbursement policies, and regulatory changes

- Lack of familiarity with National Correct Coding Initiative (NCCI) edits

- Employment of outdated or inaccurate "cheat sheets" that incorporate codes

- Coding from incomplete health records

- Use of a record abstract, charge sheet, or superbill instead of the complete health record to assign codes

- Selection of a code for a payable diagnosis instead of assignment of the correct code for the diagnosis documented in the health record

- Use of office visit E/M codes for preventive medicine services in violation of CPT coding guidelines

- Incorrect use of modifiers

- Unclear or outdated policies and procedures

## Data Collection

The following data elements should be collected as part of the evaluation and monitoring of coding accuracy:

- Patient demographic information, such as medical record number, account number, admission and discharge dates, payer, age, discharge status, attending physician, surgeon

- Payer

- Date that the record was originally coded

- Original principal and secondary diagnosis codes

- Reviewer's principal and secondary diagnosis codes

- Original procedure codes

- Reviewer's procedure codes

- Impact on case designation (that is, did the error affect DRG, APC, or home health resource group classification?)

*basis for audit tool*

- Impact on reimbursement

- Quality errors

- Root cause of the coding error (for example, lack of adherence to official coding guideline, missed documentation, inconsistent documentation, incomplete documentation, and clerical error)

- Original and reviewer's discharge disposition (for reviews of acute care hospital inpatient records)

- Health record documentation supporting reviewer's codes (note whether documentation was likely to have been present at the time the record was originally coded, for example, a discharge summary dictated after the record was coded)

- Citation or reference to support reviewer's coding changes (for example, *Coding Clinic for ICD-9-CM* citation and reference to a specific guideline from the *ICD-9-CM Official Guidelines for Coding and Reporting*)

- Coding professional

- Reviewer

### Retrospective versus Prospective Review

Every healthcare organization will need to decide whether retrospective and/or prospective record reviews of coding accuracy will be conducted. If violations of civil, criminal, or administrative law are identified during a retrospective review, this information must be reported to the federal government. Any problems identified during a retrospective review should be reported promptly to the corporate compliance officer who, in conjunction with legal counsel, can determine the extent of liability and whether the matter should be reported to government authorities. Any identified overpayments should be refunded to the affected payer with a letter of explanation. A retrospective review offers an opportunity to identify and investigate practice patterns or deviations from national norms before becoming the target of a government investigation. The organization's internal investigation may reveal a reasonable explanation for the variation, which will be useful in the event of a government investigation.

Before conducting a retrospective audit, an organization should carefully consider the benefits and drawbacks and the necessary actions if the audit results identify a possible problem involving overpayments. When a problem has been discovered, it cannot be ignored. The problem will need to be investigated to determine the extent and the appropriate corrective action, including refunds of overpayments, that must be taken. It is advisable that the organization consult its legal counsel prior to initiating a retrospective audit. If it is determined that a retrospective audit is appropriate, such as in situations in which coding problems involving overpayments are suspected, legal counsel can advise as to the retrospective time period that should be covered by the audit in view of the facts and applicable statutes of limitations.

When a prospective review is performed, a sample of records should be reviewed after they have been coded, but before the claims have been submitted to the payer. The advantage of a prospective review is that errors can be corrected and corrective action plans initiated for any identified systematic problems before the submission of erroneous claims, thus avoiding the need to refund overpayments.

### Internal versus External Review

Coding evaluation and assessment can be conducted either internally or by an outside firm. A combination of these approaches may work best when an organization does not have qualified staff available who work independently from the actual coding function. For example, regular ongoing monitoring can be conducted by internal staff and a less frequent formal audit (perhaps annually) by an outside organization. It is recommended to have at least the baseline and periodic audits conducted by someone outside the organization. It is difficult for an internal staff member to maintain the necessary objectivity to conduct an audit. Also, outside auditors have a broader scope of knowledge to identify potential problems. The frequency of an external review depends on the organization's case volume and internal risk assessment. A good external audit of the organization's operations, documentation, and claim submission process can help it evaluate its risk objectively and will produce sound recommendations for implementing a proactive approach to correct any identified problems. An external review often helps promote physician education and awareness and focus on documentation issues and training of coding professionals.

Regardless of whether the assessments are conducted internally or externally, it is imperative that the review be conducted by an expert in the area being audited. Auditing/monitoring of coding should be performed by an objective entity with adequate training and experience in coding. For example, a corporate compliance officer who is not an HIM professional or a department director who has not been actively coding for several years does not possess the requisite expertise to review coding accuracy. Individuals performing coding assessments should be familiar with the functions, processes, and rules and guidelines pertaining to coding and health record documentation. They should have several years of coding experience in the applicable coding system(s) and healthcare setting and the appropriate credentials. The reviewer also should be required to demonstrate a practical application of auditing skills and data quality assessment competence.

Organizations can broaden the skills of their coding staff by implementing a peer review monitoring program, whereby coding professionals review each other's work. However, implementation of such a program should not serve as the only method of review. Interrater reliability can be measured when the coding professionals recode each other's records. This method is not effective in identifying all types of errors such as those errors or misunderstandings occurring among all the coding professionals. For an organization with few academically trained and/or certified professionals, use of an outside firm for all auditing and monitoring activities may be the only viable option to ensure compliance and maintain acceptable coding accuracy.

## Analysis of Results

After variations have been identified, in-depth reviews can be conducted to determine the reason(s). When problems are identified through the auditing and monitoring process, focused reviews can be conducted that examine a higher volume of cases in these areas on a more frequent basis. Focused reviews aimed at the OIG's identified target areas also should be conducted to determine whether the organization has any problems in these areas. Areas suggesting a need for focused review also can be identified by comparing DRG or code distribution data over time or with local, state, or national figures. Additionally, focused reviews can be designed based on problem areas identified via other mechanisms, such as claims denial patterns or under-reimbursed services. Whenever deviations are discovered, the causes should always be investigated. Cause analysis may be conducted using many different quality tools (for example, root cause analysis, process mapping, fish-bone [Ishikawa] diagram). Analysis tools are available from a variety of sources. An organization's quality improvement department may be able to provide analysis tools. Sample cause analysis tools are also available in the Appendices of the HPMP Compliance Handbook (Texas Medical Foundation Health Quality Institute 2005).

When an in-depth review confirms that a variation truly is a problem, steps will need to be taken to initiate corrective action and prevent recurrence.

Results of ongoing monitoring activities can be used to help focus the audit and investigation processes, including sample selection. Appropriate refinements can be made to data collection and analytic processes for future reviews.

Feedback on the results of auditing and monitoring activities should be presented to appropriate individuals such as coding staff and physicians. Severity of illness and acuity data should be shared with physicians, administration, and staff. Statistics by individual coding professionals or type of setting should be maintained and, when necessary, the coding professional and the supervisor should work together to develop an action plan to improve coding accuracy. In addition, progress in improvements in coding accuracy should be tracked.

The results of the coding reviews should be used to identify any problem areas that may require more frequent or intensive review (for example, a higher volume of records to be reviewed such as 100 percent of a specific diagnosis code). The results of auditing and monitoring activities should be used to identify gaps in knowledge or weak areas, and appropriate training should be provided to address these deficiencies. Depending on the nature of the problem areas, the training might be aimed at the coding staff or the physicians.

Areas of vulnerability in relation to compliance identified through the monitoring process should be examined regularly until it is clear the problem has been corrected. When monitoring discloses that deviations were undetected in a timely manner because of deficiencies in the compliance program, appropriate modifications to the program must be implemented. A comparison of audit results with previous audits should be conducted to identify whether any identified problems have increased, decreased, or remained the same.

When a review of DRG assignment accuracy is conducted (either internally or by an outside company), lower-weighted as well as higher-weighted DRG adjustments should be submitted to the Medicare contractor. The submission of only higher-weighted DRG adjustments may be viewed as a willful intent to defraud the payer rather than correction of claims for appropriate reimbursement.

Auditing and monitoring processes should encompass claims submitted to both private payers and government programs. Whenever a review identifies errors that resulted in receipt of incorrect reimbursement (either an overpayment or underpayment), the claim should be resubmitted with the corrected code assignments to the affected payer according to that payer's policy for claim resubmission. If any errors are discovered that resulted in an overpayment, the difference must be refunded to the affected payer. In addition, appropriate documentation and an explanation for the reason for the refund should be included. Refunds for identified overpayments must be returned to the payer even when the time frame for claim resubmission has expired. Also, any errors should be corrected in internal databases and indexes so that correct and consistent code sets are maintained for each encounter or episode. (See figure 5.5 for suggestions regarding auditing and monitoring methodologies.)

## Documentation of Process and Results

All auditing and monitoring activities should be documented. (See figure 5.6.) Documentation should include results by the individual coding professional and by the coding professionals as a group or by clinical specialty, if applicable. Errors should be classified by both type and severity. (See figure 5.7.) Any trends related to availability of documentation at the time of coding should be noted, as well as any trends related to the root cause of the coding error. Examples of trends by root cause include an official coding guideline or a coding rule or convention.

Results of auditing and monitoring activities (even when no problem is identified) should be reported to the HIM compliance specialist. In turn, that person should submit a written report of findings to the corporate compliance officer, who then should share the reports with the following:

- The organization's senior management

- The compliance committee

- The medical staff, if appropriate

- The corporate compliance officer for the parent organization (when the organization reporting the audit findings is owned by a larger corporate entity)

## Use of Benchmark Comparisons

Organizations should use comparative data to benchmark utilization and billing patterns with national, state, and regional norms. Comparative data can be used to assist an organization in evaluating indicator results and determining whether an area should be examined further. Comparative data are available from a number of sources, including Centers for Medicare and Medicaid Services (CMS), QIOs, state data commissions, professional associations such as hospital associations, medical societies, and private companies. CMS's MEDPAR data are available from CMS, and this is an excellent source of national Medicare benchmark data (CMS n.d.). Improbable combinations of codes, unusual trends (including changes in internal patterns), or variations from national, state, or regional norms may indicate areas requiring focused health record review. (See figure 5.8.)

**Figure 5.5.   Guidelines for the auditing and monitoring of HIM functions**

*audits &
monitors for
AdM plan*

The following guidelines are only suggestions and are not intended to serve as an all-inclusive list.

- Compare diagnosis and procedure codes with health record documentation. If coding is performed without a complete health record, review the coding accuracy after the record is complete to determine if an incomplete record is affecting coding accuracy adversely.

- Compare diagnosis codes with procedure codes for consistency.

- For CPT E/M code assignment, compare the required components of the reported code with the documentation in the health record to ensure that the code level assigned is substantiated.

- For organizations operating under the outpatient PPS, compare the E/M code assignments with the criteria developed by the organization and the health record documentation for the following reasons:

  —To assess the accuracy of the code assignment

  —To ensure that the organization's system for mapping facility services to the E/M code levels is being followed

  —To determine whether supporting documentation is present in the health record

- Compare the diagnostic information provided by the ordering physician or practitioner for diagnostic tests with the diagnosis codes reported on the claim and, if possible, with the reason for the ordered test documented in the physician's office health record.

- Review medical necessity denials for the following reasons:

  —To determine the accuracy of diagnostic information reported on the claim (Do the diagnosis codes match the diagnostic information provided by the ordering physician or practitioner and documented in his or her office record?)

  —To verify the accuracy of the billed tests (Were the tests that were billed the same as the tests that were ordered and performed?)

  —To ascertain whether an ABN was issued, and if not, to identify the reason(s) why not

- When multiple CPT codes have been assigned, verify that they are not components of a larger, comprehensive procedure that could be described with a single code.

- For Medicare patients, compare the reported CPT codes with the applicable NCCI edits.

- Work with physicians to develop a mechanism for comparing the diagnosis and procedure codes assigned by the physician's office and the facility for the same encounter.

- Perform periodic chart-to-bill audits by reviewing representative samples or records coded by different coding professionals or involving different physicians. This may indicate problem areas requiring more intensive review and, possibly, corrective action.

- Evaluate claim denials, claim rejections, and code and DRG changes from the Medicare contractor, QIO, and private payers.

  —Ensure that the APCs assigned by the Medicare contractor and the provider organization are in agreement and investigate any discrepancies.

  —Appeal all denials believed to be inappropriate, even if only small amounts of money are involved.

  —Verify that denials based on the NCCI edits are based on current edits and not on a deleted one.

  —Cite any official sources that support the accuracy of the organization's code assignment.

  —Follow up on the issue until a response has been received by the payer.

**Figure 5.5.**  *(Continued)*

---

   —Educate the coding staff if review of the denials, rejections, and code changes indicates a pattern of inaccurate coding.

   —Monitor claims rejections for patterns of errors and initiate corrective action when a pattern is identified.

   –Are modifiers not being used or being used improperly?

   –Are codes being unbundled inappropriately?

   –Are duplicate codes being assigned by both the HIM department and ancillary departments?

   —Correct any errors in coding and billing practices to prevent future claim denials. High denial rates or repeated coding and billing errors may increase the organization's risk of being audited.

- Perform trend analysis of practice patterns by examining the organization's internal coding and DRG patterns over time and doing the following:

   —Look for significant changes in the organization's case mix or coding practices. Sudden increases in an organization's case-mix index or a case-mix index that is high relative to other hospitals with a similar mix of patients and services may serve as a red flag to fraud investigators. Some fluctuation in the case-mix index is to be expected, but a sharp and sustained increase may be considered suspect.

   —Identify any DRGs that show substantial increases in the number of cases assigned to them. Compare the DRG distribution, ranked by volume, over the past three years and identify any DRGs that have changed ranking significantly for further, in-depth study. This intensive review should include identifying the reason for the change in ranking.

   —Select individual DRGs and compare the previous year to the current year.

   —Look at families of related DRGs such as "with CC" and "without CC" pairs or high-risk DRG pairs, examining the case distribution within a family over time.

- Compare utilization and billing patterns with national, state, and regional norms by doing the following:

   —Look at the organization's highest- and lowest-volume DRGs and APCs. Compare these DRGs and APCs in terms of volume with norms for the region, state, and nation.

   —Look at changes in the volume of patients assigned to particular DRGs and APCs.

   —Compare the organization's case distribution within a family with regional, state, and national averages.

- Analyze trends—both over time and against regional, state, and national averages—for CPT procedure codes and APCs. For physician practices, compare the frequency of various levels of E/M codes with other physician practices, particularly those in the same specialty.

- Analyze trends for evidence of inappropriate upcoding.

- Examine any identified variations from norms or over time to determine causes. Variations do not necessarily indicate improper coding practices, so all possible causes should be considered. HIM professionals should take the lead in identifying variations, determining the validity of the coding practices represented by the data, producing explanations for the variations (or at least verifying that they are not due to improper coding), and documenting circumstances resulting in unexpected variations.

- Determine whether the correct discharge status is being reported, particularly for patients transferred to another acute care hospital or to a postacute setting. For patients who will be receiving home health care upon discharge from the acute care facility, confirm that a written plan of care for the provision of home health services is documented in the health record. Look for a pattern of discharge status corrections made by the Medicare contractor.

**Figure 5.6.   Information to document when auditing or monitoring**

- Date of review
- Identity of evaluator
- Number of cases reviewed
- Number of errors identified
- Number of errors affecting reimbursement
- Financial impact after balancing overcoding and undercoding
- Identification and categorization of trends by such things as DRG or APC, diagnosis, procedure, physician, coding professional, documentation issue, or discharge disposition
- Review methodology
- Review personnel
- Conclusion
- Action taken
- Follow-up conducted

**Figure 5.7.   Examples of error categorization for a hospital inpatient Medicare coding audit**

- Principal diagnosis
- Addition of secondary diagnosis that is not a complication and comorbidity (CC)
- Addition of secondary diagnosis that is a CC
- Deletion of secondary diagnosis that is not a CC
- Delection of secondary diagnosis that is a CC
- Addition of procedure that is not an operating room (OR) procedure
- Addition of procedure that is an OR procedure
- Change in diagnosis code affecting DRG assignment
- Change in diagnosis code not affecting DRG assignment
- Change in procedure code affecting DRG assignment
- Change in procedure code not affecting DRG assignment

**Figure 5.8.   Factors to consider when monitoring coding accuracy**

**Reliability:** The degree to which the same results are achieved (for example, when different individuals code the same health record, they use the same codes.)

**Validity:** The degree to which the codes accurately reflect the patient's diagnoses and procedures

**Completeness:** The degree to which the codes capture all the diagnoses and procedures reflected in the health record

**Timeliness:** The time frame in which the health records are being coded

The PEPPER (Program for Evaluating Payment Patterns Electronic Report) reports available from QIOs provide summary statistics of hospital administrative claims data on CMS target areas. Hospitals can use PEPPER reports to compare their own data across time and to compare their performance with other hospitals in their state. Data are provided to hospitals in a flexible format to help prioritize areas in which to focus auditing and monitoring efforts with the goal of identifying and preventing payment errors. Some of the CMS target areas in the PEPPER reports should look familiar, as they have been identified by the OIG and others as compliance risk areas. These target areas include the following:

- One-day stays
- One-day stays in DRGs 127, 143, 182/183, 296/297
- DRGs with CC pair
- DRG 14
- DRG 79
- DRG 89
- DRG 243 (medical necessity of admission)
- DRG 416
- Seven-day readmission to same facility or elsewhere
- Three-day qualifying skilled nursing facility admission

## Monitoring the Physician Query Process

The use of queries should be monitored for trends, and education should be provided to physicians on proper documentation of a diagnosis when a pattern of poor documentation is identified. Education is key to improvement and will result in better documentation up front and a reduction in the need to query the physician and then, if necessary, amend the record. Educational programs should include information on the effect documentation has on reimbursement as well as continued patient care. Educational sessions may provide insight into improvements that could be made in documentation capture processes to facilitate better health record practices.

Periodic reviews of the use of queries should include an evaluation of what percentage of the query forms are eliciting negative and positive responses from the physicians. A high negative response rate may indicate that members of the coding staff are being overzealous and not using the query process judiciously. A high positive response rate may indicate widespread poor documentation habits that need to be addressed. It also may indicate that the absence of certain reports, such as the discharge summary or operative report, at the time of coding is forcing the coding staff to query the physician to obtain the information they need for complete code selection. In this instance, it might make more sense, in terms of turnaround time and productivity, to wait for completion of these reports, particularly if they are the primary source for the final diagnoses or the only source of operative session details.

Patterns of poor documentation that have not been addressed through education or other corrective action are signs of an ineffective compliance program. Ideally, complete and accurate physician documentation should occur at the time care is rendered. The need for a query form following patient discharge results from incomplete, conflicting, or ambiguous documentation, which is an indication of poor information capture of patient conditions and events. Therefore, query form usage should be the exception, not the norm. The OIG noted in its *Compliance Program Guidance for Hospitals* that "accurate coding depends upon the quality of completeness of the physician's documentation" and "active staff physician participation in educational programs focusing on coding and documentation should be emphasized by the hospital" (OIG 1998, 8995, fn 43).

Organizations should take swift action when an individual physician commits ongoing errors in documentation and it is apparent that query forms as an educational tool have not been effective in changing the physician's behavior. This represents a serious compliance problem, and frequent use of query forms is a red flag for auditors that documentation problems are persistent and the compliance program has not been effective in correcting these problems.

The query format should be monitored to ensure that the queries are not leading the physicians to agree to the reporting of additional diagnoses or procedures that are not supported by the health record documentation for the express purpose of higher reimbursement. Patterns of inappropriately written queries may need to be referred to the facility's compliance officer if it appears that overpayment may have resulted as a direct result of this process.

Recurring violations of a facility's own policies and procedures related to the use of physician queries also should be addressed.

Appropriate use of the form, analysis of trends, and follow-up education for identified patterns of documentation deficiencies should lead to a decrease in the need to use a query form. The query process can be used to move the institution and its clinical staff closer to an ideal world in terms of patient care and documentation quality through improvement of future documentation practices, medical error and patient safety monitoring, and quality review.

## Auditing Compliance Program Effectiveness

In order for a compliance program to be effective, it must be evaluated continually in a proactive manner through auditing and monitoring and primarily focus on preventing regulatory requirement violations as well as responding to problems. It is not enough to have a compliance program—the organization must be able to demonstrate that its program is effective. Several federal documents have noted the importance of demonstrating the effectiveness of a compliance program. The Federal Sentencing Guidelines state that a program must be effective in preventing and detecting criminal conduct. According to the OIG's *Compliance Program Guidance for Hospitals,* the desired outcome of an effective program is to promote adherence to applicable federal and state law, and the program requirements of federal, state and private health plans (OIG 1998). The Government Accounting Office (GAO) stated in a 1999 report to Congress that the "principal measure of a compliance program's effectiveness is its ability to prevent improper Medicare payments" (GAO 1999, 3).

Hospitals should regularly review the implementation and execution of their compliance program elements. This review should be conducted at least annually and should include an assessment of each of the basic elements individually, as well as the overall success of the program. This review should help the hospital identify any weaknesses in its compliance program and implement appropriate changes.

The adage "actions speak louder than words" applies in such situations. An organization must demonstrate that it does what its written program states that it does. If the organization does not plan to implement a procedure until a future date, its compliance program should not indicate that this procedure is currently being carried out. The attributes of each individual element of a compliance program must be evaluated in order to assess the program's effectiveness as a whole. Appropriate changes in the program should be made to address any identified weaknesses.

A common method of assessing compliance program effectiveness is measurement of various outcome indicators (such as billing and coding error rates, identified overpayments, and audit results). However, the OIG noted in the Supplemental Compliance Program Guidance for Hospitals that they have observed that exclusive reliance on these indicators may cause an organization to miss crucial underlying weaknesses. They recommend that hospitals examine program outcomes and assess the underlying structure and process of each compliance program element. The OIG identified a number of factors observed in effective compliance programs. These factors can be applied to both the overall compliance program as well as the HIM compliance program. They include consideration of the following:

- Are policies and procedures clearly written, relevant to day-to-day responsibilities, readily available to those who need them, and reevaluated on a regular basis?

- Does the organization monitor staff compliance with internal policies and procedures?

- Has the organization developed a risk assessment tool, which is reevaluated on a regular basis, to assess and identify weaknesses and risks in operations?

- Does the risk assessment tool include an evaluation of federal healthcare program requirements, as well as other publications, such as OIG's compliance program guidance documents, work plans, special advisory bulletins, and special fraud alerts?

- Does the organization provide qualified trainers to conduct annual compliance training for its staff, including both general and specific training pertinent to the staff's responsibilities?

- Has the organization evaluated the content of its training and education program on an annual basis and determined that the subject content is appropriate and sufficient to cover the range of issues confronting its employees?

- Has the organization kept up-to-date with any changes in federal healthcare program requirements and adapted its education and training program accordingly?

- Has the organization formulated the content of its education and training program to consider results from its audits and investigations; results from previous training and education programs, trends in hotline reports; and OIG, CMS, or other agency guidance or advisories?

- Has the organization evaluated the appropriateness of its training format by reviewing the length of the training sessions; whether training is delivered via live instructors or via computer-based training programs; the frequency of training sessions; and the need for general and specific training sessions?

- Does the organization seek feedback after each session to identify shortcomings in the training program, and does it administer post-training testing to ensure attendees understand and retain the subject matter delivered?

- Has the organization documented who has completed the required training?

- Has the organization assessed whether to impose sanctions for failing to attend training or to offer appropriate incentives for attending training?

- Is the audit plan reevaluated annually, and does it address the proper areas of concern, considering, for example, findings from previous years' audits, risk areas identified as part of the annual risk assessment, and high volume services?

- Does the audit plan include an assessment of billing systems, in addition to claims accuracy, in an effort to identify the root cause of billing errors?

- Is the role of the auditors clearly established and are coding and audit personnel independent and qualified, with the requisite certifications?

- Has the organization evaluated the error rates identified in the annual audits?

- If the error rates are not decreasing, has the organization conducted a further investigation into other aspects of the compliance program in an effort to determine hidden weaknesses and deficiencies?

- Does the audit include a review of all billing documentation, including clinical documentation, in support of the claim?

- Are detected deficiencies thoroughly and promptly investigated?

- Are corrective action plans developed that take into account the root causes of each potential violation?

- Are periodic reviews of problem areas conducted to verify that the corrective action plan that was implemented successfully corrected existing deficiencies?

- When a detected deficiency results in an identified overpayment, is it promptly reported and repaid to the payer?

- Are disciplinary standards enforced consistently across the organization?

Evaluating how a compliance program performs during the organization's day-to-day operations is a critical indicator of effectiveness. Do patterns of errors or other identified problems indicate that employees do not understand policies and procedures or coding rules and guidelines? Organizations should consider periodically testing the staff about regulatory rules and guidelines to determine its level of knowledge and comprehension of regulatory requirements, pertinent compliance issues, and the relationship of regulations to the staff's own job tasks. An effective method of evaluating comprehension is to present hypothetical scenarios of situations experienced in daily practice and to assess the responses. Evaluation of the effectiveness of the training programs also should be conducted. The organization should answer the following questions:

- How frequently are staff and physicians trained? Are employees tested after training?

- Have documentation practices improved as a result of physician education?

- Do the training sessions and materials adequately summarize the important aspects of the organization's compliance program?

- Are training instructors qualified to present the subject matter and field questions with appropriate answers?

Effective auditing and monitoring is evidenced by how an organization determines the parameters of its reviews. Questions an organization should consider in regard to these parameters include the following:

- Does the audit program encompass all payers and all aspects of proper billing? For example, does a coding audit address both the assignment of correct codes and the presence of complete and accurate documentation, or only the code assignments?

- Are results of past audits, preestablished baselines, or prior deficiencies reevaluated?

- Are identified problems corrected?

- Are steps taken to correct patterns of poor documentation?

- Are auditing techniques valid, and are audits conducted by objective, qualified reviewers?

Results of auditing/monitoring activities should be used to revise the compliance program itself in order to improve its effectiveness.

Maintaining documentation of all compliance activities is absolutely key to demonstrating effectiveness of any compliance program. The federal government considers an ineffective program, or one that exists only on paper, as being worse than no compliance program at all.

A guide titled *Evaluating and Improving a Compliance Program: A Resource for Health Care Board Members, Health Care Executives, and Compliance Officers,* issued by the Health Care Compliance Association (HCCA), suggests that evaluating the effectiveness of a compliance program can be achieved by measuring the efforts that an organization commits to its compliance program and the outcomes that those efforts achieve. The efforts include the time, money, resources, and commitment that an organization puts into building and improving a compliance program. Outcomes are the impact that these efforts have on the level of compliance. According to the HCCA guide, as the compliance program matures, the principal measure of effectiveness moves from effort to outcomes. The measures of effectiveness outlined in the HCCA guide are focused on the following five indicators (HCCA 2003):

1.  Policies and procedures

2.  Ongoing education and training

3.  Open lines of communication

4.  Ongoing monitoring and auditing

5.  Enforcement and discipline

For example, measures for evaluating the effectiveness of the ongoing education and training component of a compliance program include the following:

**Effort**

- Organizational policies require employees to receive periodic training and education regarding the organization's compliance program.

    —Percentage of employees who receive training regarding the organization's compliance program promptly following commencement of employment

    —Percentage of employees in higher risk roles who receive specific, job-related education designed to reduce the incidence of noncompliance in the department or function at intervals established by the provider

- Content of the education and training addresses the operation of the compliance program and the substantive legal issues that most directly impact the organization's risk and the employee's duties.

    —Organization has engaged in an assessment of its most significant risks by reviewing applicable OIG guidance, fraud alerts and work plans, through consultation with healthcare counsel or other experts, or by some other mechanism (consistent with the organization's size and resources) reasonably calculated to identify its principal risks.

    —Organization has a process to monitor changes in laws and regulations relating to its greatest risk areas and modifies education content as appropriate.

- Organization assesses the effectiveness of its education efforts by using tests, which evaluate employee comprehension and measure impact on job processes, or some other mechanism designed to ensure the training is effective.

    —Failure to fulfill compliance education requirements is grounds for an employee's discipline up to and including termination.

**Outcome**

- Organization has documentation that training and education of employees has occurred.
- Organization and its compliance officer have documentation that proves that policies and procedures and the Code of Conduct have been distributed to all applicable employees.
- There is documentation in employee files showing discipline for employees who do not complete training or who do not return the receipt of the Code of Conduct.

It is recommended that organizations review the HCCA guide, tailor the measures of effectiveness for their HIM compliance programs, and incorporate these measures into the auditing and monitoring component of the compliance program. The HCCA guide is available on the HCCA Web site: www.hcca-info.org (HCCA 2003).

To demonstrate that its compliance program is effective, every healthcare organization must include an evaluation and measurement of effectiveness as a component of its program. This is also true of an HIM compliance program.

## References

Centers for Medicare and Medicaid Services. n.d. Medicare Provider Analysis and Review (MEDPAR) File. Available online from http://www.cms.hhs.gov/IdentifiableDataFiles/05_MedicareProviderAnalysisand ReviewFile.asp.

General Accounting Office. 1999 (April). Medicare: Early evidence of compliance effectiveness is inconclusive. GAO/HEHS-99-59. Available online from www.gao.gov/archive/1999/he99059.pdf.

Health Care Compliance Association. 2003. *Evaluating and Improving a Compliance Program: A Resource for Health Care Board Members, Health Care Executives, and Compliance Officers.* Minneapolis: HCCA. Available online from http://www.hcca-info.org/content/navigationmenu/compliance_resources/evaluation_ improvement/evaluation_improvement.htm.

Office of Inspector General. 2005 (Jan. 31). Supplemental Compliance Program Guidance for Hospitals. *Federal Register* 70(19): 4858–76. Available at online from http://oig.hhs.gov/fraud/docs/complianceguidance/ 012705HospSupplementalGuidance.pdf.

Office of Inspector General. 1998 (Feb. 23). OIG Compliance Program Guidance for Hospitals. *Federal Register* 63(35): 8987–98. Available online from http://oig.hhs.gov/authorities/docs/cpghosp.pdf.

Office of Inspector General. n.d. Office of Audit Services, RAT-STATS program. Available online from http://www.oig.hhs.gov/organization/OAS/ratstat.html.

Russo, R. 1998. *Seven Steps to HIM Compliance.* Marblehead, MA: Opus Communications.

Texas Medical Foundation Health Quality Institute. 2005 (December). Hospital Payment Monitoring Program Compliance Workbook. Available online from http://www.tmf.org/hpmp/tools/workbook/index.htm.

# Chapter 6
# Impact of Electronic Health Records on HIM Compliance

*Sue Bowman, RHIA, CCS*

## Addressing Electronic Health Records Issues in HIM Compliance Programs

A Nationwide Health Information Network's (NHIN) greatest potential for deterring fraud will come in its advanced implementation, with fully interoperable electronic health records (EHRs) and integrated advanced fraud-control tools. Four states are envisioned through which the NHIN will evolve (Hanson and Cassidy 2006):

- **The status quo,** as it is anticipated to be in 2006 after implementation of the Medicare Part D prescription benefit. In this state, there is no NHIN. Some EHRs and electronic transactions such as e-prescribing exist, but with the exception of claims and prescription databases, there is little aggregate clinical data and no interoperability.

- **Early NHIN.** In this state, electronic clinical transactions such as laboratory results and e-prescribing become widespread. EHR adoption increases, but there remains little EHR interoperability among providers.

- **Intermediate NHIN.** This state features interoperability with intelligent coding tools that search for fraud. A record locator system facilitates the exchange of clinical records among providers. Clinical vocabularies are in widespread use, ICD-10 has been implemented, and intelligent coding tools are used for claims generation.

- **Advanced NHIN.** Advanced analytics exist in this state. Interoperability enables the aggregation of rich clinical and financial databases to which advanced analytic techniques are applied to detect patterns of fraud.

---

Portions of this chapter were adapted from two AHIMA practice briefs (*Update: Maintaining a Legally Sound Health Record* and *Delving into Computer-Assisted Coding*) and from two Foundation on Research and Education (FORE) reports. See reference list for full citations.

Many of the sound coding and documentation practices that are used in a paper-based environment also apply to an electronic environment. However, the use of EHRs has introduced new functionalities and processes that have led to new compliance challenges. Healthcare organizations must conduct a risk assessment, evaluate EHR product design and functionalities to assess compliance with federal and state laws and regulations, and develop policies/procedures for appropriate use of the EHR system. The risk assessment should include a review of HIPAA regulations and state and federal laws and a survey of all departments to understand how each uses the system.

As healthcare organizations implement EHR systems, the following issues should be addressed in their HIM compliance programs.

## Copy and Paste Functionality

The "copy and paste" functionality available in EHR systems eliminates duplication of effort and saves time, but it must be used carefully to ensure accurate documentation. It poses several risks, including the following:

- Pasting the note to the wrong encounter or the wrong patient record
- Lack of identification of the original author and date
- Acceptability of copying and pasting the original author's note without his or her knowledge or permission
- Duplication of inapplicable information (relevant to the original encounter but not the current one)
- Incorporation of misleading or erroneous documentation due to loss of context that was available to users in the original source
- Inability to accurately determine services and findings specific to a patient's encounter
- Inaccurate automated code generation

The primary issue with the copy and paste functionality in the EHR is one of authorship—who is the author and what is the date of origination for a copied entry? For example, if documentation is copied from a previous encounter and pasted into the current encounter, without a reference to the original document, it will not be clear to the coding professional, auditor, clinical staff, or anyone else reviewing the record that this information relates to a previous encounter. In addition to the implications for patient care, this could pose serious compliance risks for the following two reasons:

1. A diagnosis or procedure might be reported on a reimbursement claim that is not relevant to that encounter (because the diagnosis or procedure was included in the copied and pasted documentation with no indication that it pertains to a prior encounter)

2. A higher-level visit code may be reported (based on information that pertains to the events of a prior encounter rather than the current encounter)

It has been noted that ambulatory EHR systems in particular hold the potential for errors of this sort, as many enable a single user to complete both documentation and coding (Rollins 2006).

Payers require documentation that is specific to and accurately reflective of each unique encounter. Medicare cites instances in which documentation of physical examinations were nearly identical on subsequent visits, even when diagnoses changed. In other instances, multiple patients had the exact same findings upon follow-up visits. Medicare warns that defaulted documentation of this kind can harm quality of care as well as result in reporting a more extensive history and physical examination than is medically necessary.

Organizations should develop policy and procedures related to copying and pasting documentation in their EHR systems. By following these guidelines and training clinical staff, providers can allow copying and pasting within certain boundaries:

- In general, the original source author and date must be evidenced in copied information. If users are allowed to copy forward from a previous entry by another person, an attribution statement referring to the original document, date, and author should be attached or incorporated where applicable.

- Copying and pasting should be considered "not OK until proven otherwise." The copy and paste functionality should be used judiciously. For example, when referring to other documentation in the record, such as another clinician's note, a reference to the other note could be entered, with a link to it, rather than copying and pasting the documentation.

- Each potential function must be evaluated for policy or procedure acceptance or rejection by a practice.

- In some settings, copy and paste may be acceptable for legal record purposes but not for others (clinical trials data, quality assurance data, pay-for-performance data).

- In the hybrid environment, audit tracking of copy and paste may not be available because it involves different systems.

- In some contexts, it is never legitimate, including settings where the actual function takes personal health information outside the security environment.

- Some systems have an intermediate step allowing information to be brought forward but require another validation step.

- As a mitigation step, boilerplate text or libraries may be devised to describe common or routine information as agreed upon by the organizational standards.

If test results are copied and pasted into an encounter note, the date of the original test results should be noted, along with the electronic system in which they reside. If information is taken from another source, such as an e-mail message the patient sent the clinician describing the symptoms or response to a medication, the information should be quoted directly and attributed to the patient and the date and source of the original information annotated.

It is important for clinicians to understand that they are responsible for the content of their authenticated notes, including information that has been copied from elsewhere.

## Use of Templates, Boilerplates, and Canned Text

EHR systems must allow limited automatic creation of information. The primary reason canned text or templates are used is to save time. When used inappropriately, they misrepresent a patient's condition, might not reflect changes in a condition, or may not accurately reflect the procedure(s) actually performed. Regardless of the format, text entries, canned phrases, or templates should follow fundamental principles for the quality of the health record entry. In both paper-based and electronic health record systems, specific language should be used to avoid vague or generalized language. Objective facts should be documented and personal opinions should be avoided. The complete facts and pertinent information related to an event, course of treatment, patient condition, response to care, and deviation from standard treatment (including the reason for it) should be documented.

Care must be taken that the use of templates, boilerplates, and canned text support clinical care and accurate documentation, not simply to expedite the process. Creation and periodic review of these tools should be based on clinically appropriate, standards-based protocol for common or routine information. Documentation using one of these methods should require an active choice in response to the interaction between the patient and provider. Template users should document pertinent positive results and delete incorrect autogenerated entries.

## Timeliness and Chronology of Entries

Procedures must be in place to define timeliness for each component of the EHR system in which there are no real-time automated links between subsystems.

The record must reflect the continuous chronology of the patient's healthcare. Tools should be provided to allow viewing of episode-based information. The chronology of events must be readily apparent in any given view.

The EHR system must have the ability to date- and time-stamp each entry as the entry is made. Every entry in the health record must have a system-generated date and time based on the current date and time. Date and time stamps must be associated with the signature at the time the documentation is finalized. The date and time of entries must be accessible to anyone reviewing the record.

EHR systems should include capabilities to monitor and track health record completion (including notification to clinicians regarding incomplete documentation and aggregated management screens and reports for HIM staff).

## Corrections, Errors, and Amendments

EHR systems must have the ability to track corrections or changes to an entry once the entry has been entered or authenticated. When correcting or making a change to an EHR entry, the original entry should be viewable, the current date and time should be entered, the person making the change should be identified, and the reasons should be noted. In situations in which a hard copy is printed from the EHR, the hard copy must also be corrected.

Every entry should be date-, time-, and author-stamped by the system. A symbol that indicates a new or additional entry that has resulted in an additional version should be viewable. It must be clear to the user that there are additional versions of the data being viewed. A preferred method is to apply a strikethrough for error with commentary and date-, time-, and author-stamp or equivalent functionality to retain original versions linked to the corrected version.

When a pertinent entry was missed or not written in a timely manner, a late entry should be used to record the information in the health record. Systems must have the ability for the documenter to enter date and time of occurrence for late entries.

As in paper-based record systems, an addendum created in an EHR should be identified as such and should include the current date and time. An addendum in an EHR should have a link to the original entry or a symbol by the original entry to indicate the amendment.

## Version Management

Organizations must address management of document versions. Once documentation has been made available for patient care, it must be retained and managed regardless of whether the document was authenticated (if authentication applies). Organizations must decide whether all versions of a document will be displayed or just the final version, who has access to the various versions of a document, and how the availability of versions will be flagged in the health record.

It is acceptable for a draft of a dictated and transcribed note or report to be changed before authentication unless there is a reason to believe the changes are suspect and would not reflect actual events or actions. Facility policy should define the acceptable period allowed for a document to remain in draft form before the author reviews and approves it (for example, 24 to 72 hours). Once a document is no longer considered a draft or has been authenticated, any changes or alterations should be made following the procedures for a late entry or amendment. The original document must be maintained along with the new revised document.

## Data Integrity: Access Control and Audit Trails

Integrity is defined as the accuracy, consistency, and reliability of information content, processes, and systems. To protect the integrity of the EHR, policies and procedures must be in place:

- Regarding the reconciliation of electronic processes (the process for checking individual data elements, reports, files)

- Regarding the assessment of potential data corruption, data mismatches, and extraneous data

- Regarding management of different iterations of documents (version control)

- Regarding the definition of when the record is complete and permanently filed

- Regarding downtime processes and ability to capture data following downtime through direct entry or scanning

Access control is the process that determines who is authorized to access patient information in the health record. In an EHR environment, access control and validation procedures must be in place to validate a person's access to the system based on role or function. For example, coding professionals need access to the complete health record for encounters they are expected to code.

Because health record documentation necessary for accurate and complete coding may be maintained in multiple information systems, it is important for the location of all of the health record documentation pertaining to a particular patient encounter to be clearly identified and access granted to the appropriate coding professional(s).

An audit trail is a business record of all transactions and activities, including access, associated with the health record. Elements of an audit trail may include date, time, nature of transaction or activity, and the individual or automated system linked to the transaction or activity. Transactions may include additions or edits to the medical record. The purpose of an audit trail is to create a system control to establish accountability for transactions and activities as well as compliance with organizational policies, procedures, and protocols related to health record access and maintenance.

Every transaction within an EHR must be retrievable through audit capability. The following transactions should be included in an audit trail report: view, write, correct, amend, and change.

In an EHR, an audit trail may be one of the following:

- Electronic file of transactions and activities (data creation, access, revision along with date and time)

- Hard-copy report of transactions and activities

- Batch file processing report

- Information system data transmission or interface report

- Exception report of unauthorized access attempts

The Certification Commission for Health Information Technology (CCHIT) has developed criteria for EHR audit functions that will be used in certifying EHR products. Issues addressed in these criteria include the system's ability to generate an audit record when auditable events happen, such as when users log in and log out or when a chart is created, viewed, updated, or deleted. Criteria also detail the standard information captured, such as date and time of the event, type of event, user identity, and success or failure of the event. But CCHIT certification alone is not a cure-all, particularly when it comes to meeting provisions of the Federal Rules of Evidence, which outline discovery and admissibility rules in legal proceedings. Organizations in the process of purchasing EHR applications should address record verification and audit concerns up front, provided HIM, compliance, legal, and internal audit staff members are involved.

As organizations look for ways to improve their record verification and audit mechanisms, it is important to recognize that it may not be possible to automate 100 percent of processes right away. Also, improving verification and auditing processes in the short term may mean changing policies or not activating certain EHR system functionalities.

EHR applications with robust verification and auditing capabilities have the potential to capture an enormous amount of data—likely more than an organization may need or can manage. In such instances, the question becomes how to capture and process the right data. To avoid information overload, organizations must balance risks and resources to capture a manageable amount of data.

It is essential that HIM professionals be involved in determination of audit require-ments in an EHR system as well as the appropriate level of audit detail for their individual organizations.

## Computer-Assisted Coding Technology

Automating coding software is generating interest for many reasons; an important one is its ability to speed the turnaround time between patient encounter and reimbursement. How-ever, automated coding has interesting potential in another important, though less-discussed, aspect of healthcare: fraud management. In combination with antifraud software, automated coding software has the potential to reduce fraudulent activity by preventing code reporting errors, increasing the accuracy of coded data, and detecting false claims. The combination is all the more relevant as the industry moves to EHRs (Garvin et al. 2006).

Current coding software products span a range of automation. Supplementary cod-ing tools increase the consistency of the diagnostic and procedural codes assigned. These products consist of tools from the very basic to the more complex.

There are many tools to assist coding professionals in the code assignment process, including bar codes, pick or look-up lists, automated superbills, logic- or rules-based encoders, groupers, imaged and remote coding applications, and hard coding via charge-master tables. More robust tools include complex prompting based on reference rules, color-coded references and edits, and software that allows coding from a remote, secure location. Additional prompts can be added onto existing software to help the coding pro-fessional fully code each case and view the reimbursement results. This software is usually referred to as coding optimization software. Codes may be inconsistently assigned because of variability of coding education and training, the degree of accuracy of the coding tools used, and error introduced into the workflow because of incomplete documentation and interrupted workflows. Through the use of coding software, the healthcare industry seeks to increase the accuracy of code assignments and minimize the potential for error in the associated processes that affect coding.

Advances in computer technology have resulted in computer applications that go a step further and actually suggest potentially applicable medical codes. Various terms are used for such systems, including automated coding, automated documentation, auto-coding, computer-generated coding, and computer-assisted coding. In AHIMA's Practice Brief titled *Delving into Computer-Assisted Coding,* **computer-assisted coding** (CAC) is defined as the use of computer software that automatically generates a set of medical codes for review, validation, and use based on clinical documentation provided by healthcare practitioners. It must be noted, however, that no product currently on the market is able to automate code assignments completely, because of the multiple variables in coding that complicate machine processing. A coding professional or clinician makes the final deter-mination of the codes reported or stored.

When combined with the EHR or electronic documents, automated coding can stream-line the way that healthcare organizations gather data and submit claims for services. It can also provide a way to analyze health data and coding patterns to perform continuous auditing prior to billing and claims submission.

Automated coding products can incorporate and analyze patient data generated from a variety of sources. They can also evaluate record-specific information. Both of these aspects can help prevent fraud in reimbursement claims. It should be noted that some basic text to code-mapping products may not provide antifraud features and may contribute to improper coding if not properly designed.

CAC can be accomplished using either **natural language processing** (NLP) or structured input. NLP is a software technology that uses artificial intelligence to extract pertinent data and terms from a text-based document and convert them into a set of medical codes to be used or edited by a coding professional. NLP uses either a statistics- or rules-based approach. With a statistics-based approach, the software makes predictions of what a proper code should include for a given word or phrase based on what statistics have shown in the past. A rules-based approach involves building up an understanding of the words and phrases used in medical documents and the codes that should be used to report these various words and phrases by way of a complex series of rules. Structured input is based on the use of menus that contain clinical terms. As an individual menu item is chosen, a narrative text phrase is produced and becomes part of the health record documentation.

The capabilities to combat healthcare fraud are possible when several types of technology are used together. The greatest potential comes from combining automated coding with NLP (using both rules-based and statistics-based approaches) with artificial neural networks (ANNs) and predictive modeling to detect fraud within an EHR. ANNs can predict the potential for fraud in a specific claim based on the data in the claim and in the EHR. ANNs do not need constant updating; they acquire data continuously by analyzing certain pieces of information. Much like the text analytics in NLP, the medical data in ANNs are analyzed for any given claim and provide a statistical estimate that the data will either match or not match the desired output. Training the system to detect fraud is improved by using examples of fraudulent cases. Once this is completed, the system uses its prior knowledge to determine if a medical claim or data is falsified. These systems can be used for both prepayment and postpayment fraud detection.

Specific performance of CAC technology in terms of coding accuracy for correct reimbursement is largely unknown. Presently, the use of CAC technology is recommended as an assistive tool for the coding professional rather than an entirely automated process without human intervention. The CAC software does an initial screening against well-defined terms and produces a preliminary set of draft codes, which are reviewed, edited, and revised by a coding professional to generate the final set of codes. The final assessment of codes remains the responsibility of coding professionals who can edit and correct the codes using their expert knowledge along with other tools and references. As CAC systems mature, it is expected that the level of human review will decrease.

Benefits of CAC include the following:

- Improved coding consistency

- More comprehensive coding

- Enhanced coding compliance

- Decreased coding/billing costs

- Faster turnaround time (resulting in decreased accounts receivable days)

- Enhanced workflow

The use of CAC technology may increase coding compliance because it can store enormous amounts of complex and ever-changing rules and regulations and it incorporates assistive tools to improve coding accuracy, including edits, prompts, quality checks, and links to online reference materials. It is anticipated that the use of CAC tools will result in more accurate, consistent, and compliant coding because this software is better equipped than humans to handle the proliferation and intricacies of coding rules and reimbursement regulations. The use of this technology offers the benefit of availability of a coding audit trail. Because coding decisions made by CAC software are based on programming and on rules and statistical calculations, the reason a particular code was selected at any given time can be reconstructed if necessary.

Although the use of CAC technology certainly offers many advantages, it also presents compliance risks that must be addressed. The use of CAC technology can result in both increased errors and decreased errors, depending on the associated processes that are undertaken with the use of the technology. CAC software logic may be incorrect or not updated on a timely basis and result in coding errors. Coding errors can also result if review and audit functions are not being performed as recommended. Because CAC-generated coding errors will be made consistently across the board, in every similar situation, a significant pattern of improperly coded claims may result.

CAC tools that rely on structured input have additional compliance risks. If not carefully designed and used with caution, documentation generated via structured templates may lead to more reimbursement than deserved for the services rendered.

As with encoding products, the design of CAC software may either facilitate or hinder the coding process. Poorly designed computer screens or inappropriate or misleading prompts and edit checks can result in decreased coding accuracy. Failure to update the software on a timely basis to reflect new or revised rules and regulations will also have a negative impact on coding accuracy.

With appropriate statistical evaluation and expert coding validation, errors can be decreased and new aggregate analysis similar to an audit can take place concurrently. This method can result in improved documentation and increased accuracy of claims. Organizations using CAC technology should develop a testing and audit plan to validate the results of the software application. Initial software integrity, subsequent updates, and machine logic should be tested using fully coded and validated documents. The findings should be documented and, as necessary, a project management plan should be created to facilitate rapid reconciliation of issues, revisions, necessary upgrades, or refinements. Acceptable confidence thresholds for various coding systems (ICD-9-CM, CPT, HCPCS level 2, etc.) should be defined to optimize the advantages of using the CAC tool and to provide a baseline for applicable specialty use.

The importance of monitoring coded data that is generated by CAC applications, and the use of this data within the context of the EHR, is an important component of an HIM compliance program. It is also important to educate compliance staff about how all of the various automated systems used within the organization work together. Multiple interfaces with many types of computer systems are currently a reality in healthcare, which can lead to compliance challenges if the systems do not communicate with one another, are not regularly updated (or are updated on different schedules), contain conflicting data, or use or incorporate incorrect edits or logic.

Audit trails are vital in order to assess the patterns of use within the EHR as well as the patterns of coding and billing. Healthcare organizations using CAC software should also conduct compliance checks to determine the accuracy of coded data and evaluate aggregate data for problematic trends when using CAC technology on a continuing basis as part of the routine compliance program.

The report titled "Automated Coding Software: Development and Use to Enhance Anti-Fraud Activities" (discussed in further detail in the following paragraphs) issued the following recommendations for users of CAC technology to reduce compliance risks:

- Use software that generates codes only after the text is developed

- Conduct compliance checks to determine the accuracy of coded data and evaluate aggregate data for problematic trends when using automated coding on a continuing basis as part of the routine compliance program

- Seek products that incorporate the following features and standards: standard coding references and coding edits, simple mechanisms to attain intraoperability with billing and abstracting systems, aggregate data evaluation capabilities in order to detect potential fraud, and audit trails

- Create accountability within the organization with regard to accuracy of claims and build positive relationships with payers to determine how to improve interactions

- Establish and enforce standard educational requirements in job descriptions for all coding and billing experts that include minimum education and continuing education requirements

- Include coding and billing professionals in decisions to purchase and implement software. The impact software has on the accuracy of coding, billing, and the beneficiaries of healthcare programs should also be evaluated so that appropriate modifications to the software, implementation, and education can take place to prevent incorrect bills.

During the software selection process, healthcare organizations should seek products with the following design characteristics:

- Use of a combination of statistics-based and rules-based automated coding to determine codes using a standardized database (as opposed to a facility-specific database) to determine initial coding standards. This should then be followed by an evaluation of coding rules by qualified coding professionals to develop associated rules. Codes should be generated only after the text has been developed.

- Audit capabilities for tracking all users of the document and the subsequent coding and billing process

- Machine learning capabilities through the use of artificial neural networks for data profiling, advanced analytic models, and ranked scoring in fraud and abuse software

- Continuous monitoring capabilities of aggregate data analysis to detect any potential patterns of abuse with the aim of reducing submission of inaccurate claims

- Standards-based software with fraud alert warnings from the OIG areas of focus, authoritative coding references (for example, *ICD-9-CM Official Guidelines for Coding and Reporting,* the American Hospital Association's *Coding Clinic for ICD-9-CM,* the American Medical Association's *CPT Assistant,* rules and conventions contained within the coding systems)

- Use of CAC systems (natural language processing or structured text) that only code treatment or services that are adequately documented

- Incorporation of simple mechanisms for attaining interoperability with billing and abstracting systems

- Incorporation of access controls to prevent or minimize opportunities for unauthorized persons (whether practitioner or nonpractitioner) from entering information about an encounter or healthcare episode that did not occur or for producing false claims for services never rendered

- Incorporation of identity authentication procedures to verify who accesses EHRs, CAC software, and medical claim submissions, as well as mechanisms to track this access

- Incorporation of document versioning, to allow identification of the fact that a document has been changed, the date(s) and time of the changes, and the ability to access earlier versions

- Coding experts who have appropriate certifications and education should be used in product development and during product support to ensure that the code sets and authoritative references are up to date.

As the HIM profession moves toward the routine use of electronic records and automated coding, it will need to maintain many traditional skills and continue many current practices, such as the use of current coding tools, working within an established compliance program, and evaluating products for accuracy. HIM professionals will also need new skills, certified products, the ability to work with aggregate data analysis, and familiarity with the use of ANNs. The role of skilled coding professionals will not be diminished but enhanced.

## Use of Health Information Technology to Enhance Fraud Prevention and Detection

Fraud has a significant impact on the U.S. health economy. Some estimates place the loss as high as 10 percent of the annual healthcare expenditure, or $170 billion. Technology can play a critical role in detecting fraud and abuse and can help pave the way toward prevention. Although technology cannot eliminate the fraud problem, it can significantly minimize fraud and abuse and ultimately reduce fraud losses.

### OIG: Use of Information Technology Presents New Compliance Risks

The *OIG's Supplemental Compliance Program Guidance for Hospitals* identified the use of information technology as presenting new compliance risks and issues that must be addressed in organizational compliance programs. It was noted that as the healthcare industry moves forward, organizations will increasingly rely on information technology. For example, the implementation of EHR systems, HIPAA privacy and security regulations, electronic claims submission, electronic prescribing, networked information sharing among providers, and systems for the tracking and reduction of medical errors will require hospitals to depend more on information technologies. Information technology presents new opportunities to advance healthcare efficiency, but also new challenges to ensuring the accuracy of claims and the information used to generate claims. It may be difficult for purchasers of computer systems and software to know exactly how the system operates and generates information. The OIG recommended that prudent hospitals take steps to ensure that they thoroughly assess all new computer systems and software that impact coding, billing, or the generation or transmission of information related to the submission of reimbursement claims.

### Reports on Use of Health Information Technology to Enhance AntiFraud Activities

The Foundation of Research and Education (FORE) of AHIMA issued two reports in 2005 detailing how health information technology can address the growing problem of healthcare fraud. The reports are the result of a six month project conducted under contract to the Office of the National Coordinator for Health Information Technology (ONC) within the U.S. Department of Health and Human Services (HHS) that involved two main tasks:

1. A descriptive study of the issues and steps in the development and use of automated coding software that enhance healthcare antifraud activities

2. Identifying best practices to enhance the capabilities of a nationwide interoperable health information technology infrastructure to assist in prevention, detection, and prosecution in cases of healthcare fraud or improper claims and billing.

The report that addressed the use of automated coding software included the following major recommendations:

- Computer-assisted coding software should use a combination of statistics-based and rules-based automated coding and a standardized national database (as opposed to a facility-specific database) to train the statistics-based engine.

- Audit trails are essential in all coding and billing software and EHR applications to ensure that codes are based on documentation by clinicians.

- Users of automated coding should have an appropriate compliance program that includes continuous data analysis to detect potential patterns of abuse prior to claims submission and payment, appropriately trained coding professionals, and use of current coding references and appropriate coding practice standards.

- Product certification for computer-assisted coding products should be instituted. Certification should be based on criteria assessing the accuracy with which health record documentation is converted to codes based on standard coding principles and guidelines.

- Payers and providers must work more closely to prevent fraud. Adherence to standard coding conventions and rules is essential, as is aggregate data analysis and continuous monitoring enabled by computerization.

- When making any software purchase, providers and payers should evaluate the potential impact on the accuracy of coding, billing, and claims processing so there are no unintended consequences. Coding experts should participate in the selection and implementation processes.

The second report, on the use of health information technology to enhance and expand healthcare antifraud activities, included the following guiding principles and recommendations:

1. **The NHIN policies, procedures, and standards must proactively prevent, detect, and support prosecution of healthcare fraud rather than be neutral to it.**

   Recommendations:

   a. Develop enterprise management and operating policies for all stakeholders that will render the NHIN inherently resistant to fraud and support fraud management.

   b. Build in as part of the NHIN infrastructure standards, procedures, and prototypes to facilitate nationwide healthcare fraud management.

   c. Certify EHR software features and functions that are required or prohibited in the NHIN infrastructure to enable effective healthcare fraud management.

2. **EHRs and information available through the NHIN must fully comply with applicable federal and state laws and meet the requirements for reliability and admissibility of evidence.**

   Recommendations:

   a. Establish standards for the electronic maintenance, submission, and disclosure of health and financial information contained in the EHR. Standards should address accuracy, completeness, accountability, access and availability, audit ability (verifiability), identification, authentication, nonrepudiation, integrity, digital certificate, digital signature, electronic signature, and public key infrastructure.

   b. Delineate data quality and electronic transmission standards.

   c. Adopt a national approach to making public key infrastructure and other data security technologies available to all constituents of the NHIN.

   d. Ensure that access to and disclosure of EHR content and other information available through the NHIN is consistent with health information privacy and security laws and other applicable laws.

3. **A standard minimum definition of a Legal Health Record (LHR) must be adopted for EHRs.**

   Recommendations:

   a. Establish national standards for the EHR to be maintained as a business record and, as such, adopt maintenance, retention, and disclosure practices for it as a business record that meets the requirements for reliable and admissible evidence.

   b. Establish national "EHR as the LHR" standards (using the current guidelines for paper health records as a generally accepted base) to address the transition from paper through hybrid to fully electronic health records.

4. **Comprehensive Healthcare Fraud Management programs must enable rather than inhibit nationwide EHR adoption.**

   Recommendations:

   a. Include fraud management features and functionality in the interoperable EHR without placing undue financial burden on the providers.

   b. Design EHR fraud management features that will not disrupt the provider workflow or interfere with the patient care process.

   c. Balance the development of fraud management programs on the NHIN with other priority interests and infrastructure design requirements, especially patient care.

5.  **Healthcare Fraud Management is the responsibility of all healthcare stakeholders.**

    Recommendations:

    a.  Disseminate definitions and guidelines to inform and address the impact and consequences of healthcare fraud on the economy, on patient health risk, and on population health risk.

    b.  Inform stakeholders of the interpretation of healthcare fraud guidelines with regard to EHR documentation and coding.

    c.  Identify (consistent with current legal requirements) when and who has the right to access relevant portions of patient records (EHRs) through the customary mechanisms of the NHIN for the purpose of effective healthcare fraud management.

6.  **Increased consumer awareness of healthcare fraud and the role health information technology and EHRs play in its reduction can improve the effectiveness of healthcare fraud management programs.**

    Recommendations:

    a.  Develop and deploy a consumer awareness program on the role of information technology in healthcare fraud and its ability to detect and assist consumers to personally minimize fraud.

    b.  Emphasize the benefits of the NHIN and EHRs in the national fight against healthcare fraud in program content and publications.

7.  **EHR standards must define requirements to promote fraud management and minimize opportunities for fraud and abuse, consistent with the use of EHRs for patient care.**

    Recommendations:

    a.  Mandate the minimum infrastructure necessary to ensure that EHR systems are maintained to facilitate ongoing fraud management programs and fraud prosecution activities.

    b.  Define the EHR system requirements to support accurate documentation of the clinical care process, minimizing the potential to facilitate fraudulent practices.

    c.  Develop NHIN IT infrastructure requirements to match or link the electronic documentation of a patient's clinical events and other relevant data files with the corresponding claims to enable healthcare fraud management.

    d.  Develop minimum NHIN IT infrastructure procedures and requirements for data management, data efficiency, data exchange, data availability, security, backup, disaster recovery, record alteration, record authentication, and record retention that can be audited and verified.

8. **Standardized reference terminology and up-to-date classification systems that facilitate the automation of clinical coding are essential to the adoption of interoperable EHRs and the associated IT enabled healthcare fraud management programs.**

   Recommendations:

   a. Adopt uniform rules, regulations, and guidelines for standardized reference terminology and up-to-date classification systems across the country.

   b. Ensure that the organizations authorized to develop, deploy, and maintain such standards and guidelines assume ongoing responsibility to:

      —Provide clarity with a specific standard or guideline as required.

      —Publish and disseminate the standards or guidelines in a manner that is generally understood.

      —Respond in a timely manner to all requests for clarification of standards or guidelines.

   c. Inform the individuals and entities choosing to participate in medical commerce that they are responsible for knowing and understanding the standards and guidelines with respect to clinical coding and classification.

9. **Fully integrate and implement fraud management programs and advanced analytics software in interoperable EHRs and the NHIN to achieve all of the estimated potential economic benefits.**

   Recommendations:

   a. Begin by building national work plans with specific timeframes for the varying levels of the NHIN's interoperability and its integration with and implementation of advanced analytics software for aggregate data analysis.

   b. Minimize the period of automated transactions without interoperability across providers.

   c. Move to an NHIN with analytic tools applied to aggregate data as quickly as possible once interoperability is achieved.

10. **Data required from the NHIN for monitoring fraud and abuse must be derived from its operations and not require additional data transactions.**

    Recommendations:

    a. Provide access to aggregate deidentified data generated in the normal operations of the NHIN, provided that the aggregation of data does not impose an obligation on the provider to generate data it would not otherwise have created for patient care.

b.  Assess the potential applicability of creating a Healthcare Information Sharing and Analysis Center (HISAC) as a component of a national fraud management program.

## References

AHIMA e-HIM Work Group on Computer-Assisted Coding. 2004 (Nov.–Dec.). Practice brief: Delving into computer-assisted coding. *Journal of American Health Information Management Association* (76)10:48A–H (with web extras).

AHIMA e-HIM Work Group on Maintaining the Legal EHR. 2005 (Nov.–Dec.). Update: Maintaining a Legally Sound Health Record—Paper and Electronic. *Journal of American Health Information Management Association* (76)10:64A–L.

American Health Information Management Association. 2005 (July). Fore Report: Automated Coding Software—Development and Use to Enhance Anti-Fraud Activities. Chicago: AHIMA.

American Health Information Management Association. 2005 (September). Fore Report: Use of Health Information Technology to Enhance and Expand Health Care Anti-Fraud Activities. Chicago: AHIMA.

Garvin, J.H., S. Moeini, and V. Watzlaf. 2006 (March). Fighting fraud, automatically: How coding automation can prevent healthcare fraud. *Journal of American Health Information Management Association* 77(3):32–36.

Hanson, S.P., and B.S. Cassidy. 2006 (March). Fraud control: New tools, new potential. *Journal of American Health Information Management Association* 77(3):24–27,30.

Rollins, G. 2006 (March). Following the digital trail: Weak auditing functions spell trouble for an electronic record. *Journal of American Health Information Management Association* 77(3):38–41.

# Part II
# Supplemental Compliance Guidance
# for Specific Practice Settings

The setting-specific chapters provide supplemental compliance information focused on certain healthcare settings. Part I provides general compliance guidance for all healthcare settings. Part I should be read before the material related to specific healthcare settings.

# Chapter 7
# Hospital Outpatient Services

*Susan M. Hull, MPH, RHIA, CCS, CCS-P, and Sue Bowman, RHIA, CCS*

## Introduction

All services paid under the outpatient prospective payment system (OPPS) are classified into groups called ambulatory payment classifications (APCs). Services in each APC are similar clinically and in terms of the resources they require. A payment rate is established for each APC and the hospital is reimbursed that amount, irrespective of the actual costs incurred in providing the services. Depending on the services provided, hospitals may be paid for more than one APC for an encounter. APC groups are based on Healthcare Common Procedure Coding System (HCPCS) codes, and correct HCPCS code assignment is essential for appropriate reimbursement. The hospital outpatient prospective payment system is evaluated annually by the Centers for Medicare and Medicaid Services (CMS) and any changes are published in the *Federal Register.* Changes may include revisions in relative weights, reassignment to different APCs, revisions to packaging guidelines, and wage index changes. HIM and coding professionals should review the appropriate *Federal Register* each year to ensure that all policies and procedures are current and appropriate.

Outpatient coding guidelines are included in Section IV, Diagnostic Coding and Reporting Guidelines for Outpatient Services, of the *ICD-9-CM Official Guidelines for Coding and Reporting,* available on the National Center for Health Statistics (NCHS) Web site at: http://www.cdc.gov/nchs/data/icd9/icdguide.pdf. Coding professionals who are new to outpatient coding should carefully review these guidelines, as they differ significantly from inpatient coding guidelines.

The implementation of the OPPS has made accurate documentation and coding critically important in the hospital outpatient setting. The OIG specifically identified the OPPS as a target in its 2004 Work Plan and has continued to address outpatient-related issues in each year's work plan since then. (See appendix B for a list of high-risk areas for fraud and abuse enforcement.)

In addition to the impact on appropriate reimbursement, accuracy in coding of hospital outpatient claims also is important because the billing data reported by hospitals will be used to revise weights and other adjustments that will affect APC payments in future years.

Whereas HCPCS codes and modifiers directly impact reimbursement, diagnosis codes are important for validating the appropriateness of the HCPCS level II code assignment and justifying the medical necessity of the services rendered. In addition, accurate reporting of information required for separate Medicare reimbursement for observation services is imperative in order to ensure that the organization is reimbursed appropriately for the services provided.

Hospitals code clinic and emergency department visits using the same Current Procedural Terminology (CPT) evaluation and management (E/M) codes as physicians. However, hospitals have been allowed to create their own internal set of guidelines to determine the proper level of visit to report for each patient. As long as hospitals are allowed to develop their own systems for reporting CPT E/M codes for emergency and clinic visits, each hospital must be able to demonstrate that it is following its own system consistently and for all patients, and that the facility's system reasonably relates the intensity of resources to the different levels of E/M codes. Reporting systems may be based on point assignment for various nursing interventions, definition of specific interventions that justify higher levels of service, or may be diagnosis based. Determining the appropriate E/M level depends on thorough documentation by physicians, nurses, and other clinical personnel. The medical record must include documentation of all observations, diagnoses, treatments, and medical decision making involved in a patient encounter. In the event of a compliance audit, the hospital will be required to show documentation in support of the levels reported, as well as consistent use of their own internal reporting system.

After CMS has implemented a standardized system for reporting emergency and clinic visits, hospitals will need to modify their compliance programs and methodology for assigning E/M levels of service to ensure compliance with the new requirements.

When processing OPPS claims, CMS uses a set of billing edits, called the National Correct Coding Initiative (NCCI) edits, to identify coding patterns that result in potential overpayments to providers. CMS developed the NCCI edits to promote national correct coding methodologies and to eliminate improper coding. These edits determine what procedures and services cannot be billed at the same time when they are furnished for the same patient on the same day. Thus, the NCCI prohibits the unbundling of procedures by ensuring that the comprehensive code is billed instead of multiple component codes and by identifying mutually exclusive code pairs that should not be billed together. These edits are part of the outpatient code editor and can be obtained at the following link: http://www.cms.hhs.gov/NationalCorrectCodInitEd/. Note that hospitals always comply with the prior quarter's edits, unlike physicians, who comply with the current quarter's edits.

Following are a number of actions hospitals can take to ensure compliance with OPPS requirements (Stewart 2001, 58–60):

- Provide training to physicians regarding their obligations for accurate and complete documentation in the health record. The goal is to improve documentation in order to capture all diagnoses and procedures performed and to ensure accurate and complete coding.

- Provide training to the HIM staff on health record review methods for appropriate assignment of ICD-9-CM and HCPCS codes and modifiers, as well as special reimbursement-related issues that depend on code assignment.

- Review the chargemaster periodically (at least annually) and update as CPT/ HCPCS codes are added or revised to ensure accurate reporting of those ancillary and other items and/or service charges generated by the chargemaster. As an ancillary department adds new services, its chargemaster should be reviewed and updated as appropriate to ensure proper reporting and reimbursement for the new services. A periodic, complete review should involve all of the departments whose services are represented on the chargemaster. It is also important that the technicians who actually perform the procedures be included in this review, as they truly know what services are being provided.

- Provide appropriate ICD-9-CM, CPT, and HCPCS level II training, tailored to the target audience, to physicians (for example, to provide guidance related to medical necessity determinations) and to ancillary department personnel (particularly those involved with chargemaster maintenance). This education should include modifier training, when appropriate. Education for the medical staff should include issues related to medical necessity, observation policies, payer rules regarding procedures performed as an inpatient versus outpatient, issues related to discontinued procedures, and, of course, specific requirements related to proper documentation.

- Provide training to registration personnel on national and local coverage determination/local medical review policy (NCD/LCD/LMRP) requirements and procedures for obtaining advance beneficiary notices (ABNs). Develop policies to obtain symptoms or diagnoses from the ordering physician for all ancillary testing or other procedures performed before the patient undergoes the test or procedure.

- Compare E/M code assignments with the criteria developed by the hospital and the health record documentation to assess the accuracy of the code assignments, to ensure that the hospital's system for mapping facility services to the E/M code levels is being followed, and to determine whether the code assignments are supported by documentation in the health record.

- Conduct periodic reviews to ensure that diagnosis codes are consistent with procedure codes and that health record documentation supports reported diagnosis and procedure codes. When multiple CPT codes have been assigned, staff should verify that the codes are not components of a larger, comprehensive procedure that could be described with a single code. CPT code assignments should be checked against the NCCI edits applicable to hospital outpatient departments (as identified in the outpatient code editor).

- Review new or revised requirements or policies issued by CMS or the Medicare contractor (fiscal intermediary and Durable Medical Equipment Regional Carrier if appropriate) and ensure that they are communicated to all affected personnel. Changes occur frequently and require vigilance to stay on top of them. For example, there are annual changes to the APCs, constantly updated instructions from Medicare, and regular updates to ICD-9-CM codes, CPT codes, HCPCS level II codes, and the outpatient code editor. Keep in mind that the code update schedules are variable, depending on the particular code set, ranging from annual, to biannual, to quarterly. HIM professionals must stay abreast of all of these changes and ensure that systems and policies/procedures are updated to reflect the changes and that affected staff receive the necessary education about these changes.

- Investigate any discrepancies between the APCs assigned by the Medicare contractor and the hospital. All denials believed to be inappropriate should be appealed, even if only small amounts of money are involved. Staff should verify that denials based on NCCI edits are based on currently applicable edits and not on deleted edits. Cite official sources that support the accuracy of the hospital's code assignment. Staff should follow up on the issue until a response has been received from the payer. If review of the denials, rejections, and code changes indicates a pattern of inaccurate coding, this information should be used to provide education to the coding staff. Claims rejections should be monitored for patterns of errors, and corrective action should be initiated when a pattern is identified. The proper usage of modifiers and NCCI edits should be evaluated, keeping in mind the differences between physician and facility usage of modifiers and NCCI edits. Also watch out for improper unbundling of services. Determine whether duplicate codes are being assigned by both the HIM department and ancillary departments (that is, services that are "hard coded" in the chargemaster as well as coded by HIM staff). This duplicate billing is most likely to occur in such departments as cardiac catheterization, interventional radiology, and gastrointestinal laboratory, where both technical and surgical codes are typically assigned for a single procedure. Any errors in coding and billing practices must be corrected to prevent future claims denials. High denial rates or repeated coding and billing errors may increase the hospital's risk of being audited by external agencies.

- Participate in the hospitalwide regular review of compliance program effectiveness. This review, which should be conducted at least annually, should evaluate both the overall success of the program and each of the basic elements. From a coding/HIM standpoint, this would include a coding/billing audit.

## Chargemaster Maintenance

The organization's policies and procedures also should address chargemaster maintenance. Because most of the codes assigned to charge line items are generated automatically by the chargemaster rather than assigned by HIM professionals, errors in the chargemaster obviously put the organization at significant compliance risk. The importance of ongoing maintenance of the chargemaster is critical because many factors that go into the charge-master are constantly changing, such as annual updates to CPT/HCPCS codes, changes in reimbursement policies, updates to charges, growth in outpatient services, advances in technology, and development of new service lines. The chargemaster must be current, complete, and compliant with payer requirements. The chargemaster must be updated constantly throughout the year to keep up with new/revised codes, code edits, and billing requirements. It is critical that each line item charge be mapped to the correct CPT or HCPCS level II code. In an EHR environment, HIM staff should continue to ensure the accuracy of the codes in the chargemaster and that maintenance updates of code changes are performed on a timely basis. Additional HIM responsibilities in an EHR environment include the following:

- Linking the codes to electronic structured documentation

- Testing and validating mapped codes and application software

A comprehensive review of the chargemaster should be performed at least annually to ensure that it is accurate, complete, and up-to-date with code revisions and regulatory changes. If issues related to the chargemaster have been identified during a compliance audit, or if a particular department or category of services has been hit particularly hard with chargemaster changes, a focused review of these services should be undertaken. Claims denials/rejections should be traced to their source and if they are determined to be the result of an error in the chargemaster, the necessary correction can be made promptly to ensure that the problem will not continue to occur.

Chargemaster maintenance should not be the responsibility of one person but, rather, should be overseen by a committee composed of representatives from administration, finance, ancillary departments on a rotating basis, billing, corporate compliance, and HIM. Proper chargemaster maintenance requires expertise in coding, billing regulations, and health record documentation requirements. The HIM representative can advise on coding rules/guidelines and which CPT and HCPCS level II codes best represent the line item charge on the chargemaster, and serve as the "expert" on code revisions. The HIM representative can assist in determining whether a service is best "hard coded" on the chargemaster or coded by HIM coding staff.

The chargemaster is never "finished." As soon as the review is completed and the charge-master has been corrected or updated, new items will be identified that need to be added or regulatory or policy changes will occur. Maintaining the chargemaster is an ongoing chal-lenge that must be supported by a defined process with written policies and procedures.

## High-Risk Areas in the Hospital Outpatient Setting

In January 2005, the Department of Health and Human Services issued the *OIG Supplemental Compliance Program Guidance* (SCPG) *for Hospitals* (OIG 2005). This document supplemented the 1998 Compliance Guidance Program for Hospitals (OIG 1998) and provided more extensive guidance in coding and reporting of outpatient services. The OIG noted that outpatient procedure coding is a compliance risk that is underappreciated by the hospital industry. Hospitals should review their outpatient documentation practices to ensure that claims are based on complete medical records and the medical records support the levels of service claimed. Coding from incomplete medical records may create problems in complying with claim submission requirements to include on a single claim all services provided to the same patient on the same day. Because incorrect procedure coding may lead to overpayments and subject a hospital to liability for the submission of false claims, hospitals need to pay close attention to coding professional training and qualifications.

Among the specific coding/HIM-related issues identified in the SCPG are the following:

- Billing on an outpatient basis for "inpatient only" procedures. The OPPS Final Rule for each year includes a list of inpatient-only procedures in the Addenda. It is the responsibility of the hospital to ensure that utilization management procedures are in place to prevent performing inpatient-only procedures on outpatients. Inclusion on the "inpatient only" list is based on the nature of the procedure, the need for at least 24 hours of postoperative recovery time or monitoring before the patient can be safely discharged, or the underlying physical condition of the patient. CMS covers inpatient procedures performed on outpatients only when they are performed to resuscitate or stabilize a patient with an emergent or life-threatening condition who expires prior to admission. In that case, the CPT code should be reported with modifier CA. When modifier CA is appended to an inpatient procedure, reimbursement is made under APC 0375 (Ancillary Outpatient Services When Patient Expires) at a payment rate of $3,217.47 (calendar year 2006). Modifier CA should be appended to only one inpatient procedure. Reporting it more than once will result in a return to provider decision.

- Submitting claims for medically unnecessary services by failing to follow local policies of the fiscal intermediaries (FIs).

- Submitting duplicate claims or otherwise not following the NCCI guidelines. It is the responsibility of the hospital to ensure that coding software edits are in place to prevent inadvertent reporting of comprehensive/component and/or mutually exclusive code pairs together.

- Submitting incorrect claims for ancillary services because of outdated CDMs. As noted above, CDMs should be reviewed regularly, but at least annually and whenever new services are added, to ensure that codes are correct, current, and reflect the services being provided.

- Circumventing the multiple procedure discounting rules. Under the hospital OPPS, although more than one APC may be assigned for a specific patient encounter, reimbursement may not be 100 percent for every APC. In fact, some APCs, although appropriately reported, may not be reimbursed at all. Because the CPT procedure code determines the APC and thus the discounting, reporting inaccurate CPT codes to avoid discounting methodologies would be perceived as potentially fraudulent billing if a pattern of abuse was identified.

- Improper E/M code selection. As noted, currently hospitals may develop their own methods for assigning E/M codes. The method must ensure that the E/M codes assigned are appropriate and accurately reflect the resource utilization involved.

- Improperly billing for observation services. Only certain ICD-9-CM diagnoses codes justify separate observation payment under the Medicare program. Reporting inaccurate ICD-9-CM diagnosis codes in order to obtain reimbursement for noncovered observation services must be avoided. See subsequent text for updated requirements for observation reporting.

- Failure to follow the OPPS rules regarding inclusion of services on a single claim provided to the same patient at the same hospital on the same day.

- Improper billing under the partial hospitalization program.

- Use of Information Technology. The use of information technology presents new compliance risks in all healthcare settings. The OIG's Supplemental Program Guidance for Hospitals notes that OPPS implementation increases the need for hospitals to pay particular attention to their computerized billing, coding, and information systems. Billing and coding under the OPPS are more data-intensive than under the inpatient prospective payment system (IPPS).

## Observation Reporting

CMS will reimburse separately for observation services to Medicare beneficiaries only when provided for treatment of asthma, chest pain, or congestive heart failure. Specific diagnosis codes that support observation services are included in the OPPS Final Rule and are available from the FI. These diagnosis codes must be reported as either the Patient Reason for Visit (FL 76) or the principal diagnosis (FL 67). Hospital observation services are reported with HCPCS level II codes. Following are the currently applicable codes:

- G0378: Hospital observation services, per hour
- G0379: Direct admission of patient for hospital observation care.

Hospitals can bill G0379 when they admit a patient directly to observation status without an emergency department, critical care, or clinic visit at the hospital on the day of or day before observation admission.

Care must be taken in reporting observation time. Medicare will reimburse observation on an hourly basis if at least eight hours of care are rendered, but generally will not reimburse for more than 24 hours of care, although CMS has stated that claims for observation hours up to 48 will be assessed on an individual basis.

Observation start and stop times are currently defined as follows:

- A beneficiary's time in observation (and hospital billing) begins with the beneficiary's admission to an observation bed.

- A beneficiary's time in observation (and hospital billing) ends when all clinical or medical interventions have been completed, including follow-up care furnished by hospital staff and physicians that may take place after a physician has ordered the patient be released or admitted as an inpatient (CMS 2005, 68693).

- No procedure with a "T" status indicator can be reported on the same day or day before observation care is provided. That is, no observation services are separately reimbursed following an outpatient surgical procedure. Any follow-up care is considered to be a part of the outpatient procedure, which includes routine recovery.

- In addition to documentation of a diagnosis supporting observation services and reporting of hours of care, the medical record must contain evidence that the patient was seen and evaluated by a physician and that risk stratification was used by the physician in assigning the patient to observation status.

- G0378 and G0379 are further defined by CMS with a new status indicator of Q, defined as "packaged service subject to separate payment based on criteria." This indicator triggers the outpatient code editor that this is a claim for outpatient observation services.

It is imperative that hospitals closely monitor their claims for observation services to ensure compliance with the regulatory requirements and reimbursement policies that were in effect at the time the observation services were furnished (not the time the claim was submitted). Given the complexity of the various requirements for Medicare reimbursement of observation services over the past several years, ensuring compliance with the reimbursement rules for observation services is no easy task. These compliance challenges are compounded by the fact that many commercial insurance companies have observation policies that differ from Medicare.

## Modifiers 25 and 59

In November 2005, the OIG issued two reports on the use of modifiers 25 and 59. Based on the OIG's review findings, hospital outpatient departments would be well-advised to incorporate the use of modifiers 25 and 59 in the auditing and monitoring component of their compliance programs in order to ensure that the use of these modifiers is in accordance with Medicare program requirements (and other payers' requirements) and is supported by medical record documentation.

Modifier 25 is defined as a significant, separately identifiable E/M service performed on the same day as a procedure or other service. To use this modifier, the E/M services must be above and beyond the services necessary to perform the procedure. Modifier 25 must be appended to the E/M code. According to the modifier 25 report, the OIG found that 35 percent of the claims reviewed should not have been paid because the E/M services were not significant, separately identifiable, and above and beyond the usual preoperative and postoperative care associated with the procedure, or the claims failed to meet basic

Medicare documentation requirements. The OIG recommended that CMS reinforce the requirements for reporting modifier 25 and emphasize that this modifier should only be used on claims for E/M services and only when these services are provided on the same day as another procedure. Most improper payments were the result of failure to furnish medical record documentation supporting the use of modifier 25. Twenty-eight percent of all providers in the sample population used modifier 25 on more than 50 percent of their claims, thus indicating unnecessary use.

Modifier 59 should be used to indicate that a procedure or service is distinct or independent from other services performed on the same day. It is used to identify procedures/services that are not normally reported together, but are appropriate under the circumstances. This may represent a different session or patient encounter, different procedure or surgery, different site or organ system, separate incision/excision, separate lesion, or separate injury (or area of injury in extensive injuries) not ordinarily encountered or performed on the same day by the same physician. When another modifier is appropriate, it should be used instead of modifier 59. Modifier 59 (or any other modifier) should not be used to bypass CCI or other edits unless the criteria for proper use of the modifier have been met.

The objective of the modifier 59 review was to determine whether this modifier is being used inappropriately to bypass Medicare's NCCI edits and to what extent Medicare contractors are reviewing the use of modifier 59. The OIG found that 40 percent of the NCCI code pairs billed with modifier 59 did not meet Medicare program requirements. Modifier 59 was used inappropriately with 15 percent of the code pairs because the services were not distinct from one another. Most of these services were not distinct because they were performed at the same session, same anatomic site, and/or through the same incision as the primary service. In the OIG's review sample, modifier 59 was used inappropriately most often with the NCCI code pair for bone marrow biopsy (CPT code 38221) and bone marrow aspiration (CPT code 38220). The use of modifier 59 was inappropriate in these instances; the services were not distinct because they were performed at the same session and through the same incision.

In 25 percent of the NCCI code pairs billed with modifier 59, the services were not adequately documented. In most of these cases, either one or both of the services billed were not documented in the medical record, or the documentation indicated that another code should have been billed for one or both of the services performed. In the remaining cases, either the documentation was insufficient to make a determination or the documentation was not provided. In 11 percent of code pairs billed with modifier 59, the claim was paid when the modifier was billed with the incorrect code. The Medicare Claims Processing Manual states that modifier 59 should be billed with the secondary, additional, or lesser service in an NCCI code pair.

As a result of the modifier 59 review, the OIG recommended that CMS encourage the Medicare contractors to conduct prepayment and postpayment reviews of the use of modifier 59. They also recommended that CMS ensure that the Medicare claims processing systems only pay claims with modifier 59 when the modifier is billed with the correct code.

See Appendix B for additional high-risk areas identified in the OIG's 2007 Work Plan.

## References

Centers for Medicare and Medicaid Services. 2005 (Nov. 10). Medicare program; changes to the hospital outpatient prospective payment system and calendar year 2006 payment rates; final rule. *Federal Register.* 70(217):68515–9040. Available online from http://a257.g.akamaitech.net/7/257/2422/01jan20051800/edocket.access.gpo.gov/2005/pdf/05-22136.pdf.

Office of the Inspector General. 2006. Work Plan, fiscal year 2007. Available online from http://www.oig.hhs.gov/publications/docs/workplan/2007/Work%20Plan%202007.pdf.

Office of Inspector General. 2005 (Jan. 31). *OIG supplemental compliance program guidance for hospitals. Federal Register* 70(19): 4858–76. Available online from http://a257.g.akamaitech.net/7/257/2422/01jan20051800/edocket.access.gpo.gov/2005/pdf/05-1620.pdf.

Office of Inspector General. 1998 (Feb. 23). Compliance program guidance for hospitals. *Federal Register* 63(35):8987–98. Available online from http://oig.hhs.gov/authorities/docs/cpghosp.pdf.

Stewart, M.M. 2001. *Coding and Reimbursement under the Outpatient Prospective Payment System.* Chicago: AHIMA.

# Chapter 8
# Compliance Considerations
# for Physician Practices

## Lynn Kuehn, RHIA, CCS-P, FAHIMA

It is unknown how many physician practices have a compliance plan in place and how many practices follow their plans. It is likely, though, that small physician practices, with limited staff and monetary resources, may overlook the positive impact inherent in a properly designed compliance program. Physicians may not understand that the purpose of a compliance plan is to ensure compliance with rules and regulations and that a well-designed plan can improve coding and billing processes, which in turn can have a positive impact on the cash flow of the practice.

## OIG Compliance Guidance for Physicians

Many unique issues face a physician practice as an effective compliance program is implemented. To prepare practices for implementation, the OIG issued the *Compliance Program Guidance for Individual and Small Group Physician Practices*. In this program guidance, the OIG specifically acknowledges "that full implementation of all components may not be feasible for all physician practices." The OIG also notes that "the extent of implementation will depend upon the size and resources of the practice" (OIG 2000, 59436). Although the intent of this program guidance is similar to that offered for hospitals, the OIG has provided the following streamlined list of seven elements for physician practices:

- Conducting internal monitoring and auditing
- Implementing compliance and practice standards
- Designating a compliance officer or contact
- Conducting appropriate training and education
- Responding appropriately to detected offenses and developing corrective action
- Developing open lines of communication
- Enforcing disciplinary standards through well-publicized guidelines

In addition to the *Compliance Program Guidance for Individual and Small Group Physician Practices,* physician practices should consult the Compliance Program Guidance for Clinical Laboratories if they operate a physician office laboratory (POL) and the *Compliance Program Guidance for Third-Party Medical Billing Companies* for more detailed guidance on the coding and billing process.

## Risk Assessment in Physician Practices

As in all healthcare settings, physician practices need to conduct a risk assessment as they implement a program. Questions to consider as physician practices assess their risk areas include the following:

- What are the most common services provided (for example, medical visits, ancillary testing, and surgical procedures)?

- Are denials for a particular service common? Or are services routinely down-coded by Medicare or another payer?

- What high-risk issues are specific to the practice? What takes the most staff time to address? Which have the highest monetary impact?

- Who performs coding for these high-risk services? Does this individual possess a respected coding certification? What ongoing continuing education has this individual received?

- Are coding and billing processes manual or automated? Is there a way to reconcile appointments and charges?

- What controls are currently in place? For example, are edits in place to identify whether a code is missing a digit? Are different people posting charges and payments?

- Are the names of all potential employees compared to the Medicare Exclusion List prior to hiring?

- Are processes already in place to address some of the risk areas?

Depending on the clinical specialty, the risk areas may vary. For example, a practice with radiology equipment needs to understand component billing and therefore has a higher billing risk than a practice with no equipment. Or, a general surgeon who performs a variety of procedures, covered by many areas of CPT coding, requires a coding professional with extensive knowledge and might have a higher coding risk than the office of an internist.

Practices that have developed compliance plans in the past should periodically reassess their level of risk by asking the following questions:

- Is there any program provision that has not been followed?

- Has it been longer than one year since the last audit?

- Are there recommendations from the last audit that have not been implemented?

- Do providers continue to bill incorrectly even after receiving education?

- Is a new service being provided that has not been addressed in the program?

- Have the CPT codes or coding rules changed significantly in the past year for services that are being provided?

Answering "yes" to any of these questions should alert the practice that renewed emphasis must be placed on the compliance program.

## Medical Record Documentation Issues for Physicians

The guiding principle of documentation in healthcare should be to document what was done and then bill what was documented, keeping in mind the old adage of "not documented, not done." The OIG noted that one of the most important physician practice compliance issues is the appropriate documentation of diagnoses and treatment (OIG 2000, 59440). The OIG provides the following examples of internal documentation principles a physician practice might use to ensure accurate health record documentation (OIG 2000, 59440):

- The health record should be complete and legible.

- The documentation of each patient encounter should include the reason for the encounter; any relevant history; physical examination findings; prior diagnostic test results; assessment, clinical impression, or diagnosis; plan of care; and date and legible identity of the observer.

- If not documented, the rationale for ordering diagnostic and other ancillary services should be easily inferred by an independent reviewer or third party who has appropriate medical training. CPT, Healthcare Common Procedure Coding System (HCPCS), and ICD-9-CM codes used for claims submission should be supported by health record documentation.

- Appropriate health risk factors should be identified. The patient's progress, response to any changes in treatment, and any revision in diagnosis should be documented.

In addition to the documentation principles, the OIG has emphasized the following:

1. The CPT and ICD-9-CM codes reported on the health insurance claim form should be supported by documentation in the physician's office health record.

2. The health record should contain all required information.

3. Centers for Medicare and Medicaid Services (CMS) and the local carriers should be able to determine who provided the services (OIG 2000, 59440).

### Physician Office Laboratories

Compliance in a POL involves two sets of regulations—the federal coding and billing regulations that cover all physician services, as well as the regulations of the Clinical

Laboratory Improvement Amendments (CLIA), which established the CLIA program. The objective of the CLIA program is to ensure quality laboratory testing. This goal is accomplished, in part, by issuing the CLIA certificates required to operate laboratories. Laboratories cannot perform testing or bill third parties for testing services without a CLIA certificate.

Following are the four CLIA certification levels, listed here in order of increasing complexity:

- **Certificate of waiver**—Issued to a laboratory that performs only tests that are waived from the CLIA regulations. These tests can be performed safely by any person who follows the package insert that accompanies the product. Examples are home glucose monitor testing or home pregnancy test kits. No laboratory training is required to perform these tests.

- **Certificate of provider-performed microscopy (PPM)**—Issued to a laboratory in which waived tests are performed and a physician, midlevel practitioner, or dentist personally uses a microscope to clarify test findings.

- **Certificate of compliance for moderately complex tests**—Issued to a laboratory after an inspection by the state CLIA agency, during which the laboratory is found to comply with all applicable CLIA requirements.

- **Certificate of compliance for highly complex tests**—Same as moderately complex testing laboratories but allows testing at the higher, highly complex testing level. This certificate is usually held by hospitals and independent laboratories rather than physician practices.

The CLIA regulations and CMS regulations work in combination. As mentioned previously, tests cannot be performed or billed without a CLIA certificate. In addition, only tests that are assigned to the POL's CLIA certification level, or a lower level, can be performed and billed. This means that a POL holding a Certificate of Compliance for Moderately Complex Tests could perform waived or PPM tests but could not perform and bill highly complex tests.

Documentation requirements for laboratory testing require the following:

- An order must be documented for each test performed.

- Results—including the date, time, and tester's initials—must be in the medical record.

- Tests must be correctly coded using CPT or HCPCS codes.

- A valid diagnosis must be documented for each laboratory test ordered.

- Advance Beneficiary Notice (ABN) rules must be followed (see the Medical Necessity section addressed later in this chapter).

- All documentation from the record must match the information submitted on the CMS-1500 claim form.

The OIG *Compliance Program Guidance for Clinical Laboratories* instructs clinical laboratories, including POLs, *not* to do the following:

- Do not use diagnostic information from earlier dates of service

- Do not create diagnosis information that has triggered reimbursement in the past

- Do not use computer programs that automatically insert diagnosis codes without documentation from the physician

- Do not make up information for claims submission purposes

This program guidance instructs clinical laboratories to do the following:

- Contact the ordering physician if diagnostic documentation was not provided.

- Periodically monitor standing orders in connection with an extended course of treatment and assign a fixed term for their use.

- Accurately translate narrative diagnoses into ICD-9-CM codes (OIG 1998, 45080–45081).

## Reimbursement Issues

Physician reimbursement is dependent on the accurate use of procedural codes, diagnostic codes, modifiers, and the proper completion of the CMS-1500 claim form.

### Coding and Billing Procedures and Tools

The diagnoses codes that describe the case should be linked with the corresponding procedure codes, and modifiers should be used appropriately. Forms used to capture clinical information (commonly known as encounter forms, charge tickets, or superbills) should be updated periodically to ensure that they elicit the data required for accurate coding. A policy or procedure should be established that describes the schedule for maintenance of these forms.

Encounter forms must be kept up-to-date with all ICD-9-CM, CPT, and HCPCS level II code changes and should be reviewed at least annually to ensure accurate content. These forms must be well designed so that they serve as tools to improve documentation and do not lead physicians inappropriately to the choice of a particular code. These forms should reflect the common diagnoses and services provided and ordered by the physician practice. Off-the-shelf forms should not be used as is but can serve as a model for the design of a customized form that is suited to the practice's unique mix of providers, services, payers, and patients. The codes and code descriptions should be complete, valid, and accurate and space should be provided to write in additional tests, procedures, and diagnoses if none of the provided choices is appropriate. The design of encounter forms should not encourage selection of the "closest" code when a different code exists that describes the diagnosis or procedure more accurately. As mentioned in chapter 3, the practice should maintain current and appropriate coding resources for use in coding and the development of encounter forms.

## Modifier 59

The OIG routinely studies issues in which there is a high probability of error, misuse, or fraud. In November 2005, the OIG issued a report on the use of modifier 59 to bypass Medicare's National Correct Coding Initiative (NCCI) edits. They found that 40 percent of the time, the use of modifier 59 did not meet program requirements, resulting in $59 million in improper payments.

Modifier 59 should be used to describe a distinct procedure or service for a beneficiary on the same day as another procedure or service, done during a different session, during a different procedure, on a different anatomic site or organ system, through a separate incision or by separate excision, for a separate lesion or for a separate injury. When it is necessary and appropriate to submit two codes, modifier 59 should be attached to the secondary, additional, or lesser service of the two codes in the code pair. The OIG found that 11 percent of the time, modifier 59 was applied to the wrong code in the code pair. These findings caused the OIG to recommend to the CMS that prepayment and postpayment reviews should be implemented for the use of modifier 59.

## Modifier 25

The OIG also issued a report on the use of modifier 25 in November 2005. When used appropriately, modifier 25 tells the payer that a significant, separately identifiable evaluation and management (E/M) service was provided on the same day as a procedure and that the E/M service was above and beyond the usual preoperative and postoperative care associated with the procedure. The OIG found that 35 percent of the claims containing modifier 25 did not meet program requirements, resulting in $538 million in improper payments. In addition, there were claims found where modifier 25 was attached to the procedure code or when modifier 25 was attached to an E/M code but no procedure code was submitted on the same day. Neither resulted in improper payment but both types of coding were noncompliant. Again, the OIG recommended to the CMS that reviews should be implemented for modifier 25.

Physician practices should place emphasis on appropriate use of both modifier 25 and modifier 59.

## Place of Service

In January 2005, the OIG released a report on an audit of 100 claims suspected of having a place of service reporting error. They found that 88 percent of the claims with suspected errors were indeed miscoded with an "Office" place of service rather than a "Facility" place of service. Services performed in the office setting are reimbursed at a higher rate under the RBRVS Medicare Fee Schedule and therefore, misrepresentation of a service as being performed in the office when not performed there is a noncompliant practice. Physician practices should evaluate how place of service codes are being assigned and how they are displayed in Box 24B of the CMS-1500 claim form or the equivalent electronic field.

# Medical Necessity

An initial discussion of medical necessity is found in chapter 3. The physician practice should implement education for physicians, staff, and patients regarding medical necessity and the need for ABNs as useful communication tools. Patients who are aware of their potential financial responsibilities ahead of time make wise decisions about the services they use and are more likely to understand why they must pay for these services.

Once the need for an ABN has been determined, the patient has been informed about the potential medical necessity issue, and the ABN has been signed, other processes must take place to achieve payment. The procedure codes for all of the services covered by the signed ABN must be submitted with a GA modifier. The ABN needs to have been signed prior to the delivery of the service and the ABN needs to be on file for later reference.

If Medicare pays for the service, the patient is only responsible for any deductible and coinsurance. If Medicare does not pay for the service, the biller must bill the charges to the patient. If the GA modifier is not applied at the time of submission, the patient is not responsible for the charges. Figure 8.1 provides a more detailed discussion of the GA modifier.

If the practice does not recognize the need for an ABN before the service is delivered but does recognize the need before the charge is submitted, a GZ modifier should be applied to the procedure codes. By applying this modifier, the practice acknowledges that an ABN should have been signed but was not. In this instance, the patient is not responsible for the charges if Medicare does not pay. Figure 8.2 provides a more detailed discussion of the GZ modifier.

**Figure 8.1.  GA modifiers**

| GA modifier | | | | |
|---|---|---|---|---|
| "Waiver of liability on file." | | | | |
| Description | When to use the GA modifier | Examples of its use | What happens if you use the GA modifier? | What happens if you do not use the GA modifier? |
| Item or service expected to be denied as not reasonable and necessary and an advance beneficiary notice was given to the beneficiary.<br><br>These are so-called "medical necessity" denials<br><br>The GA modifier also may be used with assigned and unassigned claims for DMEPOS where one of the following Part B "technical denials" may apply:<br>• prohibited telephone solicitation,<br>• no supplier number,<br>• failure to obtain an advance determination of coverage. | When you think a service will be denied because it does not meet the Medicare program standards for medically necessary care and you gave the beneficiary an advance beneficiary notice.<br><br>You are required to include the GA modifier on your claim anytime you obtain a signed ABN, or have a patient's refusal to sign an ABN witnessed properly in an assigned claim situation (except an assigned claim for one of the specified DMEPOS technical denials).<br><br>Use a GA modifier on an assigned claim if you gave an ABN to a patient but the patient refused to sign the ABN and you did furnish the services. (In these circumstances, on all unassigned claims, as well as an assigned claim for a specified DMEPOS technical denial, use the GZ modifier.) | All instances in which you deliver an ABN to a Medicare patient and services are furnished.<br><br>For example, after having a patient sign an ABN, you furnish a service covered by Medicare but likely to be denied as "too frequent" by Medicare. | The claim will be reviewed by Medicare like any other claim and may or may not be denied. The carrier will NOT use the presence of the GA modifier to influence its determination of Medicare coverage and payment of the service.<br><br>If Medicare pays the claim, the GA modifier is irrelevant.<br><br>If the claim is denied, the beneficiary will be fully and personally liable to pay you for the service, personally or through other insurance.<br><br>Medicare will not pay you for the service since your giving an ABN to the patient is prima facie evidence that you knew Medicare probably would not pay for the service. | The claim will be reviewed by Medicare like any other claim and may or may not be denied.<br><br>If the claim is denied, the beneficiary will be held not liable and you will be held liable. Medicare will not pay you nor allow you to collect from the beneficiary. In order to remedy this situation, you will need to appeal Medicare's action limiting the beneficiary's liability.<br><br>The question of an abusive billing pattern could arise. It is possible that fraud and abuse implications may arise out of your omission of the fact of having had an ABN signed by the patient under these circumstances, especially if there is a consistent pattern of such omissions (viz., a pattern of failure to include the GA modifier when it is applicable). |

Source: Becker 2002, CMS n.d.

Medicare requires that one of two standardized ABN forms be used, one for laboratory and one for all other services. The laboratory form is available on the CMS website at new.cms.hhs.gov/BNI/Downloads/CMSR131L.pdf, and the general form is available at new.cms.hhs.gov/BNI/Downloads/CMSR131G.pdf. It should be noted that ABNs are not required for services that are considered noncovered services. These charges are always the responsibility of the patient and should not be billed to Medicare.

## Auditing in Physician Practices

Auditing can serve several purposes. Many practices use auditing to determine if there are problems associated with their processes. Additionally, audits can be used to study areas that are known to draw attention to a practice or trigger an audit from an external organization. Audits can also be used to track improvement over time.

The basic definition of an audit is a prospective or retrospective process to identify variations from an established baseline or required method. Retrospective audits are completed after the service has been billed. Prospective audits are done after the care has been rendered and is documented, but is not yet billed.

**Figure 8.2.  GZ modifier**

| GZ modifier | | | | |
|---|---|---|---|---|
| "Item or service expected to be denied as not reasonable and necessary."  (No signed ABN on file.) | | | | |
| Description | When to use the GZ modifier | Examples of its use | What happens if you use the GZ modifier? | What happens if you do not use the GZ modifier? |
| Item or service expected to be denied as not reasonable and necessary* and an ABN was not signed by the beneficiary.<br><br>These are the so-called "medical necessity" denials.<br><br>The GZ modifier also may be used with assigned and unassigned claims for DMEPOS where one of the following Part B "technical denials" may apply:<br>• Prohibited telephone solicitation,<br>• no supplier number,<br>• failure to obtain an advance determination of coverage. | When you think a service will be denied because it does not meet Medicare program standards for medically necessary care and you did not obtain a signed ABN from the beneficiary.<br><br>When you gave an ABN to a patient who refused to sign the ABN and you, nevertheless, did furnish the services, use a GZ modifier on <u>unassigned</u> claims for all physicians' services and DMEPOS; and also on <u>assigned</u> claims for which one of the DMEPOS technical denials is expected.<br><br>If you wish to indicate to the carrier that one of the above situations exists, in your opinion, then you may elect to include the GZ modifier on your claim. | When you would have given an ABN to a patient but could not because of an emergency care situation, for example, in an EMTALA covered situation in an emergency department, or in an ambulance transport.<br><br>When a patient was not personally present at your premises and could not be reached to timely sign an ABN, for example, before a specimen is tested.<br><br>When you realize too late, only after furnishing a service, that you should have given the patient an ABN. | The claim will be reviewed by Medicare like any other claim and may or may not be denied. The carrier will NOT use the presence of the GZ modifier to influence its determination of Medicare coverage and payment of the service.<br><br>If Medicare pays the claim, the GZ modifier is irrelevant.<br><br>If the claim is denied, the beneficiary generally will not be liable to pay you for the service. However, even though the beneficiary is found not liable, if you are also found not liable with respect to an unassigned claim, or an assigned claim denied for one of the DMEPOS technical denial reasons specified, you may be allowed to collect from the beneficiary.<br><br>Medicare may or may not hold you liable depending on whether you knew that payment would be denied when you furnished the service. In cases in which you gave an ABN to the patient, or attempted to, but could not obtain a beneficiary signature, most likely Medicare will hold you liable. | You never need to use the GZ modifier when you expect Medicare to pay.<br><br>You are always free to elect not to use a GZ modifier.<br><br>The claim will be reviewed by Medicare like any other claim and may or may not be denied.<br><br>NOTE: The GZ modifier is provided for physicians and suppliers who wish to submit a claim to Medicare, who know that an ABN should have been signed but was not, and who do not want <u>any</u> risk of allegation of fraud or abuse for claiming services that are not medically necessary. By notifying Medicare, by the GZ modifier, that you expect Medicare will not cover the service, you can greatly reduce the risk of a mistaken allegation of fraud or abuse. |

Source: Becker 2002, CMS n.d.

**Triggers for an External Audit**

A physician practice that consistently reports higher-level E/M codes than other practices in the same specialty stands a good chance of catching the attention of fraud investigators. Organizations may consider comparing the frequency of the use of specific E/M codes between different time periods (for example, two years or two six-month time periods). They also may compare the use of critical care codes between two time periods to identify variations. Physician practices should benchmark their E/M utilization profiles against regional or national norms and other physicians in the same specialty. Keep in mind that when a physician practice has a low Medicare patient population, Medicare benchmark data should not be used for a comparative analysis. Rather, comparative data for the same specialty should be used. For example, when comparing a pediatrician's E/M utilization profile to a regional or national benchmark, benchmarking data for pediatric practices should be used. Benchmarking data are available from a variety of sources, including the CMS, private payers, professional associations, and through Internet searches.

Benchmarking is useful for the following:

- Identifying aberrant practice patterns
- Tracking changes in practice patterns
- Uncovering potential concerns of undercoding or overcoding
- Identifying potential overutilization of a particular E/M code level
- Identifying education needs
- Determining focus areas for audits

The distribution of E/M utilization can be analyzed for indications of underuse or overuse of specific code levels. Typically, a normal E/M utilization distribution displays as a bell curve as in Figure 8.3, although the peak of the curve may vary significantly by specialty. Additional investigation is needed if there is variance between the E/M pattern indicated by the utilization analysis and that indicated by the audit findings. For example, investigation is needed if audit results show that selected code levels are appropriately supported by the health record documentation, yet the practice pattern is a diagonal line rather than a bell curve. These results would indicate overutilization of levels I and II, and underutilization of levels IV and V. The physician(s) could be underdocumenting and undercoding.

When comparing physicians' E/M utilization patterns to benchmarks, comparisons can be made between (this is not an all-inclusive list):

- The physician practice as a whole to Medicare nationally
- An individual physician to others of that specialty in the practice
- An individual physician to Medicare regionally or nationally
- New providers to the physician practice as a whole

**Figure 8.3.   Bell curve of established patient office visits**

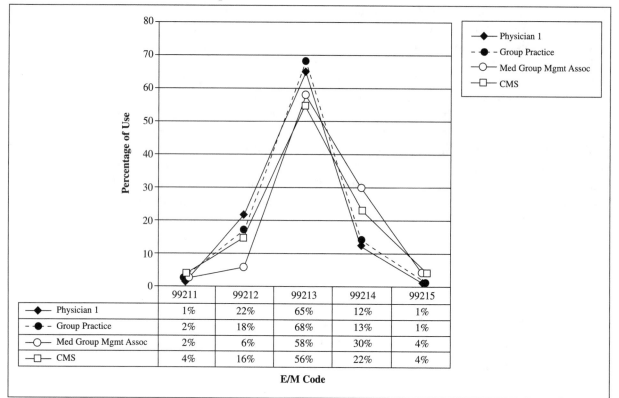

| | 99211 | 99212 | 99213 | 99214 | 99215 |
|---|---|---|---|---|---|
| ◆ Physician 1 | 1% | 22% | 65% | 12% | 1% |
| ● Group Practice | 2% | 18% | 68% | 13% | 1% |
| ○ Med Group Mgmt Assoc | 2% | 6% | 58% | 30% | 4% |
| □ CMS | 4% | 16% | 56% | 22% | 4% |

**E/M Code**

Although E/M utilization pattern analysis is a useful tool for uncovering potential problems in E/M code assignment, conclusions should not be drawn based solely on the pattern analysis. An aberrant coding pattern may reflect unique characteristics of the practice's patient population and/or mix of services provided.

The more a medical practice understands and abides by documentation requirements and CPT principles, the more it minimizes the risk of adverse consequences from external review. Because of concerns about "upcoding" of physician service levels, it helps to be cautious. See figure 8.4 for a list of problems that may cause a focused payer review (Skurka 2001, 52).

### Baseline Audits

Physician practices should conduct a baseline audit that examines the claim development and submission process. This audit will help identify elements within the process that may contribute to noncompliance or that should be the focus for education. The OIG recommends that the audit be conducted based on claims submitted during the initial three months after implementation of the education and training program to give the physician practice a benchmark against which to measure future compliance effectiveness.

**Figure 8.4.   Problems that cause focused payer reviews**

The more a medical practice understands and abides by documentation requirements and CPT principles, the more it minimizes the risk of adverse consequences from external review. But because of concerns about "upcoding" of physician service levels, it helps to be cautious. Following is a list of problems that may cause a focused payer review:

- **Using the same code over and over.** A physician can easily trigger an audit by using the same level of code repeatedly—for example, using 99213 for office visits, 99223 for hospital admissions, and 99244 for office consultations. A pattern such as this is easy to detect and shows the physician is not discriminating [levels of care] within the coding system

- **Inconsistencies within partners in a group.** A statistical comparison of partners in a practice shows inconsistent physician education about coding guidelines.

- **Upcoding/undercoding.** In some instances, physicians consistently tend to select higher-level codes. This presents data that is hard to believe and may trigger an audit or review. Two codes the federal government will focus on are 99214 (established patient office visit, level 4) and 99233 (subsequent hospital care, level 3, highest level). It is critical that organizations review their current use of these codes for appropriateness. Undercoding may not trigger an audit but results in lost revenue and creates data quality concerns. For example, some physicians use lower-level codes because they do not want to "bother" with the documentation requirements of the higher levels. This presents a false picture of patient severity and the associated physician work and may actually decrease reimbursement amounts in the future.

- **Modifiers.** Using modifiers correctly can help support documentation and claims in unusual or specific circumstances. When they are used incorrectly—for example, to force a claim to pass edits in place to reject services—modifiers can create a compliance liability. In the physician setting, modifier 25 is especially problematic because it may allow payment for a visit and a procedure when the two services are really not distinct from each other.

- **Diagnoses issues.** Using nonspecific diagnoses or terminology increases the risk of audit for providing unnecessary services. Encourage physicians to use specific diagnoses and document all complications and comorbidities when completing a patient record and ordering specific tests or treatments.

**Source:** Reprinted from Skurka 2001, p. 52.

## Periodic Audits

Periodic audits should be performed to determine whether claims are coded accurately and that they appropriately reflect the services provided. These reviews can also determine whether services or items provided are reasonable and necessary and that health records contain sufficient documentation to support the codes and charges reported on the claim. The OIG recommends that these periodic audits be conducted at least once a year (OIG 2000, 59437). Target areas to consider as topics for a physician practice audit include the items listed in figure 8.5.

## E/M Coding Audits

E/M audits should be completed using both the 1995 and 1997 Documentation Guidelines for Evaluation and Management Coding, published by CMS. These guidelines provide the documentation requirements associated with each level of history, examination, and medical decision making. Either version of the guidelines may be used. Physicians should be trained on both versions and should understand when each version is most beneficial to them for use in determining code assignment.

When performing a review of E/M coding, all of the documentation for the date of service in question should be reviewed. This review may include a health history completed by the patient, handwritten notes by the nurse, and written as well as dictated notes by the

**Figure 8.5.   Target areas for a physician practice audit**

- Accuracy of E/M code assignment (including proper use of consultation and critical care codes)

- Accuracy of application of the New Patient definition

- Accuracy of procedure code assignment (CPT codes other than E/M)

- Accuracy of diagnosis code assignment (ICD-9-CM codes)

- Quality of health record documentation (for example, does the documentation support the codes assigned? Does the documentation accurately reflect the patient encounter, including the clinical condition and services provided?)

- Consistency between diagnosis and procedure for encounter

- Consistency between diagnosis and treatment plan

- Consistency between date on documentation and the claim form

- Validation of consultation requirements (If the consultation is coded, is there documentation of a request in the record? Is there a separate, written consultation report that was sent back to the requestor?)

- Presence of signature by author of health record documentation

- Review of the practice's top 10 denials or top 10 services

- Evaluation of the use of nonspecific codes to determine if a more specific code would be appropriate

- Validation of data-entry accuracy

- Confirmation that all orders were written and signed by a physician

- Confirmation that all tests ordered by the physician were actually performed and documented and that only these tests were billed

- Accuracy of modifier assignment

- Accuracy of ABN completion, filing, and modifier assignment

- Accuracy of Place of Service code assignment

- Compliance with the PATH guidelines for physician documentation (medical student and resident supervision in the office setting)

- Consistency of all data elements between all documentation related to the encounter (record documentation, encounter form, CMS-1500 claim form, remittance advice, and computerized patient account) physician. An audit that includes only physician documentation or dictated reports may result in erroneous variances in the E/M code level.

During an E/M audit process, it is never useful to merely indicate that some codes were "too high" or "too low." Instead, the review should show how increased history, increased physical documentation, or additional documentation of decision making make it necessary to move patients to higher code levels. This review gives physicians more specific guidance on areas that may not be well documented in the record.

An acceptable level of E/M assignment accuracy should be decided upon for the practice. Although 100 percent accuracy is the ultimate goal, an accuracy threshold should be established for review purposes. Performance below that level should require mandatory education.

### Physician at Teaching Hospitals (PATH) Documentation Audits

Physicians can serve in the role of teaching physician in the office setting as well as in the hospital when they are associated with a graduate medical education (GME) program. The Medicare regulations for supervising physicians in teaching settings allows teaching physicians in a primary care setting to bill for the work of the resident in the absence of the teaching physician. E/M codes 99201–99203 and 99211–99213 can be billed under this Primary Care Exception as long as the program is registered and appropriate supervision is provided to the resident. The CMS clarified the teaching physician rules in Transmittal 1780, dated November 22, 2002. There is additional information concerning Teaching Physician Services in Transmittal 811 of the CMS Manual System released January 13, 2006, and implemented February 13, 2006. The documentation requirements for teaching physicians are specific as to content, and verification of their appropriate use should be part of a compliance program for a practice in which physicians work with a GME program and serve as teaching physicians.

### Shadow Audits

Not all audits are done by collecting data from written documents. Shadow audits involve the pairing of a documentation expert (usually a coding professional or compliance specialist) with a physician in the examination room. After receiving permission from the patient, the documentation expert observes the interaction between physician and patient and notes the questions asked, examination completed, and the treatment plan that is determined. At the end of the visit, the physician completes the documentation and both parties compare their findings of a chosen E/M level. This type of audit can help the physician understand what documentation should be present, based on the observations made by the compliance specialist.

### Steps in the Audit Process

The practice must first answer the question of who will complete the audit. There are advantages and disadvantages to the use of both internal and external auditors, as discussed in chapter 3. Another option may be to use a partnership of auditors with each bringing their skill set to the work. This partnership works well when a coding professional and biller work together to audit a billing process from service delivery to final payment. An external auditor can also be engaged specifically to train internal staff in the audit function.

Figure 8.6 details the 10 steps in the process for audits completed by physician practice staff.

There are two additional, initial process steps for audits completed by an external reviewer. These steps include the development of a Letter of Understanding or other contract mechanism under which the external reviewer will perform the work and an introductory meeting to introduce the reviewer to all physicians and staff to enlist their cooperation during the review. The remainder of the review process is the same whether completed internally or externally.

## Sample Selection

Identifying the population of cases from which a sample will be chosen can be done in several ways. Two effective ways are to use all of the claims (or services) for which a physician has received payment during a period of time, such as one month or one quarter, or to select all of the claims from risk areas or areas of potential billing vulnerabilities that were determined during the risk assessment. Cases should then be randomly selected from the chosen population.

For physician practices, the OIG recommends that a basic guide for the sample size of periodic random audits is two to five health records per payer or five to 10 health records per physician. If the audit comprises all service types (office, hospital, consultations, skilled nursing facility [SNF], and others), a larger sample size per physician is desirable.

For ease in review, cases should be chosen from the current coding year so that the codes, coding guidelines, forms, and processes are still in effect at the time of the review.

## Audit Forms

Many audit tools can be found online. Sample audit tools can be found on the CD-ROM included with this book. Additionally, sample audit forms for E/M coding and emergency

**Figure 8.6.   The 10 steps for physician practice audits**

| | |
|---|---|
| **Step 1:** | Selection of the audit topic |
| **Step 2:** | Selection or creation of an audit tool to collect data for the review |
| **Step 3:** | Identification of the audit population from which the sample will be drawn |
| **Step 4:** | Identification of the sample cases, drawn randomly from the population |
| **Step 5**: | Accumulation of the required documents for each case in the sample |
| **Step 6:** | Collection of the data from the accumulated documents |
| **Step 7:** | Summarization of collected data and formulation of recommendations |
| **Step 8:** | Presentation of findings and recommendations to practice leaders |
| **Step 9:** | Implementation of recommendations and/or education |
| **Step 10:** | Assignment of a follow-up audit date |

services coding are available to AHIMA members through the AHIMA Body of Knowledge on the Communities of Practice Web site.

There are review forms on the CD-ROM that can be used for auditing E/M codes using the 1995 guidelines and the 1997 guidelines. These forms can also be used for teaching the application of the documentation requirements for each level of history, examination, and medical decision making. Both forms provide a mechanism for categorizing types of errors and calculating the monetary impact associated with those errors. A review form is also provided for reviewing documentation created in a physician office laboratory and the billing of those services.

The scoring sheet provided allows the reviewer to assign point values to different elements of the review, based on the importance of the element in the practice's compliance plan. The summary sheet provides a cover sheet for all audit documentation, including dates and physicians included in the sample, findings, recommendations, and the planned audit follow-up date.

### Audit Follow-up and the Re-audit Process

Findings and recommendations from an audit should be implemented, including staff and physician education regarding the findings. The topic should be reevaluated after an appropriate interval. If a reevaluation is being performed six months or one year later, results of the first review should be evaluated and cases selected accordingly. If a physician scores particularly well in the first review, fewer cases (perhaps five to seven) can be reviewed the next time around.

If a physician scores poorly in a review and corrective action has been taken, the same number of records should be reviewed during the re-audit. Records should be selected from the time period following the corrective action or after the educational process has taken place. All of these processes are part of the cycle of improving the quality of coded data and working toward 100 percent compliance with rules and regulations.

## Monitoring for Improvement

As the name indicates, monitoring is spot-checking to ensure that improvements are still working as implemented, no new issues have developed, or indicators are being used to check that accuracy or error rates are within acceptable levels.

Monitoring can be done based on knowledge of the practice's risk areas or on issues raised by others. The OIG publishes the areas that it intends to study each year in their OIG Work Plan. The OIG regularly studies areas of suspicion of error, misuse, or fraud. After initial studies are complete, the OIG may continue to monitor the same topic over several years to watch for improvement in results.

For 2007, the OIG intends to study the following areas related to the physician office setting:

- **Billing service companies,** their relationships with physicians, and whether the relationships have any impact on physician billing practices

- **Physician pathology services** in physician offices, how these services are ordered, the physicians providing the service, and their relationship to outside pathology companies

- **Cardiography and echocardiography services** to determine whether physicians billed accurately for professional and technical components of these services

- **Therapy services** provided by physical and occupational therapists, whether they are reasonable and medically necessary, adequately documented and certified by physician certification statements

- **Payment to providers of care for initial preventive physical examination,** whether the specific documentation requirements have been met, and whether these services were billed correctly

- **Part B mental health services** provided in the physician's office, whether they were medically necessary and billed in accordance with the Medicare requirements

- **Wound care services,** whether they were medically necessary, billed in accordance with Medicare requirements, and whether there are adequate carrier controls to ensure appropriate payments

- **"Incident to" services,** the extent to which the services met Medicare standards for medical necessity, documentation, and quality of care

- **Eye surgeries,** whether cataract and LASIK eye surgery were billed in accordance with Medicare requirements, and whether there are adequate carrier controls to ensure appropriate payments

- **Place of service accuracy** on ambulatory surgical center and hospital outpatient department claims

- **Evaluation and management services** during the global surgery period and whether physicians received separate payments for these services

- **Psychiatric services** provided in an inpatient setting and whether individual and group sessions were billed properly

- **Reimbursement for polysomnography** appropriate billing and the factors contributing to the rise in Medicare reimbursement for polysomnography in recent years

- **"Long-distance" physician claims** associated with home health and SNF services, where the physician and beneficiary addresses are a significant distance apart and claims are made over an extended period of time

- **Violations of assignment rules** by providers, the extent to which providers are billing beneficiaries in excess of amounts allowed by Medicare requirements, and beneficiary awareness of their rights and responsibilities regarding potential billing violations

- **Advanced imaging services** in physician offices; the appropriateness of imaging services such as MRI, PET, and CT scans; the reason for growth of these services in recent years; and billing patterns in certain geographic areas and practice settings

Internally, physician practices can monitor performance by using data reports, patient billing complaints, billing problems associated with new services, and services that have a high billing risk or the number of claim denials.

## Data Quality Issues

In addition to monitoring individual claims or the steps in the claims development process, data reports can be monitored to provide a different view of the coding and billing process. As charges are entered onto patient accounts, a computer system creates a database of information. This database has many names, such as encounter database, charge history, or service records. Regardless of the name, the database contains valuable information that should be evaluated (Kuehn 2006, 306).

### Qualitative Analysis

Many reports produced from the database can provide insight into the quality of the coding, data entry, and billing functions. Monitoring the quality of these processes involves using reports that identify the patient, the date of service, the physician name, and other specifics of the visit. One example of this is a charge summary report, also called a data entry report or a batch report. This document shows all of the billing entered for the practice for a single day and may be a separate report for each person completing the data entry process. This report helps identify data entry errors, missing charges, incorrect physician numbers, incorrect place of service codes, or incorrect linking of diagnoses to procedures (Kuehn 2001, 2).

Another useful report is a claim history report that shows all of the procedure codes, diagnoses, and charges for one patient over time. When the practice has more than one coding professional, this report can provide evidence of potential interrater reliability problems among the coding professionals. Interrater reliability is established when two or more coding professionals obtain the same coded data from the same or similar documentation (Kuehn 2001, 2).

If the computer system does not produce a report that is usable in this monitoring effort, the same concept can be tested by printing the CMS-1500 forms associated with repeat visits by the same patient and comparing the entries on all of the claims. If inconsistencies appear, then the associated record should be compared with the claims to determine which entries are valid. If no inconsistencies are noted, no record review is needed and review efforts can be directed elsewhere.

## Quantitative Analysis

Another type of monitoring is evaluation of aggregate data, or quantitative analysis. This monitoring can be done on either diagnostic or procedural data. Reports are generated showing the number of times a particular code has been used, usually showing the codes in numerical order along with the standard code description. To help make the data easier to interpret, narrowing the report to a single specialty or clinic can be helpful. It is also helpful to display data from October 1 to September 30 rather than January 1 to December 31, which covers time periods when two sets of codes could be valid. This diagnostic report can help determine when nonspecific codes are being overutilized or when codes are being submitted without the necessary fourth or fifth digits.

A report of procedural codes should be run for a single month or a calendar year. This report can alert the reviewer to problems with illogical code submissions. Two classic examples are CPT code 15851, Removal of sutures under anesthesia (other than local), other surgeon, being submitted as an office charge or CPT code 88150, Cytopathology, slides, cervical or vaginal, manual screening under physician supervision being reported when only the Pap smear was collected. In both instances, staff or physicians who have not been trained in the use of the CPT coding system frequently choose these codes based on an index entry or because they misunderstand the meaning of the description.

Other problems are CPT code 99070, which should not be used (but rather billed with a specific HCPCS code for the supply), using codes after December 31 that are no longer valid in the new year, and failure to use "partner" codes such as vaccine administration along with the immunization code (Kuehn 2001, 3). Without monitoring the code usage of a practice, these types of errors can go undetected.

## Education and Training for Physicians and Staff

Physicians and staff should receive education and training on the following topics related to compliance:

- Background of fraud and abuse enforcement

- OIG target areas

- Consequences of noncompliance

- Relationship between documentation and coding

- Appropriate use of CPT and ICD-9-CM coding systems

- The 1995 and 1997 Documentation Guidelines for E/M coding, both theory and application

- Reimbursement policies

- Medical necessity issues

- Pertinent audit results (positive and negative)

- Annual review of new and deleted codes and the importance of using only valid codes from up-to-date coding references

Chapter 3 contains a thorough discussion of the qualifications for coding positions. In addition to these general qualifications, it should be noted that the Certified Coding Specialist—Physician-based (CCS-P) credential is the most appropriate AHIMA credential for the physician practice. The American Academy of Professional Coders (AAPC) awards a Certified Professional Coder (CPC) credential, which can also be appropriate in the physician practice. All staff should be provided the opportunity to receive continuing education in both their field of study and in compliance by in-house programs, on-line courses, or seminars.

## Special Challenges for Physicians in Implementing Compliance Programs

The largest challenge for an independent physician practice is the adoption of the compliance concept. Solo or small physician practices frequently believe that they are too small to find themselves under government scrutiny. However, each practicing physician in this country has an equal chance of a random audit and some physicians may trigger an audit by their coding and billing practices.

Many physician practices are not independent practices but are owned by a larger entity or are part of a large healthcare system. The OIG suggests that when a physician practice is in this situation or works with a physician practice management company, independent practice association, physician-hospital organization, management services company, or third-party billing company, the physician practice can then incorporate the compliance standards and procedures of those entities into its own standards and procedures. Only appropriate material should be incorporated and this material should be tailored to the physician practice.

Physicians should be asked to view the implementation of a compliance program and the associated auditing and monitoring in the same light as periodic preventive medicine visits with a physician. There is both value in knowing that there are no problems and value in treating any discovered problems early in their development to promote long-term health of the practice. In addition, allocation of ongoing funding should be justified by quantifying both the revenue increase from missing charges found during a review and the amount of potential audit liability determined from identifying overcoding.

## Summary

Honest mistakes do occur. The goal of implementing a compliance program should be to develop a culture that strives for 100 percent proper coding, billing, and application of government rules and regulations. In the physician practice, auditing and monitoring can not only detect and correct mistakes, they can help prevent future problems in the practice.

## References

Becker, J. 2002. GA Modifier. Document posted to AHIMA LCDs/LMRPs Community of Practice, Community Resources (proprietary content). Available online from https://www.ahimanet.org/COP/LocalCoverageDecisionsLMRPs?CFID=5466476&CFTOKEN=70106793.

Becker, J. 2002. GZ Modifier. Document posted to AHIMA LCDs/LMRPs Community of Practice, Community Resources (proprietary content). Available online from https://www.ahimanet.org/COP/LocalCoverageDecisionsLMRPs?CFID=5466476&CFTOKEN=70106793.

Campbell, J. 2002 (Oct.). Key compliance strategies for the physician practice. *Proceedings from the AHIMA 2002 National Convention, San Francisco.* Chicago: AHIMA.

Centers for Medicare & Medicaid Services. n.d. GA and GZ Modifiers. Available online from cms.hhs.gov.

Centers for Medicare & Medicaid Services. 2002 (Nov. 22). Carriers Manual, Part 3—Claims Process, Transmittal 1780. Available online from cms.hhs.gov/Transmittals/Downloads/R1780B3.pdf.

Centers for Medicare & Medicaid Services. 2006 (Jan. 13). Pub 100-04 Medicare Claims Processing, Transmittal 811. Available online from http://www.cms.hhs.gov/transmittals/downloads/R811CP.pdf.

Kuehn, L. 2001 (Oct.). Unlock the information secrets in your billing database. *Proceedings from the AHIMA 2001 National Convention, Miami.*

Kuehn, L. 2006. *CPT/HCPCS Coding and Reimbursement for Physician Services.* Chicago: AHIMA.

Office of Inspector General. 2006. Work Plan, fiscal year 2007. Available online from http://www.oig.hhs.gov/publications/docs/workplan/2007/Work%20Plan%202007.pdf.

Office of Inspector General. 2000 (Oct. 5). OIG compliance program for individual and small group physician practices. *Federal Register* 65(194):59434–52. Available online from oig.hhs.gov/authorities/docs/physician.pdf.

Office of Inspector General. 1998 (Aug. 24). OIG compliance program guidance for clinical laboratories. *Federal Register* 63(163):45076–87. Available online from oig.hhs.gov/authorities/docs/cpglab.pdf.

Office of Inspector General. 1998 (Dec. 18). OIG compliance program guidance for third party medical billing companies. *Federal Register* 63(243):70138–52. Available online from oig.hhs.gov/fraud/docs/complianceguidance/thirdparty.pdf.

Skurka, M.A. 2001. Navigating the physician services maze. *Journal of American Health Information Management Association* 72(7):51–58.

# Chapter 9
# Long-Term Care Facilities

*Carmilla Marsh, RHIA*

In long-term care, both nursing facilities and skilled nursing facilities are included in the overall description. Nursing facilities participate in the Medicaid program and skilled nursing facilities (SNFs) participate in the Medicare program. It is not unusual for a long-term care facility to be dually certified for participation both in Medicaid and Medicare programs. SNFs are reimbursed based on a Prospective Payment System (PPS) called the Resource Utilization Group (RUG) III Classification System for all costs related to the services furnished to beneficiaries under Part A of the Medicare program. The per diem daily rate is determined based on the RUG III classification assigned to the resident. Medicaid reimbursement systems vary from state to state and many states are now using a version of the RUG-III classification for payment systems.

Effective January 1, 2006, based on the 2005 RUG Refinements, Version 5.20 of the Resource Utilization Groups III (RUG-III) added a new model. The new model expanded RUG III to include three distinct models, a 53 group, a 44 group, and a 34 group. The 53 group model adds nine new groups for high cost residents who qualify both for Rehabilitation Plus Extensive Services. The 53 group model was implemented for payment in Medicare SNFs beginning January 1, 2006. The RUG classification is derived from 108 items on the Minimum Data Set (MDS). Payment for each resident will vary based on the required Medicare assessments, which are completed at specified intervals. See figure 9.1 for a sample assessment schedule.

The RUG-III Classification system (53 group) has the following eight major categories:

- Rehabilitation plus Extensive

- Rehabilitation

- Extensive Services

- Special Care

- Clinically Complex

- Cognitively Impaired

- Behavior Problems
- Reduced Physical Function

One important consideration in the classification system is the scoring of activities of daily living (ADLs). An ADL score is calculated for all assessment classifications and is one of the determining factors regarding placement into a RUG-III category. The ADL score is calculated based on late loss ADLs: bed mobility, transfer, eating, and toilet use. The ADL scores range from 4 to 18. A score of 4 represents the most independent resident, while a score of 18 reflects a very dependent resident.

Classification using any of the three RUG-III models (34 group, 44 group, and 53 group) can be hierarchical or index maximizing.

## Hierarchical Classification

Hierarchical classification is used in some payment systems, in staffing analysis, and in many research projects. In the hierarchical approach, you start at the top and work down through any one of the RUG-III models, and the classification is the first group for which the resident qualifies.

**Figure 9.1.   Medicare Assessment Schedule**

| Medicare MDS Assessment Type | Reason for Assessment (AA8b Code) | Assessment Reference Date | Grace Days for A3a | Days Authorized for Coverage and Payment | Medicare Payment Days |
|---|---|---|---|---|---|
| 5 day** | 1 | Days 1-5* | 1-3 days | 14 | 1-14 |
| 14 day | 7 | Days 11-14 | 1-5 days | 16 | 15-30 |
| 30 day | 2 | Days 21-29 | 1-5 days | 30 | 31-60 |
| 60 day | 3 | Days 50-59 | 1-5 days | 30 | 61-90 |
| 90 day | 4 | Days 80-89 | 1-5 days | 10 | 91-100 |

## Index Maximizing Classification

Index maximizing classification is used in Medicare PPS and in some Medicaid payment systems. For a specific payment system, there will be a designated Case Mix Index (CMI) or ranking assigned to each RUG-III group. Index maximizing classification is accomplished by determining all groups for which a resident qualifies and selecting the group with the highest index. The CMIs are assigned based on dollar-weighted nursing and/or rehabilitation therapy minutes. There are differences in the wage rates between rural and urban facilities that affect the ordering of the CMIs.

Accuracy in MDS coding is critically important in long-term care for a variety of reasons, including, but not limited to, better quality of care and accurate reimbursement. Documentation in the clinical record must support the coding on the MDS or facilities face the risk of retrospective review and loss of reimbursement. In addition, because the billing for Medicare recipients is based on the MDS assessments, facilities face an added risk of submitting a false claim if the information submitted for Medicare billing does not accurately reflect the RUG assignment based on the MDS assessment for the resident.

## SNF Consolidated Billing

In the Balanced Budget Act (BBA) of 1997, Congress mandated that payment for services provided to beneficiaries during a Medicare-covered SNF stay be included in a bundled prospective payment made through the fiscal intermediary to the SNF. The consolidated billing requirement confers on the SNF the billing responsibility for the entire package of care that residents receive during a covered Part A SNF stay except for specifically excluded services. A list of the excluded services can be found online at: http://www.cms. hhs.gov/SNFConsolidatedBilling/.

This requirement makes it necessary that facilities establish policies, procedures, and auditing protocols to ensure that all services are being billed correctly to the Medicare Fiscal Intermediary. Several audit tools specific to long-term care are included on this book's CD-ROM.

In February 2006, a report was issued by the Office of Inspector General (OIG), "A Review of Nursing Facility Resource Utilization Groups" (OEI-02-02-00830), which details the inspection results from 272 claims when compared to documentation in the medical record (OIG 2006a). The purpose of the inspection was to determine the extent to which RUGs on claims submitted by nursing facilities were different from those generated based on evidence in the medical record. Based on a comparison of the MDS to the rest of the medical record, 26 percent of RUGs on claims submitted by SNFs (71 of 272 claims) were different from the RUGs generated based on documentation in the rest of the medical record. Twenty-two percent of claims (59 of 272) had a RUG with a higher associated payment rate than the one generated from documentation in the medical record, which potentially could represent overpayments. Twelve of 272 patients (4 percent) had a RUG with a lower payment rate than the one generated based on evidence in the medical record, which potentially could represent underpayments. To determine the potential effects of these differences on total Medicare payments, the inspectors calculated the net difference between the payment amounts for the RUGs on the claims submitted by nursing facilities and the payment amounts for RUGs generated from evidence in the medical record. The net difference represented $542 million in potential Medicare overpayments for fiscal year 2002, when projected to all claims with RUGs generated from a 5-day, 14-day, or 30-day MDS assessment. This review was directed toward the 108 items on the MDS that are used to classify residents into the RUG Classification System. The inspection did not look at medical necessity or other supporting documentation except for the 108 items as coded on the MDS. Eleven items were identified as being the most frequently inconsistent with documentation in the rest of the medical record. Four of these items were related to therapy documentation and the remaining seven were related to ADL scoring. A complete copy of the report can be accessed online from the OIG Web site (2006).

It is clear from this report that accuracy of MDS documentation is critically important to long-term care facilities. MDS documentation represents a significant compliance risk and one that all facilities will need to assess and monitor on a regular basis. Some facilities will find it difficult with limited resources and time to conduct regular screening and audits to determine whether medical records and claims agree. For some facilities, the answer may well be to engage an outside contractor to perform audits and assist them in establishing a corrective action plan if necessary. Other facilities may find that they have the resources to conduct audits and establish procedures to ensure the accuracy and consistency of documentation and claims information.

Specific policies and procedures need to be established to facilitate accurate billing and appropriate documentation in the medical record. At a minimum, the items listed in figure 9.2 should be considered.

## OIG Work Plan for 2007

Each year the OIG publishes a work plan that is designed to address areas of vulnerabilities of the Department of Health and Human Service (HHS) programs and activities and promotes improvement in efficiency and effectiveness. In reviewing the mission activities of the four components of OIG, considerable focus is given to identification of systemic weaknesses that could lead to fraud, waste, or abuse.

In Medicare Nursing Homes, specific areas identified for 2007 include the following (OIG 2006b):

- **Skilled Nursing Facility Rehabilitation and Infusion Therapy Services:** Through medical review, OIG will analyze whether rehabilitation and infusion services provided to Medicare beneficiaries in an SNF were medically necessary, adequately supported, and provided as ordered.

- **Skilled Nursing Facilities' Involvement in Consecutive Inpatient Stays:** OIG will determine whether SNF care provided to Medicare beneficiaries with consecutive inpatient stays was medically reasonable and necessary. An inpatient hospital stay must precede all SNF stays. This study will focus on beneficiaries who experience three or more consecutive stays, including at least one SNF facility stay. OIG will examine the extent and nature of consecutive Medicare hospital inpatient stays.

**Figure 9.2.   Specific policies and procedures need to be established to facilitate accurate billing and appropriate documentation in the medical record**

1.   Audit procedures should be established and concurrent audits performed routinely both on the MDS and the corresponding medical records according to an established time schedule. Audits need to be both qualitative and quantitative.

2.   Method of written communication should be implemented to ensure that timely information is being provided to the billing office in preparation for the billing to be completed. This information should include corrections to the MDS that may necessitate an adjustment bill submission.

3.   Procedures should be established and implemented for a sampling of bills to be audited and compared to the medical record to ensure consistent and accurate documentation and billing.

4.   Specialty audits should be performed on areas in the MDS that have proven to have a high error rate, for example, therapy and ADLs.

5.    Competency tests should be administered to MDS Coordinators and other members of the Interdisciplinary Team who participate in completion of the MDS assessments.

6.   Initial and ongoing training programs should be carried out to ensure that staff are knowledgeable and compliant with MDS coding and medical record documentation.

7.   Monitoring and auditing of Medicare records need to evaluate whether the technical requirements are met in addition to the required documentation to support medical necessity.

8.   An individual should be designated as responsible for monitoring physician certification and recertification requirements to ensure that required documentation is present before Medicare is billed.

9.   Therapy certifications/recertifications should be signed prior to billing.

10.  MDS Activity Report should be provided to the billing office for verification that MDS RUG Classification matches the RUG Classification assigned by the state.

- **Enforcement Actions Against Noncompliant Nursing Homes:** OIG will continue examination of the effectiveness of CMS and State enforcement actions taken against noncompliant nursing homes. Under contracts with CMS, States conduct surveys at least every 15 months to certify that nursing facilities meet the required standards for the Medicare and Medicaid programs. OIG will assess whether CMS and its fiscal intermediaries appropriately process denial of Medicare payment remedies for facilities that are noncompliant with Federal program standards.

- **Skilled Nursing Facility Payments for Day of Discharge:** Medicare regulations mandate that the day of discharge is not a day of billable services for SNFs. OIG will determine if Medicare is inappropriately paying SNFs for services on the day of discharge.

- **Skilled Nursing Facility Consolidated Billing:** The OIG plan will determine whether controls are in place to preclude duplicate billing under Medicare Part B for services covered under the SNF PPS and assess the effectiveness of the common working file edits that were established in 2002 to prevent and detect improper payments. Under the PPS, a skilled nursing facility has Medicare billing responsibility for virtually all of the Medicare coverage services that its residents receive. As a result, the outside suppliers must receive payment from the SNF, rather than the Medicare Part B carrier.

- **Nursing Home Residents MDS Assessments and Care Planning:** OIG will examine the type, frequency, and severity of nursing home deficiencies related to MDS assessments and care planning. The concern in this area is that previous studies have shown increased deficiencies related to comprehensive assessments, care planning, and the provision of services in accordance with the care plan. OIG will also examine methods the state survey agencies use in identifying assessments and care plans that do not address individualized needs of residents.

- **Imaging and Laboratory Services in Nursing Homes:** OIG will determine the extent and nature of any medically unnecessary or excessive billing for imaging and laboratory services provided to nursing home residents. A sample of services and utilization patterns will be reviewed and examined in nursing homes.

- **Implementation of Medicare part D in Nursing Facilities:** OIG will assess the implementation of Medicare Part D in nursing homes. Prior to the implementation of Part D, nursing homes generally contracted with one long-term care pharmacy to provide drugs for all of their residents eligible for both Medicare and Medicaid. As part of this study OIG will determine how dual eligible nursing home residents are selecting and enrolling in Medicare prescription drug pans and whether these residents are receiving the drugs they need under Part D.

- **Submission of Skilled Nursing Facility No-Pay Bills:** This review will determine whether SNFs submit "no-pay bills" as required. No-pay bills are submitted to Medicare without a request for reimbursement to track beneficiaries' benefit periods. OIG will determine the extent to which failure to submit no-pay bills contributes to inappropriate calculations of Medicare SNF eligible benefit periods, as well as the amount of inappropriate Medicare payments due to this practice. Additionally the OIG will identify whether measures are in place to ensure that no-pay bills are submitted.

- **Inappropriate Psychotherapy Services in Nursing Facilities:** The purpose of this review is to determine the extent to which psychotherapy services are provided and medically necessary for Medicare beneficiaries residing in nursing facilities and the extent of inappropriate payments for these services.

Nursing homes need to carefully review the OIG Work Plan and incorporate into their Quality Improvement/Quality Assurance Program the necessary procedures to address those areas in which they are most at risk. In addition, the data generated in Quality Measure/ Quality Indicator reports provide a valuable source of information for areas, which potentially place the facility at risk for deficiency citations, substandard care, and ultimately negative outcomes of care. Interestingly, two areas that are included in the top 10 list of deficiency citations are assessment and care planning. Both of these areas are also identified in the OIG work plan, which makes it essential that they be addressed by long-term care facilities.

# Potentially High Risk Areas for Compliance in Long-Term Care Facilities

In long-term care (LTC) facilities (nursing and skilled), the following areas have consistently been identified as areas where potential or known problems exist. These areas, if not addressed through monitoring and corrective action, have the potential for increased risk in deficiency citations during the survey process. In addition, problems not corrected can contribute to increased risk for legal action and poor outcomes of care. It is imperative that facilities establish policies, procedures, and protocols that routinely monitor these areas to ensure compliance with appropriate standards of care.

## Abuse and Neglect Investigation and Reporting

Elder abuse and neglect have increasingly become the focus of civil, criminal, and administrative actions in LTC facilities. Federal regulations define elder abuse as the "willful infliction of injury, unreasonable confinement, intimidation, or cruel punishment with resulting physical harm, pain or mental anguish" (CMS 2005a). LTC facilities are required to develop and implement written policies and procedures that prohibit mistreatment, neglect, and abuse of residents and misappropriation of resident property (CMS 2005a). Federal and state laws make it a crime to abuse and neglect residents in LTC facilities, and regulations mandate that facilities and individuals report actual or suspected abuse or neglect. Facilities must be alert and sensitive to signs and symptoms of abuse or neglect and must take aggressive and proactive action to prevent the potential for abuse and neglect. Each LTC facility must implement a comprehensive program to identify and determine incidents of abuse and neglect. At a minimum, the program must contain the following components:

1. **Screening** of potential employees for a history of abuse, neglect, and mistreatment. Screening should include checking an individual's status with the appropriate licensing or certification board and performing criminal background checks and abuse registry inquiries.

2. **Training** employees through orientation and ongoing inservice training sessions about abuse, neglect, and mistreatment.

3. **Prevention** procedures to provide residents, families, and staff with information about to whom they should report incidents of abuse.

4. **Identification** procedures to assess and identify signs and symptoms of abuse and neglect.

5. **Investigation** of any alleged report of abuse and neglect.

6. **Protection** of all residents in the facility from harm such as preventing accidents and elopements during an investigation and throughout their stay in a facility.

7. **Reporting and responding** to all alleged violations and substantiated incidents of abuse and neglect to state agencies, licensing boards, and certification authorities and conducting in-depth analyses of incidents in order to implement strategies to prevent further occurrences.

## Pressure Ulcers

LTC facility residents are often frail and elderly and need to be carefully assessed and monitored to prevent pressure ulcers from occurring. Pressure ulcers can lead to debilitating conditions and sometimes death. Critical steps in pressure ulcer prevention and healing include the following:

- Identifying the individual resident at risk for developing pressure ulcers
- Identifying and evaluating the risk factors and changes in the resident's condition
- Identifying and evaluating factors that can be removed or modified
- Implementing individualized interventions to attempt to stabilize, reduce, or remove underlying risk factors
- Monitoring the impact of the interventions
- Modifying the interventions as appropriate

It is important to recognize and evaluate each resident's risk factors and to identify and evaluate all areas at risk of constant pressure.

Key to success in the area of pressure ulcer prevention and/or treatment is a complete assessment, which helps the facility identify residents at risk of developing pressure ulcers and identify the presence of pressure ulcers. The information gleaned from the assessment allows the facility to develop and implement a comprehensive care plan that reflects each resident's identified needs.

Each facility should have a system/procedure to ensure that assessments are timely and appropriate; interventions are implemented, monitored, and revised as appropriate; and changes in condition are recognized, evaluated, reported to the practitioner, and addressed. The quality assessment and assurance committee may help the facility evaluate the existing strategies to reduce the development and progression of pressure ulcers, monitor the incidence and prevalence of pressure ulcers within the facility, and ensure that facility policies and procedures are consistent with current standards of practice.

## Falls

Falls in LTC facilities are a constant source of concern, because residents who sustain falls are at risk for fractures or other serious injuries that may lead to decline and other comorbidities, reduced quality of life, and even death. In addition, facilities are at risk for deficiency citations and potential legal action. Each facility must have a system and procedure that identifies residents at risk for accidents and/or falls and adequately plans care and implements procedures to reduce or prevent accidents/falls. In some situations, it will be impossible to prevent falls due to resident choice in not following appropriate interventions that would allow the prevention of the accident/fall. In these situations, it is critically important that facilities put into place a plan to reduce the potential for injuries in the event that a fall occurs.

## Elopement

Elopement in LTC is often defined as a resident's departure from the premises without the knowledge of staff or family. Because most residents who reside in LTC facilities are physically and/or cognitively impaired, elopement can have very serious implications in terms of injury or death. There are many instances of elopement in which residents have suffered from extreme heat or cold and when later found, were dead or in serious condition requiring hospitalization. An elopement event for an LTC facility carries great risk in terms of potential legal liability as well as deficiencies from state survey agencies, and may create an immediate jeopardy situation for the facility. An assessment for elopement potential should be completed for each resident at the time of admission and periodically throughout the resident's stay. Appropriate care planning should address and incorporate interventions to deter or prevent elopement.

## Restraints

Restraint use in LTC facilities is often associated with a potential for decline in functioning for the individual resident. Residents cannot be restrained for discipline or staff convenience. Physical or chemical restraints can be used to treat medical symptoms, but residents have the right to refuse treatment. Before residents are restrained, the facility must determine the presence of a specific medical symptom that requires the use of restraints and how the use of restraints would treat the medical symptom, protect the resident's safety, and assist the resident in attaining or maintaining his or her highest practicable level of physical and psychosocial well-being. Each facility must follow a systematic process of evaluation and care planning prior to using restraints. Ongoing assessments are also needed to ensure the continuing need for the use of a restraint. The interdisciplinary team must address the risk of decline associated with restraint usage and make sure the care plan reflects appropriate interventions to minimize decline and to gradually reduce the use of restraints.

## Sentinel Events

A sentinel event is often defined as an undesirable event that could cause harm or death to a resident. In LTC, three distinct areas have been identified for the capture of data items on the MDS: dehydration, fecal impaction, and low-risk pressure ulcers. These sentinel events will be thoroughly and completely investigated by state surveyors, who will determine whether the event was avoidable or unavoidable. Appropriate assessment with proactive interventions outlined in the care plan can often reduce the potential for these events and improve the overall quality of life for each resident. In the event that a resident develops dehydration, fecal impaction, or a low-risk pressure ulcer, it is necessary for the facility to document the risk factors involved and what the facility did to prevent the occurrence. The documentation should reflect why a sentinel event was unavoidable based on the resident's disease state and/or noncompliance with appropriate interventions.

## Inaccurate MDS Assessments

Accuracy in assessment information is critically important in LTC facilities, because the information obtained through the assessment process serves as a road map to the care planning process. Inaccurate assessments result in inaccurate care plans, which contribute to decline in functio ning, potential deficiency citations, and increased potential for legal liability.

## Care Planning

Care planning is a critical function in LTC. Failure to develop appropriate and comprehensive plans of care can lead to significant civil, criminal, and administrative liability for both LTC facilities and individual healthcare professionals, particularly when residents suffer harm due to a lack of care, or inappropriate or incomplete care or treatment. Care plans should be developed by an interdisciplinary team, and residents and family members should be consulted and included in the care planning process. Care plan development should be initiated immediately following admission and evaluated in an ongoing fashion to make sure the interventions outlined in the care plan are being carried out on a daily basis to ensure that residents maintain and achieve their highest functional level. Care plans must contain measurable objectives and realistic timeframes so that residents can meet the proposed goals. Care plans should be reviewed and revised routinely as changes in status occur with individual residents, but in no case less often than quarterly. Revision of care plans reflects the facility's efforts to provide appropriate and consistent quality of care.

## Medication Errors

According to a report conducted by the Institute of Medicine (2000),

> For every dollar spent on drugs in nursing facilities, $1.33 is consumed in the treatment of drug related morbidity and mortality, amounting to $7.6 billion for the nation as a whole, and of which $3.6 billion has been estimated to be avoidable.

Numerous circumstances and situations can create medication errors, including incorrect transcription of an order, incorrect dispensing of medications, and incorrect administration. Facilities need a systematic process for reporting medication errors. The quality assurance and assessment committee should investigate and analyze medication errors and develop corrective action plans for prevention. Strategies for safe medication administration must be implemented and incorporated into the risk management and quality assurance processes. These strategies must also be a part of every facility's training and orientation program.

## Medication Availability Under Medicare Part D

With the implementation of a prescription drug benefit on January 1, 2006, facilities now face potential situations in which medications are not covered by a particular prescription drug plan without medical exceptions, prior authorizations, step therapy, or other exceptions (CMS 2003). The potential for delayed approval, dispensation, and delivery of medications to a resident are very real under this new system. This places the facility in a precarious position, as residents may experience decline if they do not have prompt access to the medications prescribed by their physician. Careful monitoring and evaluation through the quality assurance committee should be routine. Procedures must be established to ensure that staff recognize and understand the appropriate steps that must be taken to facilitate medication delivery to facility residents.

## Documentation

Documentation is a critical tool that allows and assists healthcare professionals in communicating about resident care in LTC facilities. This tool proves compliance with regulatory requirements. Documentation provides evidence of care and the resident response to that care, and it is the critical link between the care a resident receives and the evaluation of that care. Documentation also facilitates continuity of care by allowing healthcare professionals to track residents' progress and response to changes or reactions to the care provided.

Incomplete, inaccurate, or lack of documentation is the basis for many legal actions that nursing facilities are facing with increasing frequency. The importance of documentation cannot be overstated. It is imperative for nursing facilities to develop processes and policies for accurate, complete, and timely documentation, and to ensure that all staff are properly trained in all aspects of documentation.

## Billing for Services that were not Provided

LTC facilities must establish policies and procedures that promote timely and accurate billing for provided services. Routine audits should be completed to ensure adherence to the policies and procedures regarding preparation and submission of bills for reimbursement. Facilities are at risk for both civil and criminal legal action when bills are inappropriately prepared and submitted for services that were not provided. Under the False Claims Act, a monetary fine can be assessed to facilities for each incident of inappropriate billing (U.S. Code 1986).

## Risk Management

In LTC facilities, it is important to design a systematic program for risk management to reduce injuries and accidents while minimizing business and personal liability. From a financial standpoint, risk management has many benefits for LTC. Many insurance companies will lower premium costs if a facility has an organized and effective risk management program in place. An effective risk management program should include, but not be limited to, the following tasks/goals:

1. Ensuring that proper risk assessments are performed consistently

2. Providing a safe environment for all residents

3. Addressing the psychological and emotional needs of each resident

4. Ensuring communication with the resident and family about care requirements

5. Educating staff about how to minimize resident injuries

6. Promptly investigating any incident that occurs and taking proactive measures to ensure the incident does not recur

7. Establishing a process for immediately reporting incidents and accidents

8. Planning and intervening to identify potential causes of incidents

9. Conducting medical record audits to ensure compliance with policies and procedures

10. Conducting routine drills of fire alarms and evacuation procedures to ensure prompt response

## MDS Management Reports

The MDS system is part of the overall MDS National Automation Project. This system provides computerized storage, access, and analysis of MDS long-term care data on patients in nursing homes across the United States. The basic functions of the MDS system are as follows:

- Receipt of MDS records from LTC facilities

- Authentication and validation of MDS records

- Feedback to LTC facilities (acknowledgement of the transmission of data and specifying the status of record validation)

- Storage of MDS records in a database repository

Report categories available to LTC facilities include the following:

1. Data Submission Reports

2. Scheduled Reports

3. CASPER Provider Reports

4. Quality Measure/Indicator Reports

These reports should be reviewed and analyzed at predetermined and as-needed time frames using an established protocol for both the facility level as well as the resident level. This analysis should logically be integrated as a part of the facility quality assurance process. The most current version of the Long-Term Care Facility User's Manual should be used as a reference for more complete information and details about MDS management reports (CMS 2006).

Each LTC facility should establish procedures for periodic audits to test and validate the accuracy of MDS data.

## Data Submission Reports

Two MDS data reports are available electronically to facility providers: the initial feedback report and the final validation report.

### Initial Feedback Report

The initial feedback report should be received shortly after the MDS file is submitted. The person submitting the MDS data file should remain online until this report is received. This report will indicate whether the MDS submission was accepted or rejected. If the file was rejected, corrections may need to be made pursuant to the CMS correction policy and the file resubmitted.

### Final Validation Report

The final validation report is generated within 24 hours of the MDS submission. The report is created after the MDS system performs data validation, timing checks, sequence checks, and calculated element validations. The report detail section indicates the type and number of errors identified in the MDS records that were submitted or if an individual record was rejected because of fatal record errors.

## Scheduled Reports

These reports are automatically generated by the state MDS system on a monthly basis and can be accessed from the MDS state server under MDS submissions. The scheduled reports will be displayed as follows:

RRmmyyyy.txt=End of Month Roster Report

QRmmyyyy.txt=MDS Questionable New Resident Report

DRmmyyyy.txt=Residents Discharged Without Return Report

CRmmyyyy.txt=MDS Residents With Change to Resident Identifiers Report

ADmmyyyy.txt=MDS New Admission Report

ARmmyyyy.txt=MDS Activity Report

MRmmyyyy.txt=MDS Missing Assessment Report

MSRmmyyyy.txt=Monthly Quality Indicator Report

## Certification and Survey Provider Enhanced Reporting

Certification and Survey Provider Enhanced Reporting (CASPER) online reports can be requested through the CASPER Reporting system, accessible via each state's Intranet MDS home page. Each facility has a unique ID and password that provides access to the site for MDS submission and management reports.

The reports listed below can be reviewed and compared to facility data, such as census reports and MDS activity, to determine the need for corrective action. The error reports can be used to identify problematic areas on the MDS where additional staff training might be needed.

MDS Online Admissions/Re-Entry Report

MDS Online Discharges Report

Duplicate Resident Report

Errors by Field by Facility Report

Error Summary by Facility Report

Error Message Report

Facility List Report

MDS Facility List – Last Production Submission Report

Roster Report

Daily Submission Statistics Report

Monthly Submission Statistics Report

Submission Statistics by Facility Report

Vendor List Report

Vendor List of Current Facilities Report

RFA Statistics by Facility Report

Errors by Facility by Vendor Report

## Quality Measure/Quality Indicator Reports

In July 2005, a new Quality Measure/Indicator reporting system was established, which replaced the old quality indicator system, and contains reports that consolidate the two sets of measures. The new system has seven reports, as follows:

- Facility Characteristics Report
- Facility Quality Measure/Indicator Report
- Quality Measure/Indicator Monthly Trend Report
- Resident Level Quality Measure/Indicator Report: Chronic Care Sample
- Resident Level Quality Measure/Indicator Report: Post Acute Care Sample
- Resident Listing Report: Chronic Care Sample
- Resident Listing Report: Post Acute Care Sample

These reports contain a wealth of information and are routinely used by surveyors to identify potential areas of concern as part of the offsite survey preparation. They should be analyzed and used by facilities to identify potential areas where improvement and corrective action are needed.

# References

Centers for Medicare and Medicaid Services. 2003. Medicare Prescription Drug, Improvement, and Modernization Act of 2003. Public Law 108-173.

Centers for Medicare and Medicaid Services. 2005a (Oct. 28). Survey, certification, and enforcement procedures: Subpart E—Survey and certification of long-term care facilities. 42 CFR 488.301. *Federal Register* 70(208): 648–933.

Centers for Medicare and Medicaid Services. 2005b (Oct. 28). Requirements for long-term care facilities. 42 CFR 483. *Federal Register* 70(208): 62065–073.

Centers for Medicare and Medicaid Services. 2006 (Jan. 29). Minimum Data Set National Automation Project. Long-term Care Facility User's Manual, Version 7.5. Available online from https://www.qtso.com/mdsdownload.html.

Institute of Medicine. 2000. To err is human: Building a safer health system. Washington, DC: National Academy Press.

Office of Inspector General. 2006a (February). A review of nursing facility resource utilization groups. Report no. OEI-02-02-00830. Available online from http://www.oig.hhs.gov/oei/reports/oei-02-02-00830.pdf.

Office of Inspector General. 2006b. Work Plan, fiscal year 2007. Available online from http://www.oig.hhs.gov/publications/docs/workplan/2007/Work%20Plan%202007.pdf.

U.S. Code. 1986. False claims. Title 31, subtitle III, chapter 37, subchapter III, paragraph 3729.

# Chapter 10
# Inpatient Rehabilitation Facilities

*Patricia Trela, RHIA*

In 1983, the Centers for Medicare and Medicaid Services (CMS) implemented an Inpatient Prospective Payment System (IPPS) for acute care hospitals that excluded specific types of hospitals. Inpatient Rehabilitation Facilities (IRFs) received a temporary exemption from the IPPS, as no correlation could be shown between the patient's diagnosis and the cost of the patient's rehabilitation care. The intensity of rehabilitation services required by patients with the same diagnosis and the cost of the services can be very different depending on the degree of residual impairment following the acute hospitalization.

IRFs were excluded from the IPPS if they met certain criteria. Services specified by the criteria that the facility must provide include the following:

- A multidisciplinary team approach to care that includes team meetings at least every two weeks and documentation in the health record of team meetings that shows the multidisciplinary approach for the rehabilitation program. For compliance, the team meetings are conducted in person. A provider review of the documentation in the health record by the individual members of the patient's rehabilitation team does not meet the requirement for a team meeting.

- Patients receive close medical supervision, and physician documentation shows the need for a physician-coordinated program by active participation and leadership of the rehabilitation team.

- Rehabilitation nursing, physical therapy (PT), and occupational therapy (OT) are provided; speech therapy (ST), social services or psychological services, and orthotic and prosthetic devices are available and provided as needed. Documentation by the individual therapy disciplines shows their involvement and participation in the rehabilitation program.

- Pre-admission screening of potential patients determines that the patients need and will benefit from the intense rehabilitation services provided by an inpatient hospital rehabilitation program. Only patients appropriate for the services provided by the IRF are admitted. Documentation of the pre-admission screening shows that pre-admission screening was performed.

- Therapy three hours a day, five days a week is provided. Therapy documentation includes the duration of each therapy session to demonstrate that the patient received a minimum of three hours of therapy, five days a week. Documentation without an indication of the duration does not support compliance with this criterion.

- At least 75 percent of the inpatient population of the IRF requires intensive rehabilitation services for one or more of 10 conditions. This criterion is commonly referred to as the "75 percent rule." (This issue is covered in more detail beginning on page 167.) This criterion was redefined in 2004 to include 13 conditions listed in figure 10.1 (CMS 2004a).

## Documentation for IRFs

Facilities that meet the above criteria and obtain an exemption from the IPPS continue to receive cost-based reimbursement. Documentation in the health record must demonstrate that the IRF is compliant with the above criteria and supports the exemption from the IPPS and the diagnosis-related groups (DRG) payment methodology.

**Figure 10.1.    13 conditions covered in the 75 percent rule**

1. Stroke
2. Spinal cord injury
3. Congenital deformity
4. Amputation
5. Major multiple trauma
6. Fracture of the femur (hip fracture)
7. Brain injury
8. Neurological disorders, including multiple sclerosis, motor neuron diseases, polyneuropathy, muscular dystrophy, and Parkinson's disease
9. Burns
*10. Active polyarticular rheumatoid arthritis, psoriatic arthritis, and seronegative arthropathies
11. Systemic vasculidities with joint inflammation
12. Severe or advanced osteoarthritis, (osteoarthrosis or degenerative joint disease) involving 3 or more major joints (elbows, shoulder, hips, or knees)
13. Knee or hip joint replacement, or both, during an acute hospitalization immediately prior to the IRF stay

*Categories 10–13 replace polyarthritis on the prior condition list; category 13 was added. Additional criteria for these four categories must be met.

## Inpatient Rehabilitation Facilities Prospective Payment System

CMS implemented the inpatient rehabilitation facilities prospective payment system (IRF PPS) that covers Medicare Part A fee-for-service patients in 2002. The IRF PPS is designed to control increasing costs to the Medicare program. Payment is based on the discharge as the unit of measure and on the characteristics of each patient admitted. Claims are assigned to a case mix group (CMG). The CMGs are a patient classification system that groups together inpatient rehabilitation patients who are expected to have similar resource utilization needs. CMS uses the CMGs to allocate payment equitably among Medicare fee-for-service inpatient rehabilitation patients. The CMG payment methodology provides greater payment for patients with lower function than for patients with higher function because services required by patients with a lower function are believed to cost more than the services required by patients with a higher function.

The system includes the patient assessment instrument (PAI), which is completed upon admission and discharge. Admission information is collected and coded during the first three days of the admission and entered into the software on day four. Discharge information is collected during the last three days of the patient's stay. The PAI includes information for classification and quality of care monitoring and includes the information necessary to assign the CMG. Following are the nine different types of information included on the PAI:

- Identification information
- Admission information
- Payer information
- Medical information
- Discharge information
- Function modifier
- Functional independence measure (FIM) instrument
- Quality indicators
- Medical needs

Medical information reported on the PAI includes the impairment group coding (IGC) and ICD-9-CM codes for the etiology of the impairment, comorbid conditions, and complications.

At this time, CMS does not require a facility to report medical needs or quality indicators, although CMS is moving closer to implementing such quality initiatives. Medical information includes an IGC, etiologic diagnosis, date of onset of the impairment, and comorbid conditions. Information collected and reported on the PAI during the first three days of the admission for the impairment group, functional independence, and age of the patient is used to classify patients into a CMG based on expected resource utilization.

The IGC assigned on admission represents the primary reason for the admission. There are 85 IGCs. The admission IGC determines the rehabilitation impairment category (RIC) that is assigned when the information on the PAI is entered into the Grouper software. There are 21 RICs. If the IGC assigned is inaccurate, the CMG could also be incorrect because the IGC determines the two-digit RIC code that becomes the first two digits of the CMG.

Assignment of the IGC is made difficult by medical record documentation that does not clearly document the impairment that will be treated. Coding professionals may encounter difficulty interpreting physician documentation that indicates patient debility, difficulty with ambulation, or impaired mobility when the documentation does not provide information about the specific condition responsible for the impairment.

The etiologic diagnosis is a condition that is unique to the PAI. The etiology represents the acute condition that led to the impairment for which the patient is receiving rehabilitation. The etiology is reported by a code for the acute condition that led to the impairment. The date of onset of the impairment also represents the date that the etiology was acute. A late effect code is reported as the etiology if the patient has completed an IRF rehabilitation program for the same impairment prior to the current admission. There should be a correlation between the etiology and the IGC.

The uniform data system for medical rehabilitation (UDSMR) was developed to further research and improve the care of rehabilitation patients. It was also an early effort to develop a system that could predict resource use that could be a basis for a prospective payment system. The FIM instrument was developed as a method of measuring the functional status of the patient and the burden of care. Reporting a principal diagnosis that indicated admission for rehabilitation did not provide the information needed for research. Information on what caused the impairment (the etiology) was needed.

Assignment of an ICD-9-CM code for the etiology can be confusing for coding professionals because the etiologic diagnosis on the IRF PAI has a different definition than the principal diagnosis, and therefore, official coding guidelines for coding the principal diagnosis do not apply. Official coding guidelines do not address etiologic diagnosis.

The date of onset of the impairment is reported to show when the impairment was identified. This date helps identify if the impairment or etiology is a recent problem or a problem that is longstanding. An inaccurate date could make an acute condition look like a chronic condition or a chronic condition appear to be an acute condition.

Comorbidities are clinical conditions present on admission. Comorbidities affect the patient in addition to the conditions reported as the etiologic diagnosis or the impairment that is reported by the IGC. Certain comorbidities can have a significant impact on the resources used and on the cost of the rehabilitation program. Comorbidities that are considered to impact the cost of the rehabilitation program are assigned to a payment tier based on the cost of resources used to treat the comorbid condition. Each CMG has four payment tiers. Comorbidities with high costs are assigned to tier 1, medium costs to tier 2, and low costs to tier 3. Cases that do not have a comorbidity that impacts the cost of care are assigned to a tier with no comorbidity. If more than one comorbidity is reported, the comorbidity that assigns the case to the highest tier is used. Multiple comorbidities do not provide additional payment.

The physician list of admission diagnoses and how these are documented can cause the coding professional to assign incorrect codes. When all diagnoses are listed as status post, the coding professional will need to determine which conditions are current and should be assigned a code and reported, and which conditions are resolved, a past history, or are no longer an active problem and should not be assigned a code. An example of potentially confusing documentation is when the physician documents status post urinary tract infection treated with Levaquin for three more days; status post hypertension; status post diabetes mellitus; status post pneumonia.

Complications are conditions that are first identified or develop after admission during the rehabilitation stay, that delay or compromise the rehabilitation program or represent high-risk medical conditions. Complications recognized the day of discharge or the day prior to discharge are not reported on the IRF PAI, as they do not have a significant impact on the cost of the rehabilitation program. Conditions identified as a complication should be reported as a complication and also as a comorbid condition, as only conditions listed as a comorbidity are included in the reimbursement calculations.

The FIM includes 18 items, 13 motor items and 5 cognitive items. These items are scored on a seven-part scale with the most dependent scored as 1 and most independent scored as 7. These items must be scored by the third hospital day and entered into the software on the fourth hospital day for assignment of the RIC.

Documentation in the health record should support all items reported on the IRF PAI. Documentation that consists of a grid with the FIM score is insufficient documentation to support the FIM score. For example, an FIM score of six for modified independence for feeding without further documentation does not explain why the patient is scored as modified independence. Documentation that indicates that the patient requires adaptive equipment such as a rocker knife provides the information that supports this score.

On discharge, the PAI is completed. Software determines the appropriate Health Insurance Prospective Payment System (HIPPS) code based on the CMG and the comorbidities assigned to payment tiers. The HIPPS code includes a letter for the payment tier and the CMG. This code is reported on the claim form with revenue code 0024 to indicate that this claim is paid under the IRF PPS. Pricer software used by the fiscal intermediary (FI) determines the payment and any change in the HIPPS code based on the length of stay or the discharge destination.

The IRF PAI should be transmitted to CMS within 10 days following discharge. Counting the day of discharge as day one, if it is transmitted after the 28th day following discharge, a penalty is assessed. Payment for the CMG will be reduced by 25 percent.

The interrupted stay policy was developed so Medicare would not have to pay an additional CMG payment when the patient returned to the IRF within a short period of time. An interrupted stay (three days or less) occurs when the patient is discharged and returns before the third midnight. Only one claim should be submitted and the dates of the interruption are reported on the claim form and the number of days of the interruption are subtracted from the length of stay (LOS). The original impairment group assignment is not changed, even if the patient returns with another impairment that will use more resources than the original impairment. The facility should report the impairment that utilizes the most resources as the discharge IGC. The discharge IGC is not used in the reimbursement calculations.

An audit by the OIG showed that IRFs are not billing interrupted stays in compliance with Medicare interrupted stay policies. The interrupted stay policy covers transfers to acute care hospitals as well as discharges to home. Additional compliance monitoring of discharges to home is advised.

Each CMG payment tier is assigned an average LOS. The number of days assigned is inconsistent and the CMG payment tier with the highest reimbursement does not always have the longest average LOS. The IRF PAI also requires code assignment for where the patient is discharged. Accurate reporting of the discharge destination is important because patients who are transferred to another facility paid by Medicare before the average LOS for the CMG do not receive the full CMG payment. Proper coding of the discharge destination is essential for appropriate reimbursement. The codes reported on the IRF PAI for the discharge destination should represent the same discharge destination as the code reported on the claim form (UB-92/UB-04 or CMS-1450). The code numbers assigned for each discharge destination listed on the IRF PAI are not all the same as the code numbers used to code the destination on the claim form.

If the discharge code reported on the IRF PAI is used on the claim form, the disposition that the FI bases payment on could be inaccurate. An IRF should monitor to be certain that the code assigned for the discharge disposition on the claim form is accurately reported by the appropriate code. Many facilities have developed software that maps the IRF PAI discharge disposition code to a code appropriate to the claim form. This could have a degree of risk as there is not a one-to-one match with all of the conditions reported on the claim form. The IRF PAI document is submitted to CMS and the claim form is submitted for payment to the FI. An inaccurate discharge destination can result in inappropriate reimbursement. For example, when the patient is discharged to home and the facility reports the discharge disposition as transfer to a skilled nursing facility (SNF) before the average LOS, the facility receives a transfer payment instead of the full CMG.

Patients who are discharged in 3 days or less are reassigned to a special CMG for short stays. The short stay CMG does not include payment tiers. Comorbidities do not improve or change the reimbursement. The IRF does not assign the short stay CMG. The facility reports a CMG and when the FI enters the information into the PRICER software, the short stay CMG is assigned for payment purposes.

The software assigns the CMG when the facility enters the IRF PAI data into the computer. Scores assigned to the FIM and the IGC determine the CMG. The ICD-9-CM codes reported as comorbid conditions determine the payment tier.

The CMG assignment is based on the IGC, the FIM motor score, and for certain CMGs, age and the cognitive score. An error in coding any of the items that assign the CMG could result in inappropriate reimbursement.

When the IRF PAI information is entered into the computer, a CMG is assigned and, based on the codes reported for comorbidities, a letter prefix is added to indicate the payment tier. This code is called the HIPPS code and must be reported on the claim form because it determines the payment. The HIPPS code reported on the IRF PAI and the HIPPS code reported on the claim form should match. An inaccurate HIPPS code reported on the claim form can result in inappropriate reimbursement.

CMS has indicated that the ICD-9-CM codes reported on the IRF PAI and the claim form do not need to match. The conditions reported are not the same and the guidelines for code assignment are not the same. The IRF PAI reports an etiologic diagnosis that is not reported on the claim form and the claim form reports a principal diagnosis that is not reported on the IRF PAI. Codes for comorbidities on the IRF PAI are not reported for conditions that are included in the etiology or the IGC. The etiology often cannot be reported on the claim form, because it has been treated and is no longer present. For example, a below knee amputation (BKA) is performed to treat gangrene of the foot. The impairment is the BKA and the condition responsible for the BKA is gangrene (the etiology). The gangrene has been amputated and is no longer present and therefore should not be reported on the claim form as it is no longer present. Conditions identified the day prior to discharge or the day of discharge are not reported on the IRF PAI, but should be reported on the claim form. Regardless of the guidelines for the IRF PAI or the claim form, codes should be accurately assigned and reported on both the IRF PAI and the claim form.

There are many opportunities for compliance with the implementation of the IRF PPS. Reimbursement depends on accurate scoring and reporting of information on the PAI. The OIG has indicated in both the 2006 and 2007 Work Plan that IRFs paid under the IRF PPS will remain a focus area. The 2007 Work Plan indicates that the OIG will audit to see if the admissions to IRFs meet specific regulatory requirements that verify that interrupted stays are billed in compliance with Medicare PPS regulation, claims for patients transferred before the average LOS are not paid as a discharge, and payments by FIs are accurate when patient assessments are entered or transmitted late.

Financial incentives to miscode information on the IRF PAI to assign the admission to a CMG with a higher relative weight and improved reimbursement might exist. It is difficult to understand how the payments and LOS for each CMG were developed, because a higher payment tier does not always result in the highest reimbursement or the longest average LOS. Compliance risks include assignment of an inappropriate impairment group, unbundling and reporting an IGC for only one of the conditions being treated following trauma instead of an IGC that represents multitrauma, or reporting a comorbidity that developed on the day of discharge. There are many opportunities to monitor compliance with the official coding guidelines, including the following examples:

- Fractures that are treated prior to admission to the IRF should not be reported as acute fractures. Fracture aftercare codes should be reported.

- Obesity (not assigned to a payment tier) should not be reported as morbid obesity (assigned to a payment tier) unless the physician documents morbid obesity.

- Codes from chapter 16 of the ICD-9-CM for signs and symptoms should not be reported if they are inherent to a confirmed diagnosis, even if the sign or symptom is assigned to a payment tier.

## The 75 Percent Rule

The DRG system provided a fixed reimbursement for short-term acute care hospitals. The hospitals found that they could increase their profit if costs were contained. Patients who could be discharged to an IRF provided the acute care hospital with an opportunity to reduce the LOS and lower their costs while still receiving the same DRG payment. Several acute care hospitals opened their own inpatient rehabilitation units where they could transfer patients sooner, lower their costs, and receive additional cost-based reimbursement for the inpatient rehabilitation stay. Consequently, there was a large increase in the number of rehabilitation beds and a change in the diagnostic mix of patients admitted to IRFs, as well as pressure to keep these beds full. Patients with diagnoses that were not included in the 75 percent rule were admitted to the IRFs in greater numbers.

Patients who would not have been admitted in 1983 were being admitted and benefiting from the services provided by the IRF. This helped keep the additional beds full, but it also included patients with diagnoses that were not compliant with the 75 percent rule. Patients recovering from orthopedic procedures (such as fractures and joint replacements) make up a greater percentage of the IRF patient population today. The 10 diagnoses that made up the 75 percent rule in 1983 do not represent the IRF population of today.

The IRFs wanted changes to the conditions included in the 75 percent rule, as conditions frequently treated at the IRF. For example, cardiac, pulmonary, and joint replacements were not included. In 2004, CMS made changes to the diagnoses included in the 75 percent rule, added criteria that must be met for some of the conditions included in the rule, and provided guidance to the FIs for monitoring compliance with the rule. Polyarthritis was subdivided into three separate categories, and a new category for joint replacement was added. CMS issued transmittals 347 and 221, which listed the IGCs and the ICD-9-CM codes that would be considered compliant with the 75 percent rule (CMS 2004a, CMS 2004b). These transmittals provide information on changes to the 10 diagnoses that had been included in the rule prior to 2004 and documented the additional criteria for certain diagnostic classes.

Active polyarticular rheumatoid arthritis, psoriatic arthritis, and seronegative arthropathies are counted in the 75 percent rule if they result in impairment of ambulation and other activities of daily living (ADLs) that do not improve after outpatient therapy of at least two individual therapy sessions for a minimum of three weeks, aimed at the involved joints. Medical record documentation for these services must be within 20 calendar days of an acute care hospital stay immediately preceding an IRF stay, or 20 calendar days preceding an IRF admission. However, the FI has the discretion to interpret and define what it considers an appropriate, aggressive, and sustained course of outpatient therapy or therapy in another less-intense setting. The goal of the therapy should be to complete rehabilitation and not to prepare a patient for surgery.

Systemic vasculidities with joint inflammation are counted if they meet the criteria that is listed for active polyarticular rheumatoid arthritis.

Knee or hip joint replacements, or both, during the hospitalization immediately prior to the IRF stay could be counted if they also meet one of the following criteria:

- The patient had bilateral knee or bilateral hip joint replacement immediately prior to the IRF admission

- The patient is extremely obese with a body mass index of 50 or greater at the time of admission to the IRF

- The patient is age 85 or older at the time of admission to the IRF

Documentation of the patient's weight on admission is necessary for the dietitian to accurately report the BMI. Physician documentation of morbid obesity is not always consistent as physicians do not agree on the criteria for morbid obesity and may not want to look at a chart to determine if the patient is morbidly obese. There is an incentive to report a code for morbid obesity, as this condition is assigned to a payment tier that provides additional reimbursement for the IRF. Patients with a single joint replacement who have not reached age 85 will qualify as meeting the 75 percent rule if the BMI is 50 or greater. Coding professionals should not calculate the BMI in order to report a code that represents the BMI. Documentation of the BMI by the dietitian or the physician should be used for code assignment.

Facilities that admit a large number of orthopedic patients could have a difficult time meeting the 75 percent rule. Compliance with these criteria is shown by documentation in the health record.

FIs are responsible for monitoring compliance with the 75 percent rule. Prior to 2005, the methods used by the FIs were inconsistent. Cases that were considered compliant by one FI might not be considered compliant by another FI.

In order to provide guidance to the fiscal intermediaries on how they should determine compliance, CMS in 2004 issued Program Transmittals 347 and 221, and in 2006, Program Transmittal 938 (CMS 2004a, CMS 2004b, CMS 2006).

Once each year, based on the IRF's cost reporting period, IRFs are required to furnish their FI with a list that identifies the hospital number assigned and the payer for each patient admitted by the IRF in a recent, consecutive 12-month period as determined by CMS or the FI. Accurate reporting of all patients and their payment source is necessary for the FI to determine compliance with the 75 percent rule.

If an IRF's Medicare Part A fee-for-service inpatient population is 50 percent or more of the total inpatient population, it is considered to reflect the IRF's total population. An admission can be counted as meeting the 75 percent rule based on the admission IGC, the ICD-9-CM code assigned for the etiologic diagnosis, or for a comorbid condition. Transmittals 347 and 938 include a list of IGCs and ICD-9-CM diagnoses codes considered to meet the 75 percent rule (CMS 2004a, CMS 2006). The FI will compare the IGC and the ICD-9-CM diagnoses codes reported on the IRF PAI with those listed in Transmittal 938 to determine if the facility presumptively meets the 75 percent rule. The FI reports the results of its review to its regional office (RO). The RO or the FI also has the option of reviewing sections of the health record to ascertain compliance. If the facility does not presumptively meet the 75 percent rule, health record documentation will be reviewed to determine compliance.

Changes to the ICD-9-CM classification system in April and October each year make it difficult to keep the list of compliant diagnoses up-to-date in hard copy. To address this issue, CMS has posted the list of compliant IGCs and diagnosis codes that are considered to meet the 75 percent rule on the CMS website.

A noncompliant facility will lose the exemption to the IPPS and will receive DRG reimbursement, which provides significantly less reimbursement than the facility would receive if paid CMG reimbursement by the IRF PPS.

The CMS transmittals provide the IRFs temporary relief from the 75 percent rule. They lowered the compliance threshold for the 10 diagnostic categories from 75 percent to 50 percent for the first year, starting with cost reporting periods in 2004. This percentage rose in 2005 to 60 percent, in 2006 to 65 percent, and will return to 75 percent in July 2007. In 2006, Congress extended the 60 percent compliance rate for an additional year. The 75 percent rate will not be implemented until July 2008, and the use of comorbidities to determine compliance will be terminated. See figures 10.2 and 10.3.

## Outpatient Rehabilitation

Outpatient therapy needs to be provided by a qualified therapist or under the therapist's supervision following a written treatment plan. Only skilled services are covered. Services that are unskilled, maintenance, or palliative in nature are not covered. The services need to require the skills of a qualified therapist, and there must be an expectation of improvement within a reasonable period of time. Maintenance services do not require the skills of a therapist and can usually be performed by the patient or an unskilled caregiver. The goal of maintenance services is to prevent a decline in function. Patients receiving maintenance services periodically may need the skilled services of a qualified provider for evaluation/reevaluation or to design a therapy program.

The treatment plan must be developed and written by a physician, nonphysician practitioner (NPP), or therapist providing the services, and it must be part of the permanent health record. The plan should include the diagnosis, functional deficits and goals and should specify the type, amount, frequency, and duration of the therapy, and the signature, date, and professional identity of the person who established the plan. Changes to the treatment plan should be written and included in the plan immediately. Changes should be signed by the physician/NPP or therapist who furnishes the services, or a registered nurse based on oral orders from the physician. The physician/NPP must review the plan as often as necessary, but at least every 30 days. Each review should be signed by the physician/NPP who performs the review.

As a condition of payment for outpatient therapy by Medicare, a physician/NPP must certify that the therapy services are skilled therapy, the services were provided while the

**Figure 10.2.   The 75 percent final rule, May 7, 2004**

| | |
|---|---|
| 07/01/04 to 06/30/05 | 50% |
| 07/01/05 to 06/30/06 | 60% |
| 07/01/06 to 06/30/07 | 65% |
| 07/01/07 | 75% |

**Figure 10.3.   2006 revised compliance rate**

| | |
|---|---|
| 07/01/06 to 06/30/07 | 60% |
| 07/01/07 to 06/30/08 | 65% |
| 07/01/08 | 75% |

patient was under the care of a physician/NPP, and the services were provided under a written plan of treatment. Certification should be obtained at the time the treatment plan is established or as soon as possible. The certification must be signed and dated by a physician/NPP who has knowledge of the case; the same physician/NPP who orders and reviews the plan of treatment must sign the certification statement.

The plan must be established, written, dated, and signed before treatment begins. It must also include credentials of the physician/NPP. It may be written on the same day as the initial evaluation and treatment by the therapist who evaluates and establishes the plan or under the verbal direction of that therapist and must be established by the close of business the next day. Services provided before the plan of care is established may be denied.

Certification is required at least within 30 days or one month from the first therapy session. Certification would be considered timely if a timely verbal order is received and documented and followed by signature within 14 days. Recertification is required every 30 days. When therapy continues for longer than one month, recertification is required. Recertification is considered late if it is signed more than 60 days after the initial certification. When recertification is late, the physician/NPP must include a reason for the delay. Services are payable even if the certification/recertification is signed late. Noncompliance with the plan of care and certification/recertification requirements is a frequent reason for denial of payment for therapy services. Services denied as a result of noncertification cannot be billed to the patient. A process for obtaining the required signatures should be developed and monitored.

CMS has provided guidance on how to report therapy modalities reported with a CPT code that includes time spent in the delivery of a modality that required constant attendance. Time begins when the therapist is working directly with the patient to provide the treatment when the patient is in the area where the treatment will be provided. The time for transporting the patient to the treatment area, waiting time, scheduling, toileting, and documentation do not count toward treatment time. One unit of service should be reported for treatment time greater than or equal to 8 minutes and less than 23 minutes. Services of less than 8 minutes should be documented, but should not be billed. The time spent providing services described by a timed code should be documented. The beginning and ending time or the duration of the service timed to the minute should be documented in the health record with a note describing the treatment.

When more than one timed CPT code is billed on a calendar day, the total number of units billed cannot be more than the total treatment time. For example, a patient may receive a total of 47 minutes of therapy, as follows:

- 9 minutes of electrical stimulation
- 10 minutes of manual therapy
- 12 minutes of ultrasound
- 16 minutes of therapeutic exercise

Only three units of therapy should be billed because the total time was less than the time required to bill four units of therapy. In this case, one unit of manual therapy, one unit of ultrasound, and one unit of therapeutic exercise should be billed. Electrical stimulation would not be billed, as it was provided for the least amount of time. To bill four units, a minimum of 53 minutes of therapy would need to be provided. Therapy that is not billed should still be documented in the medical record.

Group therapy is therapy provided at the same time to two or more patients by a therapist. The patients can be performing the same activity or different activities. Constant attendance by the therapist is required, but one-on-one patient contact is not required.

Repetitive Part B services that are billed to the FI need to be billed monthly or at the conclusion of treatment (CMS 2004c).

Repetitive Part B services billed under the following revenue codes include:

- Physical Therapy—Revenue Codes 0420–0429

- Occupational Therapy—Revenue Codes 0430–0449

- Speech Pathology—Revenue Codes 0440–0449

Outpatient therapy claims are often inappropriately reported. Inadequate documentation is one of the most frequent reasons therapy claims are denied. At a minimum, documentation that should be included in the health record includes a plan of care signed by a physician and a description of the services provided.

Documentation that will support the claim includes physician orders, initial therapy evaluation, notes that include individual modality/procedure minutes, an updated treatment plan or reevaluation. Claims also are denied when treatment logs do not identify the patient or the modality or when group therapy is billed on the same day as individual therapy and documentation does not identify it as a separate therapy session. Certification becomes a problem when the date on the certification does not match the dates on the claim or when the signature on the certification is late and there is no documentation to explain why the signature was late. Other reasons claims are denied include when the copies of the health record documentation are of poor quality, the documentation is illegible, or the documentation is not signed by the therapist performing the service. Health records submitted to support a claim must contain sufficient information to show that the services are coded correctly, are reasonable and necessary at the start of care, and remain reasonable and necessary during the course of treatment.

When multiple services are provided on the same day, modifier 59 should be reported to show that a medically necessary distinct service was provided. For example, the patient received 30 minutes of individual therapeutic exercise in the morning. In the afternoon, the patient returned and received 15 minutes of group therapy. Modifier 59 should be reported with the code for group therapy to show that it was a distinct service that was provided at a different time.

Modifier 59 should not be used routinely. Misuse of the modifier 59 could result in an intensive medical review for the provider. It is inappropriate for a provider to append modifier 59 just to get a bill paid.

Manual therapy and therapeutic activities performed during the same 15 minute time period are mutually exclusive and should not be reported with modifier 59. Modifier 59 should only be used when these two services are performed in different 15 minute time periods.

## References and Resources

Centers for Medicare and Medicaid Services. 2006 (May 5). The inpatient rehabilitation facility prospective payment system (IRF PPS). Pub 100-04: Medicare claims processing, transmittal 938, change request 5016. Available online from http://new.cms.hhs.gov/transmittals/Downloads/R938CP.pdf.

Centers for Medicare and Medicaid Services. 2004a (Oct. 29). Inpatient rehabilitation facility (IRF) classification requirements. Pub. 100-04: Medicare claims processing, transmittal 347, change request 3503. Available online from http://new.cms.hhs.gov/transmittals/Downloads/R347CP.pdf.

Centers for Medicare and Medicaid Services. 2004b (July 1). Medicare IRF classification requirements. Pub 100-04: Medicare claims processing, transmittal 221, change request 3334. Available online from http://new.cms.hhs.gov/transmittals/Downloads/R221CP.pdf.

Centers for Medicare and Medicaid Services. 2004c (Dec. 17). Hospital billing for repetitive services. Pub 100-04: Medicare claims processing, transmittal 407, change request 3633. Available online from http://new.cms.hhs.gov/transmittals/Downloads/R407CP.pdf.

Medicare Payment Advisory Commission. 2006 (March). Report to Congress: Medicare payment policy. Section 4D: Inpatient rehabilitation facility services. Available online from medpac.gov.

# Chapter 11
# Home Health Services

*Therese Rode, RHIT, HCS-D*

Implementing a compliance program in a home health environment presents many challenges. Accurate, up-to-date health records are essential for providing high-quality care, facilitating reimbursement, and protecting the home health agency (HHA) against potential accusations of fraud and abuse.

Home health providers are overwhelmed by the burden of documentation necessary in order to comply with the prospective payment system (PPS), home health prospective payment system (HH PPS) and Outcome and Assessment Information Set (OASIS) requirements.

The need for accountability, accurate health record data, and information to support medical necessity, homebound status, and the ICD-9-CM codes reported continues to increase. Monitoring and auditing of documentation to ensure that the data submitted justifies the home care encounter is the only logical step to protect an HHA.

In this chapter the various requirements and challenges of maintaining compliance in a home health agency will be discussed.

## Outcome and Assessment Information Set

OASIS is a clinical assessment tool that evaluates patients and measures outcomes through the use of 79 demographic, clinical, and functional data elements.

OASIS serves two major purposes. First, the Medicare PPS uses the OASIS data elements to determine into which Home Health Resource Group (HHRG) a beneficiary falls. Second, OASIS provides a mechanism to monitor and report quality indicators. The goal of the OASIS tool is not to develop a comprehensive assessment instrument, but rather to provide a set of data elements necessary for measuring patient outcomes as a result of an encounter with home health.

Under PPS, agencies receive a payment for each 60-day episode of care. The base payment for each episode for the year 2005 was $2,264.28. The base payment is adjusted by placing the beneficiary into one of 80 HHRGs. The HHRG represents the clinical and functional severity of a beneficiary's condition and recent use of other health services (MO175). MO175 is calculated under the "service" domain for OASIS data collection/reporting. The base rate is also affected by wage adjustment factors. This allows for a payment variance depending on the demographic area and wage differences.

After completion of the OASIS assessment and the Plan of Care (485), the initial episode payment or the Request for Anticipated Payment (RAP) is submitted, and the HHA will receive 60 percent of the estimated case-mix adjusted episode payment. When the final bill is submitted for the initial 60-day episode, the HHA will receive a final payment equal to 40 percent of the actual case-mix adjusted episode.

On subsequent recertification, the HHA will receive payment in a 50/50 split.

Under HH PPS, a case-mix adjusted payment for a 60-day episode is made using HHRGs. This case-mix system uses 79 identified data elements from the OASIS assessment instrument. Although HHRGs differ from DRGs in that they use the OASIS data elements, both require accurate ICD-9-CM code assignments. It is unethical and fraudulent to report a diagnosis code on the claim that is not supported by documentation in the health record simply because it is "payable."

## OASIS Data Elements

The OASIS data elements are organized into three dimensions to capture the clinical, functional, and service (CFS) utilization factors that impact case mix. The score value in each dimension measures the impact of the data element on the total resource use. The number of total points assigned within each dimension varies, depending on the relevant data elements for the patient.

The diagnoses in the clinical dimension must be the primary diagnosis or, for certain limited manifestations, the first secondary diagnosis, in order to influence the HHRG assignment. A list of the diagnoses impacting the HHRG assignment (also called case mix or payment diagnosis codes) can be found in tables 8A and 8B in the final rule for the HH PPS (HCFA 2003).

Cases in which patients experience a significant change in condition (improvement or deterioration) during an episode of care are eligible for a payment rate adjustment. The health record documentation, OASIS, and the plan of care must be consistent with each other and appropriately reflect the patient's change of condition.

## Home Health Resource Group Score

The HHRG score, which impacts reimbursement, is derived from 23 elements identified from the CFS domains on the OASIS assessment. The clinical domain is calculated from 16 data elements reported, which includes not only the ICD-9-CM codes reported in MO230, MO240, and MO245 (if applicable), but also the following:

- IV Infusion therapy
- Vision

- Wounds

- Pain

- Pressure and stasis ulcers

- Dyspnea

- Urinary and bowel incontinence

- Ostomies

- Behavior problems

Diabetic, orthopedic, neurologic, burn, and trauma diagnoses also impact the clinical dimension.

The functional domain score is based on the patient's ability to perform activities of daily living (ADLs), transferring, and mobility. (ADLs include dressing, bathing, and toileting.) The service domain reports any hospital, rehabilitation, or skilled nursing facility from which the patient has been discharged in the past 14 days, as well as whether or not the patient is expected to receive 10 or more therapy visits within the 60-day episode. The HHRG score is determined by adding up the points for each of the CFS utilization categories, which are then compared to the scoring chart. Although it is possible to calculate the HHRG manually, the HHRG score is formulated through Grouper software based on the MO elements addressed above. The software will group the patient into one of 80 possible HHRGs.

The HHRG score is not directly reported on the UB-92/UB-04 Medicare billing form but is represented in the form of a Health Insurance Prospective Payment System (HIPPS) code. Each HHRG has a set of eight possible HIPPS codes that carry the same case weight but provide more specific data based on the answers reported on the OASIS.

Each of the CFS factors has severity levels. Currently, there are four clinical severity factor levels, five functional severity factor levels, and four utilization severity factor levels. There are 80 possible combinations of severity levels in the three severity sets. There are 640 (80 × 8) possible HIPPS codes.

## Health Insurance Prospective Payment System

The HIPPS code is derived as follows:

1. The first character reported on the HIPPS code for home health is always an "H," to represent home health.

2. The second through fourth positions on the code are alphabetical and represent the score derived from the CFS categories after the OASIS assessment has been completed.

3. The fifth position of the HIPPS is always a numeric character. Codes with a fifth digit other than "1" indicate an incomplete OASIS assessment. (See appendix 11A [pp. 205–217] for a listing of the HHRG and HIPPS codes).

HIPPS codes are calculated from Grouper software and are based on responses to 79 specified OASIS elements. The HIPPS are determined based on the answers derived from the CFS utilization factors reported on the OASIS assessment.

## Reimbursement Under the Home Health Prospective Payment System

The Centers for Medicare and Medicaid Services (CMS) implemented HH PPS as a result of the Balanced Budget Act of 1997. The implementation was in response to the rapidly growing home health spending under a cost-based system. With PPS, HHAs receive a unit of payment that reflects a national 60-day episode rate with applicable adjustments. That payment is designed to reflect the clinical, functional severity, and service utilization of a beneficiary's condition.

The HH PPS payment is determined in advance of the services being rendered and is fixed for the fiscal year to which it applies. Reimbursement is based on codes reported, not charges submitted.

The actual cost of providing the service is not a factor in determining reimbursement. The provider, rather than the payer, is responsible for cost control. In the past, although the reimbursement determined for HH PPS utilized historical data that included OASIS data elements and ICD-9-CM codes, the data reported were not always accurate. When HHAs were first mandated to complete the OASIS, the HHA was limited to reporting three digits of an ICD-9-CM code. Reporting only three of possibly a five-digit code diminished the accuracy of the data. HHA did not always have a clear understanding of ICD-9-CM official coding and reporting guidelines, and prior to the implementation of the Health Insurance Portability and Accountability Act (HIPAA) code and transaction set in October 2003, HHAs were not allowed to report OASIS codes. This forced HHAs to oftentimes report the patient's disease or injury, which had been resolved with the hospital stay. Also, HHAs did not always have clarification as to the intent of a specific OASIS element.

Medicare continues to reassess HH PPS using the data reported today to determine appropriate reimbursement in the future. Medicare is looking to include a pay for performance payment system. Pay for performance will be very difficult for HHAs because OASIS elements reported focus on the patient's outcome and not the outcome of the caregiver to care for the patient.

## Start of Care and Resumption of Care

HHA is reimbursed a set rate based on the codes reported on the claim form. Reimbursement will be based on a 60-day episode of care (certification period). The initial 60-day episode of care (called "start of care" or SOC) begins with the first billable, medically necessary, skilled visit performed by a registered nurse, physical therapist, or speech therapist. Medicare does not accept occupational therapy to perform the first skilled assessment visit at the SOC, nor may the first visit be made by a Home Health Aide. The initial certification period ends on (including) the 60th day after the SOC date. Recertification is required for each 60-day episode of care subsequent to the first day of care as long as the patient continues to qualify for the home health benefit.

If it is determined that the patient requires and meets Medicare criteria for the home health benefit, the HHA will complete a follow-up OASIS assessment no sooner than five days prior to the end of the previous certification and no later than the date the recertification expires. This assessment, as do all OASIS assessments, depicts the patient in a "snapshot" of time. The elements are reported based on the patient's condition at the time the assessment is completed. The OASIS user's manual provides guidelines, requirements, and instructions for completing the OASIS assessment. Chapter 8, attachment B, provides examples and guidelines for completing the OASIS assessment. The manual can be downloaded at http://www.cms.hhs.gov/OASIS/ (CMS 2005a).

Completion and transmittal of an OASIS assessment is required upon SOC and recertification (every 60 days), transfer to an acute facility, after the patient is discharged from the acute care setting (if home health is ordered and the patient continues to qualify), and if the patient experiences a significant change in condition (SCIC) (either improvement or deterioration that is not expected).

If a patient is transferred to an acute care setting for longer than 24 hours, then a transfer OASIS assessment is required. If the patient is discharged from the acute care setting prior to the end of the certification period and continues to require home health, then the assessing clinician will complete a resumption of care (ROC) OASIS. If the patient's hospital stay extends past the certification period, the HHA must discharge the patient. The patient would then be readmitted with a new SOC OASIS if the patient continued to require home health services. Once it is determined that a patient no longer requires home health services, the clinician will complete a discharge OASIS. All OASIS assessments required must be electronically locked and transmitted to the state to prevent alterations after submission.

## Medical Record Issues

Regardless of whether an organization's records are paper, electronic, or hybrid, forms need to be developed to reduce compliance risks and to assist the clinician in addressing critical data elements to support a patient's condition, homebound status, and medical necessity. The clinician needs to clearly and concisely document the clinical skills rendered and assessment performed (such as pain, abuse, and neglect), the modalities performed, progress toward the individual patient's established goals, and the outcomes of those goals.

The documentation on each visit note needs to stand on its own merit. The services rendered must be legible, clear, and concise. "A litmus test for an accurate and up-to-date health record is whether an alternative care provider can review the record on a given day and obtain a clear, consistent picture of the patient's status, care plan and goals, and the care and services provided" (Scichilone 2004, 18).

As an HHA moves to an electronic or hybrid record, the timely filing of paper documentation should become less of an issue. Although some of the challenges with the paper record should be eliminated with the electronic or hybrid record, new challenges to safeguard and ensure the integrity of the record will become apparent. The new questions that will have to be answered are listed in figure 11.1.

**Figure 11.1.   Safeguarding a medical record in an electronic environment**

- Who has access to the electronic record?
- How is this record safeguarded against tampering or unauthorized entries?
- How is documentation corrected once the clinical note is locked?
- Is there a timeframe established in which documentation can be corrected?
- Who can make entries in the record?
- Who reviews the electronic OASIS assessment, initial evaluation, and Plan of Care (POC) prior to approval? How is this reviewed? If omissions or inconsistencies are identified, how is the clinician notified and how is this corrected?
- Who monitors for timely submission of consents, authorizations for payment, and HIPAA Notice of Privacy Acknowledgement forms?
- What monitoring mechanism is in place to ensure timely entry of documentation?
- What monitoring mechanism is in place to ensure that the data entered in the electronic note complies with agency and regulatory guidelines?
- Who can print the electronic documentation and under what circumstances?
- Has the clinician reported time and travel consistent with the visit notes?
- Are audit trials consistent?
- Is there a mechanism in place to ensure that electronic notes are not "cut and pasted" and that each visit entry can stand on its own merit?
- How is the entry of patient data in the wrong patient's electronic record identified?
- How are these wrong entries corrected?
- What are the patient safety risks due to this occurrence?
- Are there monitoring mechanisms in place to guard against this occurrence?
- How is an electronic record protected if a record must be sequestered?

New or modified policies and procedures need to be developed and communicated to all staff to ensure that the patient documentation is protected in an electronic environment with the same diligence as in the paper environment. As health information managers, we need to do the following:

- Ensure the security of patient information

- Develop processes to ensure that visit notes are completed in a timely manner in accordance with established policies

- Develop policies to delineate who can access and enter data into the electronic record

- Develop processes to safeguard against patient information being entered in the wrong patient's electronic record, including the following processes:

  —What steps are taken and when this occurs

  —Standardize how corrections are made in the electronic record—where they are to be made and who can make them

- Develop processes as to who can print electronic records in order to safeguard the confidentiality of the patient's record. Printing policies are for more than safeguarding confidentiality; if clinicians print and then document on the paper rather than in the electronic system, problems may occur

- Develop policies and processes to monitor access to patient information

Data entered and completed in an electronic record remains part of the patient record in which the data was entered (even if the data now states it is for historic use only) and can never be deleted. Processes need to be in place to ensure that the data entered in the wrong patient record is safeguarded from improper disclosure. (This process is called redacting and attached to the correct patient record.)

Sound documentation practices should be instituted. The standards for appropriate documentation remain the same no matter the medium in which the data is reported. Legal health record requirements vary from state to state and in some instances do not include electronic health records. An agency will need to refer to their state requirements for guidance. There is a good possibility that state requirements with regard to electronic health records will be changing significantly over the next decade. AHIMA's e-HIM workgroups and practice counsels are in the process of providing guidance in the area of legal electronic health records.

Documentation should record the activity leading to the record entry, the identity and discipline of the individual providing the service, and any information needed to support medical necessity and other applicable reimbursement coverage criteria. All entries to the record must be made only by individuals allowed to make entries and must be signed and dated by the author of the entry. Section 484.48 of the Medicare *Conditions of Participation* requires clinical records to contain pertinent past and current findings in accordance with accepted professional standards.

## Medical Necessity Issues

Medical necessity is the concept that procedures are only reimbursed as a covered benefit when they are performed for a specific diagnosis or specified frequency. The Medicare conditions of participation (COPs), State Operations Manual, and the Fiscal Intermediary (FI) reference guide all define medical necessity. Additionally, insurers may develop their own payment policies regarding medical necessity.

A plan of care (POC) must be certified by a physician who is a doctor of medicine, osteopathy, or podiatric medicine. Periodic clinical reviews, both prior and subsequent to billing for services, should be conducted to verify that patients are receiving only medically necessary services. HHAs should examine the frequency and duration of the services they perform to determine, in consultation with a physician, whether the patient's medical condition justifies the number of visits provided and billed.

Policies and procedures should be developed and implemented to verify that beneficiaries have received the appropriate level and number of services billed. The importance of documenting the services performed and billed should be stressed to clinicians.

When an HHA cannot comply with the frequency of visits ordered by the physician, it is critical to document the reason and the notification to the physician of record responsible for the patient's care that the frequency ordered cannot be met.

To qualify for home health benefits under Medicare, the patient must meet the following four qualifying conditions:

1. The HHA must be Medicare certified.

2. The patient must be homebound. Homebound is defined by the following criteria:

   - The ability to leave home requires major effort.

   - The patient cannot leave home without assistance.

   - The patient may leave the home for medical care, or for short, infrequent nonmedical reasons such as attending religious services, adult day care, or to get a haircut.

3. The patient's physician must determine medical necessity and sign the POC that is specific to the patient's needs.

4. The patient requires skilled clinical services. These services must be reasonable and necessary and provided on an intermittent basis, and are not solely needed for venipuncture for obtaining blood samples (unless the patient is being provided with another qualifying skilled service). Skilled services include the following:

   - Physical therapy

   - Speech language therapy

   - Continuing occupational therapy: At the start of an established POC, occupational therapy cannot be a qualifying skilled service. However, when one of the above-listed qualifying services has initiated the POC and the qualifying service discharges the patient, the occupational therapist then becomes the qualifying service and may continue.

Additionally, the following conditions must be met:

- The HHA must ensure that a qualifying skilled service is not establishing the POC merely to open the case for occupational therapy.

- Homebound status must be documented in the patient record frequently enough to reflect the patient's current condition, and at a minimum of once every certification period. The medical record documentation must support the patient's homebound status in clear, specific, and measurable terms.

- The homebound status must be obvious from a reviewer's standpoint. Simply documenting the use of a cane or walker in the POC does not reflect the homebound status. Many beneficiaries who use a cane or a walker are not homebound.

Documentation in the medical record should reflect how the medical condition restricts the patient's ability to leave home.

- Documentation in the medical record **must clearly indicate** that it is a considerable and taxing effort for the beneficiary to leave home. Documentation such as "short of breath" and "poor endurance" is not sufficient. Acceptable documentation would include "short of breath after ambulating five feet and needs to rest" (CMS 2005b).

## HHS OIG Work Plan

HH PPS has presented some new compliance risks for HHAs. The HHS Office of Inspector General (OIG) continues to focus its attention on fraud and abuse within the home care setting.

Each year the OIG issues a Work Plan that describes the activities of the component organizations. The operating components of the OIG are as follows:

- Office of Audit Services
- Office of Evaluations and Inspections
- Office of Investigations
- Office of Counsel to the Inspector General

According to the OIG, a compliance plan must have the following basic requirements:

- Written policies, procedures, and standards of conduct
- Designation of a compliance officer and a compliance committee
- Conduct of effective training and education
- Development of effective lines of communication
- Enforcement of standards through well-publicized disciplinary guidelines
- Prompt response to detected offenses and development of corrective action

CMS, the Government Accountability Office (GAO) and the Medicare Payments Advisory Commission (MedPAC) were concerned that HHAs would limit visits to patients which may compromise the patient's outcome and the quality of care provided because of the change from a cost-based system to being reimbursed for an episode of care. This change in reimbursement methodologies raised questions about the quality and outcomes for home health patients.

In January 2006, the OIG issued their findings on the "Effect of the Home Health PPS on the Quality of Home Health Care" (OE1-01-04-00160). The objective was to determine if hospital readmissions and emergency department visit rates for Medicare beneficiaries discharged from hospitals to home health care have changed since the implementation of HHA PPS, in October 2000. The data used for their finding were Medicare claims data and data on beneficiaries' clinical and functional characteristics to measure the rate of readmissions to hospitals and the rate of visits to hospital emergency departments. The data analyzed were over a consistent 3-month period (April–June) for the years 2000, 2001, 2002, and 2003.

The outcome of this study was that hospital admission rates remained unchanged (about 47 percent) throughout the four years reviewed. The emergency department visits increased minimally from 29 percent to 30 percent during the same period. The study further showed a slight increase in emergency department visits for beneficiaries with at-risk diagnoses, including renal failure and heart failure. The rates for visits caused by preventable adverse events remained low—less than 1 percent.

The results indicated that the change in payment systems did not lead to an increase in either hospital admissions or emergency department visits.

What the study also showed was that beneficiaries with specific diagnoses, such as renal failure, pulmonary disease, and multiple sclerosis, had higher hospital readmission rates (4 to 5 percent increase) and more emergency department visits (4 percent increase).

Due to the outcomes of the study, the recommendation was to continue to monitor indicators of quality in home health. In addition, CMS has announced plans to link claims data to the OASIS data with the hope that the project will demonstrate how complete and accurate OASIS data alone can be.

CMS remains concerned about patient safety and preventing adverse events in the home and intends to increase its focus on patient transitions and coordination of care between care settings for postacute care.

The 2007 OIG Work Plan for HHAs will focus on the issues detailed in figure 11.2.

The area of focus of HHAs needs to include clear, precise documentation to support the skilled services rendered and the care provided followed the order established in the patient's POC or subsequent verbal orders. The clinician must document verbal orders received from the physician and any telephone calls made to the physician to update them on their patient's condition or status. HHAs need to ensure that the skilled services provided meet Medicare guidelines and clearly justify medical necessity as well as the patient's homebound status.

If a patient is reported to be a high threshold therapy patient (MO825) with 10 visits or more, the documentation must support this increase in visits. Medicare will review cases where 10, 11, or 12 therapy visits are made to ensure that the extra visits were necessary and that the same results in the patient condition could not be accomplished by the ninth visit.

## Assessing Risks

In order to assess the risks of noncompliance, it is critical that an HHA develop a multi-departmental team to identify how a visit translates into a bill. This team should develop a flowchart of how information and documentation travel through the agency processes from the time the referral was obtained until the time the patient is discharged and the chart is completed. See figure 11.3 for issues to address while assessing risks.

**Figure 11.2.   2007 OIG work plan for HHAs**

Home Health Outlier Payments:

The OIG will determine whether outlier payments to HHAs are in compliance with Medicare regulations. The outlier payment is intended to be a loss-sharing mechanism for costly cases.

An outlier payment is made for an episode for which the estimated cost exceeds a threshold amount for each case-mix group.

OIG will evaluate the frequency of outliers and whether they cluster in certain HHRGs or geographical areas.

OIG plans to determine whether or not the current outlier methodology is equitable to all HHAs.

Enhanced Payments for Home Health Therapy:

The OIG will determine whether HHA therapy services met the threshold for higher payments in compliance with CMS regulations.

The OIG will analyze the number and the duration of therapy visits provided per episode period.

If the HHA reports "yes" in MO825 indicating that 10 or more therapy visits will be made, reimbursement may be increased up to an additional $2,000. (Physical Therapy, Occupational Therapy, and Speech Therapy visits are all combined to answer this question.) This significant increase in reimbursement opens an HHA to further scrutiny by CMS and could increase an agency's potential for upcoding and potential fraud.

Cyclical Noncompliance in Medicare Home Health Agencies

OIG will examine trends and patterns in HHA survey and certification deficiencies.

OIG will also identify whether any HHAs show patterns of cyclical noncompliance with certification standards and whether CMS applies appropriate sanctions to noncompliant HHAs.

HHA will be held accountable for correcting any noncompliance identified through surveys or through additional documentation requests (ADRs). The OIG will also look for patterns of noncompliance in all areas identified.

Accuracy of data on the Home Health Compare Web site

OIG will determine the accuracy and completeness of information on the Medicare-certified HHA Web site.

This Website provides beneficiaries and their families with information on all CMS certified home health agencies.

The OIG will examine how CMS identifies and updates missing and incorrect information on the database.

Accurately Coding Claims for Medicare Home Health Resource Groups

The OIG will determine the extent to which Medicare HHAs accurately code the HHRG in the OASIS.

The OIG will determine the extent to which the HHRGs are improperly coded and the level of inappropriate payments made as a result of any miscoding.

Home Health Rehabilitation Therapy Services

The OIG will determine the extent to which rehabilitation therapy services were provided by appropriate staff and were medically necessary.

The OIG will determine if the patient's POC identified the need for the amount and level of therapy that the patient received.

The OIG will determine the amount of reimbursement received by HHA due to medically unnecessary HHA therapy.

Source: OIG 2006.

**Figure 11.3.   Risk Assessment Checklist**

- What information is obtained on intake?
- Who obtains the information?
- How is the information communicated?
- Who are your referral sources?
- Does the information contain the name and telephone number of the physician who will have oversight of the patient after hospital discharge and is agreeing to sign the POC and subsequent orders for the patient? (Note the referring physician could be a hospital physician who will not be following the patient after discharge from the hospital and will be unwilling to sign the certification orders.)
- Does your intake department access the HIQH database in order to verify the beneficiary's eligibility prior to admission?
- If an overlap with another agency is identified, who is the designated staff person who will call the other agency to resolve the overlap prior to admitting the patient to service?
- If an overlap is discovered after admission, who informs both agencies involved and how is the overlap resolved?
- How do you ensure that all patient visits are covered by the appropriate staff?
- If you have a scheduling department, what process is used to track patients to ensure visits are made per physician orders?
- What are the timelines in your agency for submitting documentation?
- Who monitors the timely receipt of documentation? Who ensures that the documentation is complete—whether electronic or paper?
- Is there a mechanism in place to ensure that consents and authorizations for payment are received and signed by the patient or personal representative?
- If visit documentation is electronic, do you have processes in place to ensure that visit notes are entered and completed within the timeframes delineated in your policies?
- Where in your flow are the paper/electronic bottlenecks?
- How quickly does the data flow to the medical record department?
- How long before the documentation is filed in the patient record?
- Who monitors timeliness and accuracy of filing? How often?
- How is this reported to management and compliance, as well as to the staff responsible?
- At what intervals are the patient records reviewed? Who is performing the review audit? What data are being reviewed? Who collects and trends the data? With whom and how is the data being shared?
- Who audits the auditors to ensure that the elements being captured are identified according to the established process?
- Who trends this data and how is this reported?
- An agency is at greater risk of noncompliance and fraud if the data being audited and the negative trends identified are not acted upon with further staff education and continued monitoring for compliance.
- If compliance risks are identified, who educates and establishes processes to ensure compliance? How is this information communicated to the staff and how is the data monitored to ensure compliance after training?
- How often is education provided to the staff? What type of monitoring/review is done after training to ensure compliance? How and to whom are the results communicated?
- Who analyzes the patient record upon discharge? What constitute a complete patient record?
- How is the identified data captured? To whom is this data communicated? How is the data shared?

Developing a multidisciplinary and multidepartmental flowchart involves input from all areas of the agency and can be a very time-consuming arduous task, but once complete, areas of risk will be obvious. Subcommittees or small multidepartmental task groups that would be responsible for reporting to a larger group may need to be formed to ensure all areas of risk that have been identified are addressed and processes or stop-gaps are formulated that will ensure compliance.

The use of laptop computers poses a multitude of risks. Policies need to be developed to ensure the security and integrity of each laptop and should include answers to the following questions:

- Where can they be stored in the office or out in the field?

- Where should they be kept in the clinician's vehicle?

- Who has access to the laptop? How is it secured in the clinician's home?

The press is full of stories of information destroyed or changed if the laptop is not protected from others (for example, children in the home). Seemingly, almost weekly the press is full of stories of laptops with health information being stolen. Although this chapter deals with compliance, it must be remembered that the agency must also comply with HIPAA privacy and security rules.

As systems change from paper to electronic, processes need to be reviewed and restructured to ensure compliance and to meet the regulatory and accreditation requirements. The health information manager must be a part of the committee that plans and effects this change. It is an ever-occurring challenge when system changes are made without notification to the affected departments. Information technology (IT) may perform upgrades or the vendor may change the program without including input from staff who will experience the effects of the change. Often employees are caught off-guard. Any change, no matter how insignificant it appears, needs to be discussed with a multidepartmental team. Change here also means consideration of the impact of processes that have been established for compliance and the education that staff must have concerning changes to ensure continued compliance.

Once processes are developed, the staff involved will need to be trained and a mechanism to monitor compliance with the new processes will need to be developed, monitored, and measured for success.

Ensuring that patient records are in compliance prior to dropping the RAP or the final claim for the episode is a huge area of risk for HHAs. Filing claims without the assurance of the accuracy of the claim submitted puts the agency at risk for allegations of fraud and abuse.

Admissions and recertification assessment data should be reviewed for identified areas of risk prior to completing the POC and locking the OASIS. This is done to ensure that the data being transmitted accurately describe the condition of the patient prior to dropping the RAP. See figure 11.4 for a list of required conditions.

In order to monitor compliance, it is suggested that the HHA conduct a random audit sampling of a minimum of 10 percent of patient episodes prior to billing the final claim for an episode to determine compliance. Some elements that should be monitored are listed in figure 11.5.

**Figure 11.4.   Conditions required for dropping a request for anticipated payment**

- Services ordered are medically necessary.
- The patient meets the criteria for homebound status.
- The OASIS and the admission documentation are consistent and support the need for the intensity of the services ordered.
- The documentation is reviewed to ensure MO175 (Inpatient facilities that the patient was discharged from in the past 14 days) was answered appropriately.
- There is documentation stating that verbal orders for authorization and approval of the POC were obtained from the physician authorized to sign the POC and that this documentation is contained in the record for each discipline ordered.
- The ordering physician on the POC and identified on the OASIS (MO072) is the same as the physician who will be responsible for following the patient and signing the POC.
- The diagnosis reported accurately represents the patient's condition and is reported in appropriate sequence and in accordance to ICD-9-CM guidelines.
- The diagnosis on the OASIS and the POC are congruent.
- The assessment documentation supports the ICD-9-CM codes reported.
- If "yes" is answered to MO825 (high threshold therapy visits), the documentation of the patient's condition supports this answer.
- If "yes" is reported in MO825 and the episode ends with less than 10 therapy visits, the HHA payment could be adjusted down $1,500 to $2,500 depending of the MSA factor.
- If "no" is reported in MO825 (high threshold therapy visits) and 10 or more therapy visits were made, the HHA cannot recapture the reimbursement lost in the Request for Anticipated form or in the final bill.
- An authorization for payment has been signed by the patient or the patient's personal representative for each discipline ordered by the physician.

**Figure 11.5.   Suggested auditing items prior to final claim**

- Documentation of receipt of a telephone call from the physician of record for authorization and approval of the POC for each discipline ordered.
- Physician has signed and dated the POC. The signed POC is filed in the record. The POC was signed in a timely manner.
- Verbal orders obtained within the episode are signed and dated by the physician who gave the order.
- There is documentation in the record that indicates that the verbal order was obtained prior to the services being rendered.
- The ICD-9-CM diagnoses codes reported on the POC, OASIS, and the claim form match. The codes are sequenced in the same order and are valid and follow official coding guidelines.
- There is documentation for each visit identified on the claim form. The claim form depicts each visit in units of time (each unit is 15 minutes). The visit was performed as ordered by the physician.
- The visits support the frequency and duration as ordered by the physician. If PRN visits are authorized on the POC, the amount and specific purpose for the PRN visits are stated on the order and the PRN visit was performed for that specific purpose.
- Were visits made not frequent enough or too frequent? Do visits have to be made nonbillable or deleted due to overfrequency, no skill service documented on the visit note, documentation does not support physician orders, or no note to support the visit billed? Is there a communication note with an explanation and a documented call to the physician when visits were not rendered per orders?
- All corrections to the documentation have been made according to regulations and agency policy.
- There is an end date for daily visits that exceed 21 consecutive days.

Any other areas of risk and/or noncompliance identified in the random audit should be included on the prebilling audit. Depending on the outcome of the random audit, a decision will need to be made as to what percentage of episodes will be audited prior to dropping the final bill for the episode.

If your agency determines that a percentage of or all final episodes will be audited prior to submitting the final claim, the agency will need to determine who is best qualified to perform this audit. What skills will be required? How will training take place? What resources are available to accomplish this task? Who will have oversight of this process?

Who will continue to audit the auditors to ensure that compliance is maintained and that the auditors review is accurate, and how will this be done? How will ongoing education take place?

Again, once areas of risk and noncompliance are identified, staff education will need to be developed and staff training presented and documented. A process will need to be put into place to monitor compliance after the training is complete.

## Preventing Overlap with Another Agency

It is not unusual for an HHA to experience an overlap of service with another HHA. An overlap can occur prior to a referral for admission (another agency is already involved in the patient's care) or any time during the episode. Often an overlap is discovered when an agency submits a final claim for an episode and discovers that its episode has been discharged by Medicare or the agency receives a call from another agency that similarly has been affected.

It is critical that an HHA check beneficiary eligibility after a referral is received to ensure that no other agency is providing skilled services to the beneficiary prior to admitting the patient to service.

The Health Insurance Query for Home Health (HIQH) is an inquiry screen developed by Medicare in order to provide HHAs with beneficiary data. The eligibility screen will allow an HHA to view the following:

- Health insurance claim numbers

- Medicare entitlement dates

- Medicare secondary payer information

- HMO information

- HH PPS episode dates (start and end date and provider number). This data will indicate if the beneficiary is already in a 60-day episode with another HHA

- HH benefit period data

- Hospice benefit period date

If another agency had admitted the patient prior to your admission, then according to CMS the other agency's admission takes priority and you must cancel your claim. If a determination cannot be made, an agency may notify the Medicare Transfer Dispute office to settle the dispute. The Transfer Dispute arbitrator will request specific documentation from both agencies. One document that is requested is a copy of the HIQH screen that was printed at the time of admission. This screen will show any involvement that the patient may have had with another agency at the time of your admission (CMS 2003).

Outpatient rehabilitation providers are also impacted by HH PPS consolidated billing and should verify the beneficiary's eligibility on the HIQH screen. Consolidated billing rules stipulate that, if services are provided and no contract exists between the HHA and the outpatient provider, the HHA is under no obligation to reimburse the provider for services (CMS 2003).

The outpatient rehabilitation provider is unable to bill for services rendered if the HIQH screen still shows the beneficiary as active with the HHA or the HHA reports a discharge date that is later than the beneficiary's start of outpatient services. If the outpatient rehabilitation facility discovers the overlap, they will need to contact the HHA to reconcile the discrepancy.

## Improper Reimbursement

There can be times when, even after consistent diligent internal audits, a patient episode can be reviewed and determination made that the episode was billed inappropriately. Sometimes the supporting documentation required to bill is incomplete, inconsistent, or missing or physician orders or the patient's condition do not support the services rendered. The HHA is required to reimburse Medicare (or any other secondary payer) for services paid for which they were not entitled to payment. If such an occurrence is identified, the HHA should perform a random sample audit to determine if this is an area of omission from their audits and the frequency of the occurrence in order to identify the need to intensify or refocus their audit.

If a violation of any compliance or regulatory mandate is discovered, the agency must perform a root cause analysis and document its findings, process changes and education given to the staff as a result of the analysis. Any episodes identified in this audit that require reimbursement to Medicare must be accounted for and repayment made. Self-reporting is critical to your integrity and solvency as an agency.

## Internal and External Audit Reviews

Each episode or each piece of documentation must be able to withstand an internal or external audit review. Each document needs to be legible and dated with the date that it was written and signed by the author along with the author's credentials (such as registered nurse–RN, physical therapist–PT, occupational therapist–OT, speech therapist-ST, or master of social work–MSW). The documentation must support the reimbursement received and justify the patient's condition and need for home care services. Physician orders must be carried out as written. Any change in the patient's condition must be documented along with notification of the change to the patient's physician and the physician's response to the change in the patient's condition.

All audit tools, trending results, process changes, and evidence of staff education needs to be maintained in order to support and justify determinations made by the agency.

If an agency is part of a large integrated healthcare system, the corporate compliance department may conduct an audit of the agency's medical records as well as the billing records. Depending on the results of their audit, the corporate compliance department will determine whether or not a more intensive audit is warranted.

The purpose of a compliance audit is to identify any discrepancies or flaws in processes, audits, or documentation practices in order to assist the agency in formulating better practices. An audit from the compliance department should be welcomed. The agency staff should be forthcoming with information and answer the auditors' questions honestly and not just tell the auditors "what they want to know." They are part of your team. Often it may feel as if the compliance auditors are dissecting your policies and procedures, processes, and documentation, and they are. But their reasoning is usually sound, and as a result of their reviews, the auditors can and will offer many educational opportunities that will assist the agency in achieving its goals of regulatory compliance. The compliance department also, through their audits, gathers the data necessary to support and defend the agency if the agency is served a subpoena for an external audit.

Whether or not an agency belongs to an integrated health system or is a small independent HHA, the agency should have a mechanism in place to perform compliance audits. If the HHA cannot provide the audit, it is recommended that an outside auditing firm be contracted to perform audits of the medical and billing records annually. Whether annual audits are performed internally or externally or a combination of both, it is critical that an audit be conducted.

If the agency is served a subpoena by the OIG, the only recourse is to comply with the mandates of the subpoena. A subpoena can be served as a result of a "qui tam"—in which an employee files an accusation with the Department of Justice that the agency is fraudulent—or by noncompliant reporting and/or billing practices.

The executive director or the head of the agency is usually the person specified on the subpoena. If the subpoena is received by another employee who is designated to receive subpoenas, that employee must hand deliver the subpoena to the person named. The individual cited on the subpoena will review the mandates listed on the court document and contact the agency's legal counsel for advice. The chief compliance officer will also be notified.

If the subpoena lists specific records that the agency must produce, the order is generally for the original records. The agency must make copies of any records or original documentation that are ordered to be delivered. A listing of all documentation requested and sent needs to be maintained. The amount of time and the employees involved in complying with the mandates of the subpoena must be tracked. The time and the salary of the personnel dedicated to complying with the subpoena needs to be reported.

Determination results from an external audit could take several years, depending on the initial findings. As a result of the audit and based on the documentation reviewed, the OIG will make a determination as to whether or not the agency was involved in fraud and/or abuse or whether the agency was paid inappropriately for services rendered.

Any amount of money that the OIG determines must be repaid to Medicare becomes public record and is subject to disclosure. Such an occurrence is not only a costly financial situation, but the resulting disclosure could severely damage the reputation of the agency or corporation, affecting referrals and potentially resulting in audits from other payers.

## Reimbursement Issues

As of June 2006, an OASIS assessment is required to be "locked" within 30 days of the assessment. Because the OASIS assessment is sent electronically, it must be locked before it is sent to the state and cannot be further altered in order to maintain integrity. Even though CMS allows 30 days, it is important to remember that the HHA must lock and transmit the OASIS assessment before a RAP can be submitted.

HHAs need to establish processes to ensure that physician orders are received and properly documented prior to billing for services. A leading reason for home health claims denials is failure to obtain physician orders in a timely manner.

Appropriate selection and reporting of ICD-9-CM codes are directly linked to proper reimbursement. Because reported codes impact the clinical dimension in the HHRGs, resulting in a direct impact on reimbursement, accurate ICD-9-CM reporting is critical. Some diagnoses affecting the clinical dimension can never be reported as the principal or primary diagnosis, according to ICD-9-CM coding rules. These diagnoses are represented by manifestation codes, and ICD-9-CM rules require the code for the etiology be sequenced first.

In those instances in which ICD-9-CM rules stipulate the proper sequencing of an etiology/manifestation pair of codes, accurate coding of both the etiology and the manifestation is required in order to ensure proper reimbursement. According to the HH PPS regulation, the manifestation codes affecting HHRG assignment, which cannot be sequenced as the first diagnosis, must be reported as the first secondary diagnosis in order to impact the clinical dimension of the HHRGs. In this circumstance, the primary diagnosis is indicated by the combination of the manifestation code (in the first secondary diagnosis field) and the code for the underlying disease (in the primary diagnosis field).

Even when the reported ICD-9-CM diagnosis codes do not impact the clinical dimension in the home health case-mix system, they support medical necessity of the home health services provided. Complete and accurate coding of the primary and secondary diagnosis also ensures the collection of accurate data for refinement of the case-mix system.

Agencies are required to determine the primary diagnosis based on the condition that is most related to the current POC. Skilled services (skilled nursing services, physical therapy, speech therapy, and occupational therapy) should be used in determining the relevancy of a diagnosis to the POC. The primary diagnosis reported on OASIS (MO230) must match the principal diagnosis reported on the claim form as well as the primary/principal diagnosis on the POC (HCFA 485, field 1). The primary/principal diagnosis may or may not be related to the patient's most recent hospital stay but must relate to the services provided by the agency. If more than one diagnosis is being treated concurrently, the diagnosis that represents the most acute condition and requires the most intensive services should be reported.

When a V code is the appropriate primary/principal diagnosis (according to the *ICD-9-CM Official Guidelines for Coding and Reporting*), and the V code replaces a case-mix diagnosis code as the primary/principal diagnosis, the case-mix diagnosis code is reported in the "payment diagnosis" field (MO245). If the patient's case-mix diagnosis involves a combination of an etiology and a manifestation code, the etiology code is reported in MO245 (a) and the manifestation code in MO245 (b).

All secondary diagnoses that are being treated or affect the patient's treatment or care, even when the condition is not the focus of care, should be reported. Diagnoses that relate to an earlier episode and have no bearing on the current POC should be excluded. The secondary diagnoses on OASIS (MO240) must match the secondary diagnosis reported on the claim form and the POC (HCFA 485).

All reported codes must be supported by physician documentation in the health record. A lack of physician documentation for codes that impact an HHRG assignment causes a serious compliance risk. Codes for conditions that are resolved or healed, or no longer affect the patient's POC, should not be reported. When clarification of a diagnosis is necessary, the physician should be contacted. When clarification of a diagnosis is received from the physician over the telephone, it should be documented in the patient's health record. A standardized physician query form may be completed and forwarded to the physician for completion. The query form provides physician documentation to clarify the patient's diagnosis or condition and may be utilized when, and if, an agency comes under scrutiny for medical necessity determination, ADR, or other government audit.

Medical reviewers at the regional home health intermediary (RHHI) review case-mix accuracy on a postpayment basis. By comparing final claims with health records, the reviewers can ensure that the requirements for home health coverage have been met and that the services provided were reasonable, necessary, and documented appropriately. They also compare the OASIS information with the health record to verify that OASIS information is supported by the documentation in the health record. When the RHHI determines that a case-mix assignment is not appropriate, it adjusts the case mix accordingly. Many causes of downcoding by the RHHIs are related to the fact that OASIS information on an assessment does not substantiate the assigned HHRG. In some instances, the documentation is in direct conflict with the HHRG assignment.

Compliance risks include upcoding or downcoding (such as improper selection of the primary diagnosis or reporting an incorrect code for the primary diagnosis) and improper sequencing (such as reporting a secondary diagnosis as the primary diagnosis or disregarding mandatory ICD-9-CM rules regarding proper sequencing). For example, incorrectly reporting the traumatic open wound ICD-9-CM codes for a postoperative wound is a compliance risk when it involves the primary diagnosis because a condition impacting the clinical dimension of HHRG assignment is being reported improperly. Coding a skin ulcer as a diabetic complication when there is no documentation linking the ulcer to the diabetes also is a compliance risk because a diabetic ulcer impacts the clinical dimension (due to the coding rule that requires the diabetes code to be sequenced first), but a nondiabetic skin ulcer does not.

Code jamming is another potential compliance risk. Code jamming involves selection of a code to ensure payment without regard to the patient's condition or services rendered. Examples that can occur include the following:

- Adding a fifth digit to create a valid code without verifying the presence of physician documentation to support the fifth digit assignment
- Reporting a more specific code than is supported by physician documentation (because certain nonspecific codes may result in claims rejections)

- Use of software programs that force a limited code selection by not displaying all possible code choices or applicable instructional notes for proper code selection

Conducting regular ICD-9-CM coding audits in which health record documentation is checked against the codes is crucial to ensure compliance with Medicare PPS. Such audits of coded data should be performed on a regular basis. In this way, errors or patterns of errors can be identified and processes can be monitored. Educating administrators, key managers, and the governing board is important to achieve full support for auditing. Managers and supervisors need to understand that coding reviews and audits can benefit the organization in the following ways:

- Improving operational efficiency
- Mitigating damages in the event of an investigation
- Protecting against certain legal exposure
- Improving overall data quality
- Ensuring reliable data for outcome-based quality management reporting

## Home Health Advance Beneficiary Notice

The Home Health Advance Beneficiary Notice (HHABN) is designed to both protect the beneficiary and to keep the beneficiary informed and involved in his or her home health care services. A significant change to the issuance of an HHABN became effective September 1, 2006 (CMS 2006).

The change was brought about as the result of a case issued by a group of homebound Medicare patients (*Lutwin v. Thompson* 2004). The plaintiffs stated that HHAs rarely consulted their physicians regarding the reduction or termination of their services and that they themselves were not informed when services were reduced and sometimes terminated. The plaintiffs wanted a "more meaningful" notice as well as rights to appeal when an HHA made a decision to reduce or terminate their services. The patients wanted more involvement in decisions that were being made about their care.

Several physicians were interviewed during the hearings. The physicians agreed that they were seldom notified by HHAs when their patients' treatment was reduced or terminated.

As a result of the court's ruling, Medicare statute now requires that HHAs provide a Notice whenever services are reduced or terminated, regardless of the reason (*Lutwin v. Thompson* 2004).

An HHABN is determined to be invalid if the following occur:

- Abbreviations are used to explain the services provided or reasons for denial of services, for example, physical therapy is abbreviated as PT, or homebound is listed as HB.
- The font is alternated or the form is reformatted.

- The form is not signed and dated by the beneficiary. Note: If the patient is physically unable to sign the HHABN, (for example, patient has 2 broken arms) but is fully capable of clearly understanding the contents and implication of the HHABN, the clinician may sign and date the notice under the direction of the beneficiary, inserting the beneficiary's name along with his or her own name—for example: "John Jones, RN, signing for Susie Smith." The signer must document that the beneficiary was present and comprehended the contents of the HHABN, but was unable to sign. The reason the beneficiary was unable to sign must be documented on the HHABN. Whenever possible, a second witness present at the time should also sign the annotation. The medical record documentation must support the description of the beneficiary's condition.

Three events will trigger an HHA to provide an HHABN to a beneficiary as well as three different forms (referred to as "option boxes" by Medicare). The selection of the appropriate form, or option box, is determined by the triggering event. The triggering events are service initiation, service reduction, and service termination.

## Service Initiation

Following are four options for service initiation:

1. If, upon admission of the patient, it is determined that the patient does not meet the criteria under Medicare guidelines for home health services, but the patient and/or patient caregiver has requested to self-pay for services (option box 1).

2. The beneficiary does not meet Medicare criteria for home health benefit but the patient/caregiver requests that the HHA bill their private insurance (option box 1).

3. The beneficiary has Medicare as secondary insurance and the patient does not meet criteria for services under Medicare guidelines (option box 1).

4. The HHA determines that the beneficiary does not meet Medicare criteria but the beneficiary requests that Medicare and/or private insurance be billed for services in order to determine eligibility and the beneficiary agrees to pay for services if Medicare and/or private insurance determines that the patient does not meet the criteria for HHA benefits (option box 1).

The beneficiary may wish to receive HHA services and wants to obtain an official decision from Medicare. In this situation, condition code 20 will be reported in form locator (FL) 24–30 of the UB-92/UB-04. Medicare review staff is required to review all claims with condition code 20. Medical record documentation will be requested through an ADR. This is often referred to as a "demand denial." The medical review staff will not call requesting missing HHABNs. The medical review staff will make a determination on the accuracy of the HHRG and HIPPS.

The HHABN would not be required if the beneficiary met the criteria for services under Medicare or if the beneficiary is seen but not admitted to the HHA.

## Service Reduction

The following five options exist for service initiation:

1. The physician determines that services ordered on admission should be reduced during the certification period because the beneficiary's progress toward meeting goals is faster than anticipated (option box 3).

2. The frequency at which supplies are ordered for the beneficiary has been reduced (option box 3).

3. Services determined at admission are reduced at recertification (option box 3).

4. Services determined at admission (or recertification) are reduced on the plan for ROC (option box 3).

5. The beneficiary is receiving a nonbillable service (such as dietitian services) in conjunction with a qualifying service and the nonbillable service is reduced (option box 3).

An HHABN is not required if the frequency or the services provided to a beneficiary increases or if the beneficiary/caregiver chooses to reduce services. However, if the HHA is increasing services for a patient who is receiving noncovered care and is self-paying for the services, the patient should be notified in advance of the increase in care and the expected increase in payment.

## Service Termination

The following four factors affect service termination:

1. The HHA determines that services will be terminated, because of the following:

   - Lack of staffing

   - Agency financial considerations

   - Employee safety

   - Patient noncompliance

2. Because the termination of services for the above reasons are not related to the beneficiary's Medicare benefit coverage, the HHA is required to complete option box 2.

3. The beneficiary's Medicare coverage has terminated, but the patient chooses to continue care (option box 1).

4. The beneficiary is discharged from the HHA prior to the signed POC (option box 1).

See appendix 11B (pp. 219–222) for more information.

If the beneficiary is transferring to another covered service or another HHA or Medicare provider, the HHABN is not required to be completed. The HHABN is also not required if all goals are met and all disciplines are discharging at the same time.

If an HHA has agreed to provide only noncovered services after the beneficiary's Medicare coverage has ended, the HHA must issue both the HHABN (option box 1) and the generic Expedited Determination Notice (this notice will be discussed later in this section).

The HHABN is not required to be completed in the following circumstances:

- The visit length is reduced, but the frequency remains the same.

- Reduction in service(s) is consistent with the orders on the original POC.

- The beneficiary requests that services be reduced or terminated.

- The reduction of services is due to an emergency or natural disaster.

- An ordered skilled visit is missed. (The reason for the missed visit and the notification of the physician should be documented.)

The HHABN must be written (preferably printed) clearly. No abbreviations can be used. The reason the HHABN is being issued must be documented in terms that can be easily understood. The clinician presenting the HHABN must explain the contents of the form as well as the implications of the content. The cost of providing services must also be clearly documented so that the beneficiary has full knowledge of the potential cost that may be incurred should he or she choose to continue service.

An HHABN is effective for 12 months. If the beneficiary chooses to continue noncovered services after that period of time, a new HHABN must be completed.

At any time when completion of an HHABN is mandated and the beneficiary refuses to sign, the HHA must document the beneficiary refusal and provide a copy of the annotated HHABN to the beneficiary.

## Notification of Planned Discharge and the Medicare Patient's Right to Appeal the Discharge Decision

As of July 1, 2005, HHAs were mandated by Medicare to provide its beneficiaries with a Notice of Medicare Provider Noncoverage a minimum of 2 days prior to anticipated discharge of all skilled services. This notice informs the beneficiary in writing of the HHA's plan to discharge all skilled services. The notice also lists the beneficiary's right to appeal to the Quality Improvement Organization (QIO) and the process of how to request an appeal should the beneficiary think that skilled services were still applicable under his or her home health benefit.

If the beneficiary requests an appeal, the HHA will be notified and asked to produce the medical records within 12 hours of the request. The QIO will review the documentation and advise both the patient and the HHA of its determination.

If the QIO finds in favor of the beneficiary, the HHA will continue to provide skilled services to the patient until such a time that the provider identifies that the beneficiary no longer meets criteria for home health benefits. Then, a second notice will be provided to the patient following the same criteria as the first. The beneficiary again has the right to appeal the decision to terminate services and would follow the same format as the first appeal.

Not all discharges from HHAs require that a notice be delivered. Circumstances that do not require an expedited appeal notice include the following:

- Patients that are seen by a practitioner but are not admitted
- Termination of some, but not all, skilled services
- Beneficiary request to discontinue care
- Unsafe situations for agency personnel or the patient
- Hospitalization or transfer to a rehabilitation facility
- Skilled nursing home placement (does not include custodial care)
- Transfer of a patient to another Medicare Certified HHA
- Beneficiary relocation
- Beneficiary noncompliance
- Death

Situations that require notification be delivered include the following:

- Treatments are no longer medically necessary for the beneficiary's illness or injury
- Teaching has been completed
- Medical condition has stabilized
- Homebound requirement is no longer met
- Physician orders are terminated
- Goals of care have been attained

Following are the exceptions to the notification delivery rules:

- The 2 days prior rule does not apply when beneficiaries are on service fewer than 2 days or in cases of unanticipated changes to coverage (physician orders discontinuation of covered services, patient announces frequent absences from home, or patient announces that the physician is sending the patient to outpatient treatment(s).
- Notices may be mailed (return receipt requested) rather than hand-delivered following telephone notification of beneficiaries, if discontinuation of coverage is

unexpected. Documentation must clearly support the reason for less than a 2-day delivery of notice.

This notice fulfills the requirement at 42 CFR 405.1200(b), if the patient meets the criteria listed above that requires that the Notification of Planned Discharge and the Medicare Patient's Right to Appeal the Discharge Decision.

This notice must be validly delivered. A valid delivery means that the beneficiary must be able to understand the purpose and contents of the notice in order to sign for receipt of the notice. The beneficiary must be able to understand that he or she may appeal the termination decision. If the beneficiary is not able to comprehend the contents of the notice, it must be delivered to and signed by the authorized representative. Valid delivery does not preclude the use of assistive devices, witnesses, or interpreters for notice delivery.

If the beneficiary refuses to sign the notice, the notice is still valid as long as the provider documents that the notice was given but the beneficiary refused to sign.

CMS requires that notification of changes in coverage for a beneficiary who is not competent be made to an authorized representative acting on behalf of the beneficiary. Notification to the authorized representative may be problematic because he or she may not be available in person to acknowledge receipt of the required notification. HHAs are required to develop procedures to use when the beneficiary is incapable or incompetent and the provider cannot obtain the signature of the beneficiary's representative through personal contact. Additional requirements are described in figure 11.6.

**Figure 11.6.   Requirements for notification of changes in coverage**

- If the provider is unable to personally deliver a notice of no coverage, then the provider should telephone the representative to advise that person of when the beneficiary's services are no longer covered.

- The beneficiary's appeal rights must be explained to the representative and the name and the telephone number of the appropriate QIO should be provided.

- The date of the conversation is the date of receipt of notice. The written notice must be sent to the personal representative the same day.

- A dated copy must be placed in the medical record. The telephone call documentation should also be place in the medical record.

- The telephone documentation will include at a minimum the following:

  —Name of the person who made the contact

  —Name of the representative contacted

  —Date and time of the contact

  —The telephone number called

- When a direct telephone call cannot be made, the notice is sent to the representative by certified mail, return receipt requested.

- The date that someone at the representative's address signs (or refuses to sign) the receipt is the date of the receipt.

- When notices are returned by the post office with no indication of a refusal date, then the beneficiary's liability starts on the second working day after the provider's mailed date.

HHAs must formulate a process that delineates who is responsible to receive the telephone call from the QIO and facilitate transmittal of the required documentation.

## Dual Notices

Situations in which both an expedited appeal notice and an HHABN are required include the following:

- All services are determined to no longer be covered by Medicare, but the beneficiary's physician has ordered continuation of services.

- The patient qualifies under the Medicare benefit for specific skilled service, but not for others (skilled nursing and occupational therapy are ordered by the physician, but the beneficiary does not qualify for occupational therapy because goals have been attained and maximum potential has been reached).

## Auditing and Monitoring

The OIG recommends that a process be established and maintained for presubmission and postsubmission review of claims (a valid statistical sample) to ensure that claims submitted for reimbursement accurately represent medically necessary services actually provided, supported by sufficient documentation and in conformity with any applicable coverage criteria for reimbursement (for example, a POC is dated and signed by the physician; the beneficiary is homebound; skilled service is required). Oversight mechanisms should be put in place to ensure that homebound status, as required by Medicare home health coverage, is verified and the specific factors qualifying the patient as homebound are properly documented. Clinical note forms that trigger a clinician to address specific requirements might help to ensure complete documentation of a patient's homebound status.

Because of the reliance of the home health PPS on OASIS data, it is imperative that measures are taken to ensure that the OASIS data are complete and accurate and that staff who complete and review the OASIS data have ongoing training in the requirements pertaining to reporting and completing the elements contained in the OASIS. Because an agency is paid based on an episode of care, there is a risk that an incentive could be created to either decrease the amount of services provided to patients or to portray patients as sicker than they really are, resulting in either overutilization or underutilization of services.

There is also a risk that an agency will answer "yes" to MO825 in order to receive a higher payment when a high threshold of therapy visits is not supported by the patient's condition or the documentation.

Because OASIS links the patient's clinical status to payment, accurate data are needed to ensure that reimbursement is appropriate for the patient's condition and the services rendered. Because the primary and secondary diagnoses are reported using ICD-9-CM codes, OASIS data must be supported by documentation in the health record.

The HHA must ensure that only current ICD-9-CM coding books are used to report codes and that the codes reported adhere to the current *ICD-9-CM Official Guidelines for*

*Coding and Reporting.* As of October 2004, ICD-9-CM codes are updated twice a year (October and April). *Coding Clinic,* which is published by the American Hospital Association (AHA) is the official publication for ICD-9-CM coding advice provided by the four Cooperating Parties (AHA, AHIMA, CMS, and the National Center for Health Statistics) and the Editorial Advisory Board. *Coding Clinic* is published quarterly and should be an accessible resource for any HHA in order to determine the correct reporting and sequencing of ICD-9-CM codes. *Coding Clinic* advice is effective upon being published. Using the advice and directions given in *Coding Clinic* will provide an HHA with support to justify its selection of ICD-9-CM codes and training provided to essential staff if involved in a compliance investigation.

Where there is a discrepancy, OASIS coding and reporting guidelines take precedence as it relates to MO245a and MO245b only. However, with the implementation of the HIPAA Coding and Transaction Data Set Rule (October 2003), there should no longer be a disparity because this regulation stipulates that all healthcare entities must conform to the *ICD-9-CM Official Guidelines for Coding and Reporting.* The OASIS "Payment Diagnosis" (MO245) had been developed to ensure that HHAs were able to continue to report case-mix diagnoses when a V code was required to be reported in MO230 and it replaced the case-mix diagnosis. Staff responsible for reporting and reviewing ICD-9-CM codes should be trained in current coding conventions. Auditing of code utilization as it pertains to the patient record needs to be established with a mechanism to trend and report any inconsistencies, omissions, or improper coding. Ongoing education should be based on the trended results identified in the audit.

Auditing and monitoring activities should encompass the quality of the health record documentation and whether the record supports the billed services. These reviews should include an assessment of the items listed in figure 11.7.

**Figure 11.7.  Auditing documentation of home health services**

---

- Were the services the physician ordered appropriately delivered? If not, is there appropriate documentation or a new physician's order to explain why?

- Are all physician orders signed and dated?

- Is there documentation to support authorization from the physician?

- Are all billed visits supported by health record documentation?

- Are visits entered within the established timeframe?

- Does the diagnostic information in the health record match the diagnosis codes reported on the OASIS assessment and the claim form?

- Does the health record documentation support the "points" assigned for the OASIS date elements that impact HHRG assignment?

- Does the primary diagnosis assigned at the SOC reflect the focus of services provided?

- Does the patient record for each billing episode substantiate the reported primary diagnosis?

- Were unreported diagnoses documented that might have affected the HHRG assignment?

- Were any coding errors identified, such as codes that do not match the patient's diagnosis, or do not reflect the specificity documented in the record, codes that are sequenced incorrectly, or codes that violate coding rules or guidelines?

---

All auditing and monitoring documentation must be maintained in order to support the claim. Data obtained from these audits should be trended to identify areas for quality improvement. An HHA is at risk for noncompliance and/or fraud if data are obtained upon audits that identify areas of inconsistency or omission and the agency does not take corrective action. If trends are identified, education and training must be put into place to correct the issues identified. The contents of the training, the staff trained, and the date the training took place must be documented. After training has been completed, the agency will need to re-audit to ensure that the areas of concern have been corrected.

Auditing of the audit is key to maintaining compliance. A random sample of episodes audited should be pulled and re-audited prior to final billing in order to ensure that all elements on the audit tool are being addressed and that the bill is adjusted when omissions are identified or in the absence of the supporting documentation to substantiate reimbursement. The results of this audit should be compiled on an ongoing basis and reported to the agency's senior management. Reports should be reviewed on a regular basis in order to identify trends and/or areas of omission or inconsistency. The report also serves to provide feedback to the auditor(s) and affords an opportunity for quality improvement. If areas of omission or inconsistency are identified in the audit, educational training needs to be provided and documented. The audit of the auditors will continue to ensure that the education provided resolved the issues identified.

## Revenue Cycle Team

Many organizations have established a revenue cycle team to reduce risk and facilitate timely reimbursement of claims. These teams are multidisciplinary and include staff from patient accounts, finance, clinical, coding, business operations, and medical records to ensure that processes are in place so that the claims that are filed meet the regulations established by the HHPPS.

As each department has its own challenges and areas of risk, this multidisciplinary team is able to look at the entire flow of processes and identify the impact that each process has on the various departments throughout the agency. The process should allow for brainstorming of issues, prioritizing the issues, selecting issues according to criticality (achieved through a consensus), formulating subcommittees to investigate and change a process if necessary, implement the process change, monitor the effectiveness and impact of the process change, and make further recommendations. The monitoring of the change is ongoing. Each subcommittee reports progress back to the main team. Issues that have been resolved are closed. The team then votes on the next issues to investigate and subcommittees are formed, and the process continues until all issues identified have been resolved.

Ensuring compliance in a home health environment requires diligent monitoring, auditing, ongoing education, being aware of any changes in coding and reimbursement guidelines or requirements, and being proactive in ongoing review and update of policies and procedures to ensure compliance with practice and policies.

Compliance cannot be the responsibility of any one person or department. It is a team effort and the entire agency is part of that team. One broken link in the chain can subject an agency to relentless audits and reviews by the OIG, the Department of Justice, or Medicare and distrust by the community that is being served. Compliance is not just about following the rules because of the threat of audit, damage to reputation, or fines. Compliance is about doing the right things for our patients because that is what is in their best interest and that is our mission.

## References and Resources

Abraham, P.R. 2001. *Documentation and Reimbursement for Home Care and Hospice Programs.* Chicago: AHIMA.

Cahaba GBA. 2006 (August). Coverage guidelines for home health agencies: Medicare fiscal intermediary. Available online from https://www.cahabagba.com/part_a/education_and_outreach/educational_materials/hh_coverage.pdf.

Cahaba GBA. 2006 (March 28). What happened to the HHABN?!? Created under contract for Centers for Medicare and Medicaid Services.

Centers for Medicare and Medicaid Services. 2006 (Aug. 4). Beneficiary notices initiative. Available online from http://www.cms.hhs.gov/BNI/03_HHABN.asp.

Centers for Medicare and Medicaid Services. 2006 (Jan. 4). Prospective payment systems: General information. HIPPS codes. Available online from http://www.cms.hhs.gov/ProspMedicareFeeSvcPmtGen/02_HIPPSCodes.asp.

Centers for Medicare and Medicaid Services. 2005a. OASIS user's manual. Available online from http://www.cms.hhs.gov/OASIS/.

Centers for Medicare and Medicaid Services. 2005b (Aug. 12). Medicare benefit policy manual, Pub. 100-2, revision 27. Chapter 7: Home health services, item 30.1: Confined to the home. Available online from http://www.cms.hhs.gov/Manuals/.

Centers for Medicare and Medicaid Services. 2005 (Aug. 11). Medicare benefit policy manual, home health services. CMS Pub. 100-02, Ch 7 30.1. Available online from www.cms.hhs.gov/Manuals/iom/list.asp.

Centers for Medicare and Medicaid Services. 2003 (March 13). Program Memorandum—Carriers. Transmittal B-03-021, change request 2619. Provider education regarding home health consolidated billing (HH CB) and provider liability, Pub. 60B. Available online from http://www.cms.hhs.gov/transmittals/Downloads/b03021.pdf.

Government Accountability Office. 2005 (Dec. 15). Information on false claims act litigation: Briefing for Congressional requesters. Document no. GAO-06-320R. Available online from http://www.gao.gov/new.items/d06320r.pdf.

Health Care Financing Administration. 2000 (July 3). Medicare program; prospective payment system for home health agencies; final rule. 42 CFR 409, 410, 411, 413, 424, and 484. *Federal Register* 65(128):41127–214.

*Lutwin v. Thompson,* 361 F.3d. 136(2d.Cir 2004).

Office of the Inspector General. 2006. Work Plan, fiscal year 2007. Available online from http://www.oig.hhs.gov/publications/docs/workplan/2007/Work%20Plan%202007.pdf

Office of the Inspector General. 2006 (March). Consultations in Medicare: coding and reimbursement. Document no. OEI-09-02-00030. Available online from http://oig.hhs.gov/oei/reports/oei-09-02-00030.pdf.

Office of the Inspector General. 2006 (January). Review of billing under the home health prospective payment system for therapy services. Document no. A-07-04-01010. Available online from http://www.oig.hhs.gov/oas/reports/region7/70401010.pdf.

Office of the Inspector General. 2006 (January). Effect of the home health prospective payment system on the quality of home health care. Document no. OEI-01-04-00160. Available online from http://oig.hhs.gov/oei/reports/oei-09-02-00030.pdf.

Scichilone, R. 2004 (June 7). AHIMA home health services coding and reporting. Handouts from Continuing Education online course, Reimbursement Methods, Lesson 3.

# Appendix 11A
# HIPPS Conversion Table

| HIPPS Conversion Table | | | | |
|---|---|---|---|---|
| The first position of every home health HIPPS code will be "H." | | | | |
| **Position 2 Clinical Domain** | **Position 3 Functional Domain** | **Position 4 Service Domain** | **Domain Level** | **Position 5 "Data Validity flag"** |
| A | E | J | = min | **1** = 2nd, 3rd, & 4th positions computed |
| B | F | K | = low | **2** = 2nd position derived |
| C | G | L | = mod | **3** = 3rd position derived |
| D | H | M | = high | **4** = 4th position derived |
| | I | | = max | **5** = 2nd & 3rd positions derived |
| | | | | **6** = 3rd & 4th positions derived |
| | | | | **7** = 2nd & 4th positions derived |
| | | | | **8** = 2nd, 3rd & 4th positions derived |
| | | N through Z | Expansion value for future use | **9, 0** |

HIPPS Code Maintenance Process (Version 2)
CMS Division of Institutional Claims Processing

| HHRG Description | Case Mix Description by Domains | HIPPS Code | Weight | Fallback HIPPS Code | Fallback code weight |
|---|---|---|---|---|---|
| **HIPPS Table for Pricer** | | | | | |
| C0F0S0-all computed | Clinical=Min,Functional=Min,Service=Min | **HAEJ1** | **0.5265** | **na** | **na** |
| 2nd position derived | | HAEJ2 | 0.5265 | na | na |
| 3rd position derived | | **HAEJ3** | **0.5265** | **na** | **na** |
| 4th position derived | | HAEJ4 | 0.5265 | na | na |
| 2nd & 3rd derived | | **HAEJ5** | **0.5265** | **na** | **na** |
| 3rd & 4th derived | | HAEJ6 | 0.5265 | na | na |
| 2nd& 4th derived | | **HAEJ7** | **0.5265** | **na** | **na** |
| All derived | | HAEJ8 | 0.5265 | na | na |
| C0F0S1 | Clinical=Min,Functional=Min,Service=Low | **HAEK1** | **0.6074** | **na** | **na** |
| *Above pattern repeats* | | HAEK2 | 0.6074 | na | na |
| *for all HHRG blocks* | | **HAEK3** | **0.6074** | **na** | **na** |
| | | HAEK4 | 0.6074 | na | na |
| | | **HAEK5** | **0.6074** | **na** | **na** |
| | | HAEK6 | 0.6074 | na | na |
| | | **HAEK7** | **0.6074** | **na** | **na** |
| | | HAEK8 | 0.6074 | na | na |
| C0F0S2 | Clinical=Min,Functional=Min,Service=Mod | **HAEL1** | **1.4847** | **HAEJ1** | **0.5265** |
| | | HAEL2 | 1.4847 | HAEJ2 | 0.5265 |
| | | **HAEL3** | **1.4847** | **HAEJ3** | **0.5265** |
| | | HAEL4 | 1.4847 | HAEJ4 | 0.5265 |
| | | **HAEL5** | **1.4847** | **HAEJ5** | **0.5265** |
| | | HAEL6 | 1.4847 | HAEJ6 | 0.5265 |
| | | **HAEL7** | **1.4847** | **HAEJ7** | **0.5265** |
| | | HAEL8 | 1.4847 | HAEJ8 | 0.5265 |
| C0F0S3 | Clinical=Min,Functional=Min,Service=High | **HAEM1** | **1.7364** | **HAEK1** | **0.6074** |
| | | HAEM2 | 1.7364 | HAEK2 | 0.6074 |
| | | **HAEM3** | **1.7364** | **HAEK3** | **0.6074** |
| | | HAEM4 | 1.7364 | HAEK4 | 0.6074 |
| | | **HAEM5** | **1.7364** | **HAEK5** | **0.6074** |
| | | HAEM6 | 1.7364 | HAEK6 | 0.6074 |
| | | **HAEM7** | **1.7364** | **HAEK7** | **0.6074** |
| | | HAEM8 | 1.7364 | HAEK8 | 0.6074 |
| C0F1S0 | Clinical=Min,Functional=Low,Service=Min | **HAFJ1** | **0.6213** | **na** | **na** |
| | | HAFJ2 | 0.6213 | na | na |
| | | **HAFJ3** | **0.6213** | **na** | **na** |
| | | HAFJ4 | 0.6213 | na | na |
| | | **HAFJ5** | **0.6213** | **na** | **na** |
| | | HAFJ6 | 0.6213 | na | na |
| | | **HAFJ7** | **0.6213** | **na** | **na** |
| | | HAFJ8 | 0.6213 | na | na |
| C0F1S1 | Clinical=Min,Functional=Low,Service=Low | **HAFK1** | **0.7022** | **na** | **na** |
| | | HAFK2 | 0.7022 | na | na |
| | | **HAFK3** | **0.7022** | **na** | **na** |
| | | HAFK4 | 0.7022 | na | na |
| | | **HAFK5** | **0.7022** | **na** | **na** |
| | | HAFK6 | 0.7022 | na | na |
| | | **HAFK7** | **0.7022** | **na** | **na** |
| | | HAFK8 | 0.7022 | na | na |
| C0F1S2 | Clinical=Min,Functional=Low,Service=Mod | **HAFL1** | **1.5796** | **HAFJ1** | **0.6213** |
| | | HAFL2 | 1.5796 | HAFJ2 | 0.6213 |
| | | **HAFL3** | **1.5796** | **HAFJ3** | **0.6213** |
| | | HAFL4 | 1.5796 | HAFJ4 | 0.6213 |
| | | **HAFL5** | **1.5796** | **HAFJ5** | **0.6213** |
| | | HAFL6 | 1.5796 | HAFJ6 | 0.6213 |
| | | **HAFL7** | **1.5796** | **HAFJ7** | **0.6213** |
| | | HAFL8 | 1.5796 | HAFJ8 | 0.6213 |

| | HIPPS Table for Pricer | | | Fallback HIPPS Code | Fallback code weight |
|---|---|---|---|---|---|
| **HHRG Description** | **Case Mix Description by Domains** | **HIPPS Code** | **Weight** | | |
| C0F1S3 | Clinical=Min,Functional=Low,Service=High | HAFM1 | 1.8313 | HAFK1 | 0.7022 |
| | | HAFM2 | 1.8313 | HAFK2 | 0.7022 |
| | | HAFM3 | 1.8313 | HAFK3 | 0.7022 |
| | | HAFM4 | 1.8313 | HAFK4 | 0.7022 |
| | | HAFM5 | 1.8313 | HAFK5 | 0.7022 |
| | | HAFM6 | 1.8313 | HAFK6 | 0.7022 |
| | | HAFM7 | 1.8313 | HAFK7 | 0.7022 |
| | | HAFM8 | 1.8313 | HAFK8 | 0.7022 |
| C0F2S0 | Clinical=Min,Functional=Mod,Service=Min | HAGJ1 | 0.7249 | na | na |
| | | HAGJ2 | 0.7249 | na | na |
| | | HAGJ3 | 0.7249 | na | na |
| | | HAGJ4 | 0.7249 | na | na |
| | | HAGJ5 | 0.7249 | na | na |
| | | HAGJ6 | 0.7249 | na | na |
| | | HAGJ7 | 0.7249 | na | na |
| | | HAGJ8 | 0.7249 | na | na |
| C0F2S1 | Clinical=Min,Functional=Mod,Service=Low | HAGK1 | 0.8058 | na | na |
| | | HAGK2 | 0.8058 | na | na |
| | | HAGK3 | 0.8058 | na | na |
| | | HAGK4 | 0.8058 | na | na |
| | | HAGK5 | 0.8058 | na | na |
| | | HAGK6 | 0.8058 | na | na |
| | | HAGK7 | 0.8058 | na | na |
| | | HAGK8 | 0.8058 | na | na |
| C0F2S2 | Clinical=Min,Functional=Mod,Service=Mod | HAGL1 | 1.6831 | HAGJ1 | 0.7249 |
| | | HAGL2 | 1.6831 | HAGJ2 | 0.7249 |
| | | HAGL3 | 1.6831 | HAGJ3 | 0.7249 |
| | | HAGL4 | 1.6831 | HAGJ4 | 0.7249 |
| | | HAGL5 | 1.6831 | HAGJ5 | 0.7249 |
| | | HAGL6 | 1.6831 | HAGJ6 | 0.7249 |
| | | HAGL7 | 1.6831 | HAGJ7 | 0.7249 |
| | | HAGL8 | 1.6831 | HAGJ8 | 0.7249 |
| C0F2S3 | Clinical=Min,Functional=Mod,Service=High | HAGM1 | 1.9348 | HAGK1 | 0.8058 |
| | | HAGM2 | 1.9348 | HAGK2 | 0.8058 |
| | | HAGM3 | 1.9348 | HAGK3 | 0.8058 |
| | | HAGM4 | 1.9348 | HAGK4 | 0.8058 |
| | | HAGM5 | 1.9348 | HAGK5 | 0.8058 |
| | | HAGM6 | 1.9348 | HAGK6 | 0.8058 |
| | | HAGM7 | 1.9348 | HAGK7 | 0.8058 |
| | | HAGM8 | 1.9348 | HAGK8 | 0.8058 |
| C0F3S0 | Clinical=Min,Functional=High,Service=Min | HAHJ1 | 0.7629 | na | na |
| | | HAHJ2 | 0.7629 | na | na |
| | | HAHJ3 | 0.7629 | na | na |
| | | HAHJ4 | 0.7629 | na | na |
| | | HAHJ5 | 0.7629 | na | na |
| | | HAHJ6 | 0.7629 | na | na |
| | | HAHJ7 | 0.7629 | na | na |
| | | HAHJ8 | 0.7629 | na | na |
| C0F3S1 | Clinical=Min,Functional=High,Service=Low | HAHK1 | 0.8438 | na | na |
| | | HAHK2 | 0.8438 | na | na |
| | | HAHK3 | 0.8438 | na | na |
| | | HAHK4 | 0.8438 | na | na |
| | | HAHK5 | 0.8438 | na | na |
| | | HAHK6 | 0.8438 | na | na |
| | | HAHK7 | 0.8438 | na | na |
| | | HAHK8 | 0.8438 | na | na |

| | HIPPS Table for Pricer | | | | |
|---|---|---|---|---|---|
| **HHRG Description** | **Case Mix Description by Domains** | **HIPPS Code** | **Weight** | **Fallback HIPPS Code** | **Fallback code weight** |
| **C0F3S2** | **Clinical=Min,Functional=High,Service=Mod** | **HAHL1** | **1.7212** | **HAHJ1** | **0.7629** |
| | | HAHL2 | 1.7212 | HAHJ2 | 0.7629 |
| | | **HAHL3** | **1.7212** | **HAHJ3** | **0.7629** |
| | | HAHL4 | 1.7212 | HAHJ4 | 0.7629 |
| | | **HAHL5** | **1.7212** | **HAHJ5** | **0.7629** |
| | | HAHL6 | 1.7212 | HAHJ6 | 0.7629 |
| | | **HAHL7** | **1.7212** | **HAHJ7** | **0.7629** |
| | | HAHL8 | 1.7212 | HAHJ8 | 0.7629 |
| **C0F3S3** | **Clinical=Min,Functional=High,Service=High** | **HAHM1** | **1.9728** | **HAHK1** | **0.8438** |
| | | HAHM2 | 1.9728 | HAHK2 | 0.8438 |
| | | **HAHM3** | **1.9728** | **HAHK3** | **0.8438** |
| | | HAHM4 | 1.9728 | HAHK4 | 0.8438 |
| | | **HAHM5** | **1.9728** | **HAHK5** | **0.8438** |
| | | HAHM6 | 1.9728 | HAHK6 | 0.8438 |
| | | **HAHM7** | **1.9728** | **HAHK7** | **0.8438** |
| | | HAHM8 | 1.9728 | HAHK8 | 0.8438 |
| **C0F4S0** | **Clinical=Min,Functional=Max,Service=Min** | **HAIJ1** | **0.9305** | **na** | **na** |
| | | HAIJ2 | 0.9305 | na | na |
| | | **HAIJ3** | **0.9305** | **na** | **na** |
| | | HAIJ4 | 0.9305 | na | na |
| | | **HAIJ5** | **0.9305** | **na** | **na** |
| | | HAIJ6 | 0.9305 | na | na |
| | | **HAIJ7** | **0.9305** | **na** | **na** |
| | | HAIJ8 | 0.9305 | na | na |
| **C0F4S1** | **Clinical=Min,Functional=Max,Service=Low** | **HAIK1** | **1.0114** | **na** | **na** |
| | | HAIK2 | 1.0114 | na | na |
| | | **HAIK3** | **1.0114** | **na** | **na** |
| | | HAIK4 | 1.0114 | na | na |
| | | **HAIK5** | **1.0114** | **na** | **na** |
| | | HAIK6 | 1.0114 | na | na |
| | | **HAIK7** | **1.0114** | **na** | **na** |
| | | HAIK8 | 1.0114 | na | na |
| **C0F4S2** | **Clinical=Min,Functional=Max,Service=Mod** | **HAIL1** | **1.8887** | **HAIJ1** | **0.9305** |
| | | HAIL2 | 1.8887 | HAIJ2 | 0.9305 |
| | | **HAIL3** | **1.8887** | **HAIJ3** | **0.9305** |
| | | HAIL4 | 1.8887 | HAIJ4 | 0.9305 |
| | | **HAIL5** | **1.8887** | **HAIJ5** | **0.9305** |
| | | HAIL6 | 1.8887 | HAIJ6 | 0.9305 |
| | | **HAIL7** | **1.8887** | **HAIJ7** | **0.9305** |
| | | HAIL8 | 1.8887 | HAIJ8 | 0.9305 |
| **C0F4S3** | **Clinical=Min,Functional=Max,Service=High** | **HAIM1** | **2.1404** | **HAIK1** | **1.0114** |
| | | HAIM2 | 2.1404 | HAIK2 | 1.0114 |
| | | **HAIM3** | **2.1404** | **HAIK3** | **1.0114** |
| | | HAIM4 | 2.1404 | HAIK4 | 1.0114 |
| | | **HAIM5** | **2.1404** | **HAIK5** | **1.0114** |
| | | HAIM6 | 2.1404 | HAIK6 | 1.0114 |
| | | **HAIM7** | **2.1404** | **HAIK7** | **1.0114** |
| | | HAIM8 | 2.1404 | HAIK8 | 1.0114 |
| **C1F0S0** | **Clinical=Low,Functional=Min,Service=Min** | **HBEJ1** | **0.6221** | **na** | **na** |
| | | HBEJ2 | 0.6221 | na | na |
| | | **HBEJ3** | **0.6221** | **na** | **na** |
| | | HBEJ4 | 0.6221 | na | na |
| | | **HBEJ5** | **0.6221** | **na** | **na** |
| | | HBEJ6 | 0.6221 | na | na |
| | | **HBEJ7** | **0.6221** | **na** | **na** |
| | | HBEJ8 | 0.6221 | na | na |

| HHRG Description | HIPPS Table for Pricer<br>Case Mix Description by Domains | HIPPS Code | Weight | Fallback HIPPS Code | Fallback code weight |
|---|---|---|---|---|---|
| C1F0S1 | Clinical=Low,Functional=Min,Service=Low | HBEK1 | 0.703 | na | na |
| | | HBEK2 | 0.703 | na | na |
| | | HBEK3 | 0.703 | na | na |
| | | HBEK4 | 0.703 | na | na |
| | | HBEK5 | 0.703 | na | na |
| | | HBEK6 | 0.703 | na | na |
| | | HBEK7 | 0.703 | na | na |
| | | HBEK8 | 0.703 | na | na |
| C1F0S2 | Clinical=Low,Functional=Min,Service=Mod | HBEL1 | 1.5803 | HBEJ1 | 0.6221 |
| | | HBEL2 | 1.5803 | HBEJ2 | 0.6221 |
| | | HBEL3 | 1.5803 | HBEJ3 | 0.6221 |
| | | HBEL4 | 1.5803 | HBEJ4 | 0.6221 |
| | | HBEL5 | 1.5803 | HBEJ5 | 0.6221 |
| | | HBEL6 | 1.5803 | HBEJ6 | 0.6221 |
| | | HBEL7 | 1.5803 | HBEJ7 | 0.6221 |
| | | HBEL8 | 1.5803 | HBEJ8 | 0.6221 |
| C1F0S3 | Clinical=Low,Functional=Min,Service=High | HBEM1 | 1.832 | HBEK1 | 0.703 |
| | | HBEM2 | 1.832 | HBEK2 | 0.703 |
| | | HBEM3 | 1.832 | HBEK3 | 0.703 |
| | | HBEM4 | 1.832 | HBEK4 | 0.703 |
| | | HBEM5 | 1.832 | HBEK5 | 0.703 |
| | | HBEM6 | 1.832 | HBEK6 | 0.703 |
| | | HBEM7 | 1.832 | HBEK7 | 0.703 |
| | | HBEM8 | 1.832 | HBEK8 | 0.703 |
| C1F1S0 | Clinical=Low,Functional=Low,Service=Min | HBFJ1 | 0.7169 | na | na |
| | | HBFJ2 | 0.7169 | na | na |
| | | HBFJ3 | 0.7169 | na | na |
| | | HBFJ4 | 0.7169 | na | na |
| | | HBFJ5 | 0.7169 | na | na |
| | | HBFJ6 | 0.7169 | na | na |
| | | HBFJ7 | 0.7169 | na | na |
| | | HBFJ8 | 0.7169 | na | na |
| C1F1S1 | Clinical=Low,Functional=Low,Service=Low | HBFK1 | 0.7978 | na | na |
| | | HBFK2 | 0.7978 | na | na |
| | | HBFK3 | 0.7978 | na | na |
| | | HBFK4 | 0.7978 | na | na |
| | | HBFK5 | 0.7978 | na | na |
| | | HBFK6 | 0.7978 | na | na |
| | | HBFK7 | 0.7978 | na | na |
| | | HBFK8 | 0.7978 | na | na |
| C1F1S2 | Clinical=Low,Functional=Low,Service=Mod | HBFL1 | 1.6752 | HBFJ1 | 0.7169 |
| | | HBFL2 | 1.6752 | HBFJ2 | 0.7169 |
| | | HBFL3 | 1.6752 | HBFJ3 | 0.7169 |
| | | HBFL4 | 1.6752 | HBFJ4 | 0.7169 |
| | | HBFL5 | 1.6752 | HBFJ5 | 0.7169 |
| | | HBFL6 | 1.6752 | HBFJ6 | 0.7169 |
| | | HBFL7 | 1.6752 | HBFJ7 | 0.7169 |
| | | HBFL8 | 1.6752 | HBFJ8 | 0.7169 |
| C1F1S3 | Clinical=Low,Functional=Low,Service=High | HBFM1 | 1.9269 | HBFK1 | 0.7978 |
| | | HBFM2 | 1.9269 | HBFK2 | 0.7978 |
| | | HBFM3 | 1.9269 | HBFK3 | 0.7978 |
| | | HBFM4 | 1.9269 | HBFK4 | 0.7978 |
| | | HBFM5 | 1.9269 | HBFK5 | 0.7978 |
| | | HBFM6 | 1.9269 | HBFK6 | 0.7978 |
| | | HBFM7 | 1.9269 | HBFK7 | 0.7978 |
| | | HBFM8 | 1.9269 | HBFK8 | 0.7978 |

| | HIPPS Table for Pricer | | | | |
|---|---|---|---|---|---|
| **HHRG Description** | **Case Mix Description by Domains** | **HIPPS Code** | **Weight** | **Fallback HIPPS Code** | **Fallback code weight** |
| C1F2S0 | Clinical=Low,Functional=Mod,Service=Min | HBGJ1 | 0.8205 | na | na |
| | | HBGJ2 | 0.8205 | na | na |
| | | HBGJ3 | 0.8205 | na | na |
| | | HBGJ4 | 0.8205 | na | na |
| | | HBGJ5 | 0.8205 | na | na |
| | | HBGJ6 | 0.8205 | na | na |
| | | HBGJ7 | 0.8205 | na | na |
| | | HBGJ8 | 0.8205 | na | na |
| C1F2S1 | Clinical=Low,Functional=Mod,Service=Low | HBGK1 | 0.9014 | na | na |
| | | HBGK2 | 0.9014 | na | na |
| | | HBGK3 | 0.9014 | na | na |
| | | HBGK4 | 0.9014 | na | na |
| | | HBGK5 | 0.9014 | na | na |
| | | HBGK6 | 0.9014 | na | na |
| | | HBGK7 | 0.9014 | na | na |
| | | HBGK8 | 0.9014 | na | na |
| C1F2S2 | Clinical=Low,Functional=Mod,Service=Mod | HBGL1 | 1.7787 | HBGJ1 | 0.8205 |
| | | HBGL2 | 1.7787 | HBGJ2 | 0.8205 |
| | | HBGL3 | 1.7787 | HBGJ3 | 0.8205 |
| | | HBGL4 | 1.7787 | HBGJ4 | 0.8205 |
| | | HBGL5 | 1.7787 | HBGJ5 | 0.8205 |
| | | HBGL6 | 1.7787 | HBGJ6 | 0.8205 |
| | | HBGL7 | 1.7787 | HBGJ7 | 0.8205 |
| | | HBGL8 | 1.7787 | HBGJ8 | 0.8205 |
| C1F2S3 | Clinical=Low,Functional=Mod,Service=High | HBGM1 | 2.0304 | HBGK1 | 0.9014 |
| | | HBGM2 | 2.0304 | HBGK2 | 0.9014 |
| | | HBGM3 | 2.0304 | HBGK3 | 0.9014 |
| | | HBGM4 | 2.0304 | HBGK4 | 0.9014 |
| | | HBGM5 | 2.0304 | HBGK5 | 0.9014 |
| | | HBGM6 | 2.0304 | HBGK6 | 0.9014 |
| | | HBGM7 | 2.0304 | HBGK7 | 0.9014 |
| | | HBGM8 | 2.0304 | HBGK8 | 0.9014 |
| C1F3S0 | Clinical=Low,Functional=High,Service=Min | HBHJ1 | 0.8585 | na | na |
| | | HBHJ2 | 0.8585 | na | na |
| | | HBHJ3 | 0.8585 | na | na |
| | | HBHJ4 | 0.8585 | na | na |
| | | HBHJ5 | 0.8585 | na | na |
| | | HBHJ6 | 0.8585 | na | na |
| | | HBHJ7 | 0.8585 | na | na |
| | | HBHJ8 | 0.8585 | na | na |
| C1F3S1 | Clinical=Low,Functional=High,Service=Low | HBHK1 | 0.9394 | na | na |
| | | HBHK2 | 0.9394 | na | na |
| | | HBHK3 | 0.9394 | na | na |
| | | HBHK4 | 0.9394 | na | na |
| | | HBHK5 | 0.9394 | na | na |
| | | HBHK6 | 0.9394 | na | na |
| | | HBHK7 | 0.9394 | na | na |
| | | HBHK8 | 0.9394 | na | na |
| C1F3S2 | Clinical=Low,Functional=High,Service=Mod | HBHL1 | 1.8168 | HBHJ1 | 0.8585 |
| | | HBHL2 | 1.8168 | HBHJ2 | 0.8585 |
| | | HBHL3 | 1.8168 | HBHJ3 | 0.8585 |
| | | HBHL4 | 1.8168 | HBHJ4 | 0.8585 |
| | | HBHL5 | 1.8168 | HBHJ5 | 0.8585 |
| | | HBHL6 | 1.8168 | HBHJ6 | 0.8585 |
| | | HBHL7 | 1.8168 | HBHJ7 | 0.8585 |
| | | HBHL8 | 1.8168 | HBHJ8 | 0.8585 |

| HHRG Description | HIPPS Table for Pricer | | | | |
|---|---|---|---|---|---|
| | Case Mix Description by Domains | HIPPS Code | Weight | Fallback HIPPS Code | Fallback code weight |
| C1F3S3 | Clinical=Low,Functional=High,Service=High | HBHM1 | 2.0684 | HBHK1 | 0.9394 |
| | | HBHM2 | 2.0684 | HBHK2 | 0.9394 |
| | | HBHM3 | 2.0684 | HBHK3 | 0.9394 |
| | | HBHM4 | 2.0684 | HBHK4 | 0.9394 |
| | | HBHM5 | 2.0684 | HBHK5 | 0.9394 |
| | | HBHM6 | 2.0684 | HBHK6 | 0.9394 |
| | | HBHM7 | 2.0684 | HBHK7 | 0.9394 |
| | | HBHM8 | 2.0684 | HBHK8 | 0.9394 |
| C1F4S0 | Clinical=Low,Functional=Max,Service=Min | HBIJ1 | 1.0261 | na | na |
| | | HBIJ2 | 1.0261 | na | na |
| | | HBIJ3 | 1.0261 | na | na |
| | | HBIJ4 | 1.0261 | na | na |
| | | HBIJ5 | 1.0261 | na | na |
| | | HBIJ6 | 1.0261 | na | na |
| | | HBIJ7 | 1.0261 | na | na |
| | | HBIJ8 | 1.0261 | na | na |
| C1F4S1 | Clinical=Low,Functional=Max,Service=Low | HBIK1 | 1.107 | na | na |
| | | HBIK2 | 1.107 | na | na |
| | | HBIK3 | 1.107 | na | na |
| | | HBIK4 | 1.107 | na | na |
| | | HBIK5 | 1.107 | na | na |
| | | HBIK6 | 1.107 | na | na |
| | | HBIK7 | 1.107 | na | na |
| | | HBIK8 | 1.107 | na | na |
| C1F4S2 | Clinical=Low,Functional=Max,Service=Mod | HBIL1 | 1.9843 | HBIJ1 | 1.0261 |
| | | HBIL2 | 1.9843 | HBIJ2 | 1.0261 |
| | | HBIL3 | 1.9843 | HBIJ3 | 1.0261 |
| | | HBIL4 | 1.9843 | HBIJ4 | 1.0261 |
| | | HBIL5 | 1.9843 | HBIJ5 | 1.0261 |
| | | HBIL6 | 1.9843 | HBIJ6 | 1.0261 |
| | | HBIL7 | 1.9843 | HBIJ7 | 1.0261 |
| | | HBIL8 | 1.9843 | HBIJ8 | 1.0261 |
| C1F4S3 | Clinical=Low,Functional=Max,Service=High | HBIM1 | 2.236 | HBIK1 | 1.107 |
| | | HBIM2 | 2.236 | HBIK2 | 1.107 |
| | | HBIM3 | 2.236 | HBIK3 | 1.107 |
| | | HBIM4 | 2.236 | HBIK4 | 1.107 |
| | | HBIM5 | 2.236 | HBIK5 | 1.107 |
| | | HBIM6 | 2.236 | HBIK6 | 1.107 |
| | | HBIM7 | 2.236 | HBIK7 | 1.107 |
| | | HBIM8 | 2.236 | HBIK8 | 1.107 |
| C2F0S0 | Clinical=Mod,Functional=Min,Service=Min | HCEJ1 | 0.7965 | na | na |
| | | HCEJ2 | 0.7965 | na | na |
| | | HCEJ3 | 0.7965 | na | na |
| | | HCEJ4 | 0.7965 | na | na |
| | | HCEJ5 | 0.7965 | na | na |
| | | HCEJ6 | 0.7965 | na | na |
| | | HCEJ7 | 0.7965 | na | na |
| | | HCEJ8 | 0.7965 | na | na |
| C2F0S1 | Clinical=Mod,Functional=Min,Service=Low | HCEK1 | 0.8774 | na | na |
| | | HCEK2 | 0.8774 | na | na |
| | | HCEK3 | 0.8774 | na | na |
| | | HCEK4 | 0.8774 | na | na |
| | | HCEK5 | 0.8774 | na | na |
| | | HCEK6 | 0.8774 | na | na |
| | | HCEK7 | 0.8774 | na | na |
| | | HCEK8 | 0.8774 | na | na |

| | HIPPS Table for Pricer | | | | |
|---|---|---|---|---|---|
| **HHRG Description** | **Case Mix Description by Domains** | **HIPPS Code** | **Weight** | **Fallback HIPPS Code** | **Fallback code weight** |
| C2F0S2 | Clinical=Mod,Functional=Min,Service=Mod | **HCEL1** | **1.7548** | **HCEJ1** | **0.7965** |
| | | HCEL2 | 1.7548 | HCEJ2 | 0.7965 |
| | | **HCEL3** | **1.7548** | **HCEJ3** | **0.7965** |
| | | HCEL4 | 1.7548 | HCEJ4 | 0.7965 |
| | | **HCEL5** | **1.7548** | **HCEJ5** | **0.7965** |
| | | HCEL6 | 1.7548 | HCEJ6 | 0.7965 |
| | | **HCEL7** | **1.7548** | **HCEJ7** | **0.7965** |
| | | HCEL8 | 1.7548 | HCEJ8 | 0.7965 |
| C2F0S3 | Clinical=Mod,Functional=Min,Service=High | **HCEM1** | **2.0065** | **HCEK1** | **0.8774** |
| | | HCEM2 | 2.0065 | HCEK2 | 0.8774 |
| | | **HCEM3** | **2.0065** | **HCEK3** | **0.8774** |
| | | HCEM4 | 2.0065 | HCEK4 | 0.8774 |
| | | **HCEM5** | **2.0065** | **HCEK5** | **0.8774** |
| | | HCEM6 | 2.0065 | HCEK6 | 0.8774 |
| | | **HCEM7** | **2.0065** | **HCEK7** | **0.8774** |
| | | HCEM8 | 2.0065 | HCEK8 | 0.8774 |
| C2F1S0 | Clinical=Mod,Functional=Low,Service=Min | **HCFJ1** | **0.8914** | na | na |
| | | HCFJ2 | 0.8914 | na | na |
| | | **HCFJ3** | **0.8914** | na | na |
| | | HCFJ4 | 0.8914 | na | na |
| | | **HCFJ5** | **0.8914** | na | na |
| | | HCFJ6 | 0.8914 | na | na |
| | | **HCFJ7** | **0.8914** | na | na |
| | | HCFJ8 | 0.8914 | na | na |
| C2F1S1 | Clinical=Mod,Functional=Low,Service=Low | **HCFK1** | **0.9723** | na | na |
| | | HCFK2 | 0.9723 | na | na |
| | | **HCFK3** | **0.9723** | na | na |
| | | HCFK4 | 0.9723 | na | na |
| | | **HCFK5** | **0.9723** | na | na |
| | | HCFK6 | 0.9723 | na | na |
| | | **HCFK7** | **0.9723** | na | na |
| | | HCFK8 | 0.9723 | na | na |
| C2F1S2 | Clinical=Mod,Functional=Low,Service=Mod | **HCFL1** | **1.8496** | **HCFJ1** | **0.8914** |
| | | HCFL2 | 1.8496 | HCFJ2 | 0.8914 |
| | | **HCFL3** | **1.8496** | **HCFJ3** | **0.8914** |
| | | HCFL4 | 1.8496 | HCFJ4 | 0.8914 |
| | | **HCFL5** | **1.8496** | **HCFJ5** | **0.8914** |
| | | HCFL6 | 1.8496 | HCFJ6 | 0.8914 |
| | | **HCFL7** | **1.8496** | **HCFJ7** | **0.8914** |
| | | HCFL8 | 1.8496 | HCFJ8 | 0.8914 |
| C2F1S3 | Clinical=Mod,Functional=Low,Service=High | **HCFM1** | **2.1013** | **HCFK1** | **0.9723** |
| | | HCFM2 | 2.1013 | HCFK2 | 0.9723 |
| | | **HCFM3** | **2.1013** | **HCFK3** | **0.9723** |
| | | HCFM4 | 2.1013 | HCFK4 | 0.9723 |
| | | **HCFM5** | **2.1013** | **HCFK5** | **0.9723** |
| | | HCFM6 | 2.1013 | HCFK6 | 0.9723 |
| | | **HCFM7** | **2.1013** | **HCFK7** | **0.9723** |
| | | HCFM8 | 2.1013 | HCFK8 | 0.9723 |
| C2F2S0 | Clinical=Mod,Functional=Mod,Service=Min | **HCGJ1** | **0.9949** | na | na |
| | | HCGJ2 | 0.9949 | na | na |
| | | **HCGJ3** | **0.9949** | na | na |
| | | HCGJ4 | 0.9949 | na | na |
| | | **HCGJ5** | **0.9949** | na | na |
| | | HCGJ6 | 0.9949 | na | na |
| | | **HCGJ7** | **0.9949** | na | na |
| | | HCGJ8 | 0.9949 | na | na |

| | **HIPPS Table for Pricer** | | | | |
|---|---|---|---|---|---|
| **HHRG Description** | **Case Mix Description by Domains** | **HIPPS Code** | **Weight** | **Fallback HIPPS Code** | **Fallback code weight** |
| C2F2S1 | Clinical=Mod,Functional=Mod,Service=Low | HCGK1 | 1.0758 | na | na |
| | | HCGK2 | 1.0758 | na | na |
| | | HCGK3 | 1.0758 | na | na |
| | | HCGK4 | 1.0758 | na | na |
| | | HCGK5 | 1.0758 | na | na |
| | | HCGK6 | 1.0758 | na | na |
| | | HCGK7 | 1.0758 | na | na |
| | | HCGK8 | 1.0758 | na | na |
| C2F2S2 | Clinical=Mod,Functional=Mod,Service=Mod | HCGL1 | 1.9532 | HCGJ1 | 0.9949 |
| | | HCGL2 | 1.9532 | HCGJ2 | 0.9949 |
| | | HCGL3 | 1.9532 | HCGJ3 | 0.9949 |
| | | HCGL4 | 1.9532 | HCGJ4 | 0.9949 |
| | | HCGL5 | 1.9532 | HCGJ5 | 0.9949 |
| | | HCGL6 | 1.9532 | HCGJ6 | 0.9949 |
| | | HCGL7 | 1.9532 | HCGJ7 | 0.9949 |
| | | HCGL8 | 1.9532 | HCGJ8 | 0.9949 |
| C2F2S3 | Clinical=Mod,Functional=Mod,Service=High | HCGM1 | 2.2048 | HCGK1 | 1.0758 |
| | | HCGM2 | 2.2048 | HCGK2 | 1.0758 |
| | | HCGM3 | 2.2048 | HCGK3 | 1.0758 |
| | | HCGM4 | 2.2048 | HCGK4 | 1.0758 |
| | | HCGM5 | 2.2048 | HCGK5 | 1.0758 |
| | | HCGM6 | 2.2048 | HCGK6 | 1.0758 |
| | | HCGM7 | 2.2048 | HCGK7 | 1.0758 |
| | | HCGM8 | 2.2048 | HCGK8 | 1.0758 |
| C2F3S0 | Clinical=Mod,Functional=High,Service=Min | HCHJ1 | 1.0329 | na | na |
| | | HCHJ2 | 1.0329 | na | na |
| | | HCHJ3 | 1.0329 | na | na |
| | | HCHJ4 | 1.0329 | na | na |
| | | HCHJ5 | 1.0329 | na | na |
| | | HCHJ6 | 1.0329 | na | na |
| | | HCHJ7 | 1.0329 | na | na |
| | | HCHJ8 | 1.0329 | na | na |
| C2F3S1 | Clinical=Mod,Functional=High,Service=Low | HCHK1 | 1.1139 | na | na |
| | | HCHK2 | 1.1139 | na | na |
| | | HCHK3 | 1.1139 | na | na |
| | | HCHK4 | 1.1139 | na | na |
| | | HCHK5 | 1.1139 | na | na |
| | | HCHK6 | 1.1139 | na | na |
| | | HCHK7 | 1.1139 | na | na |
| | | HCHK8 | 1.1139 | na | na |
| C2F3S2 | Clinical=Mod,Functional=High,Service=Mod | HCHL1 | 1.9912 | HCHJ1 | 1.0329 |
| | | HCHL2 | 1.9912 | HCHJ2 | 1.0329 |
| | | HCHL3 | 1.9912 | HCHJ3 | 1.0329 |
| | | HCHL4 | 1.9912 | HCHJ4 | 1.0329 |
| | | HCHL5 | 1.9912 | HCHJ5 | 1.0329 |
| | | HCHL6 | 1.9912 | HCHJ6 | 1.0329 |
| | | HCHL7 | 1.9912 | HCHJ7 | 1.0329 |
| | | HCHL8 | 1.9912 | HCHJ8 | 1.0329 |
| C2F3S3 | Clinical=Mod,Functional=High,Service=High | HCHM1 | 2.2429 | HCHK1 | 1.1139 |
| | | HCHM2 | 2.2429 | HCHK2 | 1.1139 |
| | | HCHM3 | 2.2429 | HCHK3 | 1.1139 |
| | | HCHM4 | 2.2429 | HCHK4 | 1.1139 |
| | | HCHM5 | 2.2429 | HCHK5 | 1.1139 |
| | | HCHM6 | 2.2429 | HCHK6 | 1.1139 |
| | | HCHM7 | 2.2429 | HCHK7 | 1.1139 |
| | | HCHM8 | 2.2429 | HCHK8 | 1.1139 |

| | HIPPS Table for Pricer | | | Fallback | |
|---|---|---|---|---|---|
| HHRG Description | Case Mix Description by Domains | HIPPS Code | Weight | HIPPS Code | Fallback code weight |
| C2F4S0 | Clinical=Mod,Functional=Max,Service=Min | HCIJ1 | 1.2005 | na | na |
| | | HCIJ2 | 1.2005 | na | na |
| | | HCIJ3 | 1.2005 | na | na |
| | | HCIJ4 | 1.2005 | na | na |
| | | HCIJ5 | 1.2005 | na | na |
| | | HCIJ6 | 1.2005 | na | na |
| | | HCIJ7 | 1.2005 | na | na |
| | | HCIJ8 | 1.2005 | na | na |
| C2F4S1 | Clinical=Mod,Functional=Max,Service=Low | HCIK1 | 1.2814 | na | na |
| | | HCIK2 | 1.2814 | na | na |
| | | HCIK3 | 1.2814 | na | na |
| | | HCIK4 | 1.2814 | na | na |
| | | HCIK5 | 1.2814 | na | na |
| | | HCIK6 | 1.2814 | na | na |
| | | HCIK7 | 1.2814 | na | na |
| | | HCIK8 | 1.2814 | na | na |
| C2F4S2 | Clinical=Mod,Functional=Max,Service=Mod | HCIL1 | 2.1588 | HCIJ1 | 1.2005 |
| | | HCIL2 | 2.1588 | HCIJ2 | 1.2005 |
| | | HCIL3 | 2.1588 | HCIJ3 | 1.2005 |
| | | HCIL4 | 2.1588 | HCIJ4 | 1.2005 |
| | | HCIL5 | 2.1588 | HCIJ5 | 1.2005 |
| | | HCIL6 | 2.1588 | HCIJ6 | 1.2005 |
| | | HCIL7 | 2.1588 | HCIJ7 | 1.2005 |
| | | HCIL8 | 2.1588 | HCIJ8 | 1.2005 |
| C2F4S3 | Clinical=Mod,Functional=Max,Service=High | HCIM1 | 2.4105 | HCIK1 | 1.2814 |
| | | HCIM2 | 2.4105 | HCIK2 | 1.2814 |
| | | HCIM3 | 2.4105 | HCIK3 | 1.2814 |
| | | HCIM4 | 2.4105 | HCIK4 | 1.2814 |
| | | HCIM5 | 2.4105 | HCIK5 | 1.2814 |
| | | HCIM6 | 2.4105 | HCIK6 | 1.2814 |
| | | HCIM7 | 2.4105 | HCIK7 | 1.2814 |
| | | HCIM8 | 2.4105 | HCIK8 | 1.2814 |
| C3F0S0 | Clinical=High,Functional=Min,Service=Min | HDEJ1 | 1.1973 | na | na |
| | | HDEJ2 | 1.1973 | na | na |
| | | HDEJ3 | 1.1973 | na | na |
| | | HDEJ4 | 1.1973 | na | na |
| | | HDEJ5 | 1.1973 | na | na |
| | | HDEJ6 | 1.1973 | na | na |
| | | HDEJ7 | 1.1973 | na | na |
| | | HDEJ8 | 1.1973 | na | na |
| C3F0S1 | Clinical=High,Functional=Min,Service=Low | HDEK1 | 1.2782 | na | na |
| | | HDEK2 | 1.2782 | na | na |
| | | HDEK3 | 1.2782 | na | na |
| | | HDEK4 | 1.2782 | na | na |
| | | HDEK5 | 1.2782 | na | na |
| | | HDEK6 | 1.2782 | na | na |
| | | HDEK7 | 1.2782 | na | na |
| | | HDEK8 | 1.2782 | na | na |
| C3F0S2 | Clinical=High,Functional=Min,Service=Mod | HDEL1 | 2.1556 | HDEJ1 | 1.1973 |
| | | HDEL2 | 2.1556 | HDEJ2 | 1.1973 |
| | | HDEL3 | 2.1556 | HDEJ3 | 1.1973 |
| | | HDEL4 | 2.1556 | HDEJ4 | 1.1973 |
| | | HDEL5 | 2.1556 | HDEJ5 | 1.1973 |
| | | HDEL6 | 2.1556 | HDEJ6 | 1.1973 |
| | | HDEL7 | 2.1556 | HDEJ7 | 1.1973 |
| | | HDEL8 | 2.1556 | HDEJ8 | 1.1973 |

| HHRG Description | Case Mix Description by Domains | HIPPS Code | Weight | Fallback HIPPS Code | Fallback code weight |
|---|---|---|---|---|---|
| | **HIPPS Table for Pricer** | | | | |
| C3F0S3 | Clinical=High,Functional=Min,Service=High | **HDEM1** | **2.4073** | **HDEK1** | **1.2782** |
| | | HDEM2 | 2.4073 | HDEK2 | 1.2782 |
| | | **HDEM3** | **2.4073** | **HDEK3** | **1.2782** |
| | | HDEM4 | 2.4073 | HDEK4 | 1.2782 |
| | | **HDEM5** | **2.4073** | **HDEK5** | **1.2782** |
| | | HDEM6 | 2.4073 | HDEK6 | 1.2782 |
| | | **HDEM7** | **2.4073** | **HDEK7** | **1.2782** |
| | | HDEM8 | 2.4073 | HDEK8 | 1.2782 |
| C3F1S0 | Clinical=High,Functional=Low,Service=Min | **HDFJ1** | **1.2922** | na | na |
| | | HDFJ2 | 1.2922 | na | na |
| | | **HDFJ3** | **1.2922** | na | na |
| | | HDFJ4 | 1.2922 | na | na |
| | | **HDFJ5** | **1.2922** | na | na |
| | | HDFJ6 | 1.2922 | na | na |
| | | **HDFJ7** | **1.2922** | na | na |
| | | HDFJ8 | 1.2922 | na | na |
| C3F1S1 | Clinical=High,Functional=Low,Service=Low | **HDFK1** | **1.3731** | na | na |
| | | HDFK2 | 1.3731 | na | na |
| | | **HDFK3** | **1.3731** | na | na |
| | | HDFK4 | 1.3731 | na | na |
| | | **HDFK5** | **1.3731** | na | na |
| | | HDFK6 | 1.3731 | na | na |
| | | **HDFK7** | **1.3731** | na | na |
| | | HDFK8 | 1.3731 | na | na |
| C3F1S2 | Clinical=High,Functional=Low,Service=Mod | **HDFL1** | **2.2504** | **HDFJ1** | **1.2922** |
| | | HDFL2 | 2.2504 | HDFJ2 | 1.2922 |
| | | **HDFL3** | **2.2504** | **HDFJ3** | **1.2922** |
| | | HDFL4 | 2.2504 | HDFJ4 | 1.2922 |
| | | **HDFL5** | **2.2504** | **HDFJ5** | **1.2922** |
| | | HDFL6 | 2.2504 | HDFJ6 | 1.2922 |
| | | **HDFL7** | **2.2504** | **HDFJ7** | **1.2922** |
| | | HDFL8 | 2.2504 | HDFJ8 | 1.2922 |
| C3F1S3 | Clinical=High,Functional=Low,Service=High | **HDFM1** | **2.5021** | **HDFK1** | **1.3731** |
| | | HDFM2 | 2.5021 | HDFK2 | 1.3731 |
| | | **HDFM3** | **2.5021** | **HDFK3** | **1.3731** |
| | | HDFM4 | 2.5021 | HDFK4 | 1.3731 |
| | | **HDFM5** | **2.5021** | **HDFK5** | **1.3731** |
| | | HDFM6 | 2.5021 | HDFK6 | 1.3731 |
| | | **HDFM7** | **2.5021** | **HDFK7** | **1.3731** |
| | | HDFM8 | 2.5021 | HDFK8 | 1.3731 |
| C3F2S0 | Clinical=High,Functional=Mod,Service=Min | **HDGJ1** | **1.3957** | na | na |
| | | HDGJ2 | 1.3957 | na | na |
| | | **HDGJ3** | **1.3957** | na | na |
| | | HDGJ4 | 1.3957 | na | na |
| | | **HDGJ5** | **1.3957** | na | na |
| | | HDGJ6 | 1.3957 | na | na |
| | | **HDGJ7** | **1.3957** | na | na |
| | | HDGJ8 | 1.3957 | na | na |
| C3F2S1 | Clinical=High,Functional=Mod,Service=Low | **HDGK1** | **1.4766** | na | na |
| | | HDGK2 | 1.4766 | na | na |
| | | **HDGK3** | **1.4766** | na | na |
| | | HDGK4 | 1.4766 | na | na |
| | | **HDGK5** | **1.4766** | na | na |
| | | HDGK6 | 1.4766 | na | na |
| | | **HDGK7** | **1.4766** | na | na |
| | | HDGK8 | 1.4766 | na | na |

| | HIPPS Table for Pricer | | | | |
|---|---|---|---|---|---|
| HHRG Description | Case Mix Description by Domains | HIPPS Code | Weight | Fallback HIPPS Code | Fallback code weight |
| C3F2S2 | Clinical=High,Functional=Mod,Service=Mod | HDGL1 | 2.354 | HDGJ1 | 1.3957 |
| | | HDGL2 | 2.354 | HDGJ2 | 1.3957 |
| | | HDGL3 | 2.354 | HDGJ3 | 1.3957 |
| | | HDGL4 | 2.354 | HDGJ4 | 1.3957 |
| | | HDGL5 | 2.354 | HDGJ5 | 1.3957 |
| | | HDGL6 | 2.354 | HDGJ6 | 1.3957 |
| | | HDGL7 | 2.354 | HDGJ7 | 1.3957 |
| | | HDGL8 | 2.354 | HDGJ8 | 1.3957 |
| C3F2S3 | Clinical=High,Functional=Mod,Service=High | HDGM1 | 2.6056 | HDGK1 | 1.4766 |
| | | HDGM2 | 2.6056 | HDGK2 | 1.4766 |
| | | HDGM3 | 2.6056 | HDGK3 | 1.4766 |
| | | HDGM4 | 2.6056 | HDGK4 | 1.4766 |
| | | HDGM5 | 2.6056 | HDGK5 | 1.4766 |
| | | HDGM6 | 2.6056 | HDGK6 | 1.4766 |
| | | HDGM7 | 2.6056 | HDGK7 | 1.4766 |
| | | HDGM8 | 2.6056 | HDGK8 | 1.4766 |
| C3F3S0 | Clinical=High,Functional=High,Service=Min | HDHJ1 | 1.4337 | na | na |
| | | HDHJ2 | 1.4337 | na | na |
| | | HDHJ3 | 1.4337 | na | na |
| | | HDHJ4 | 1.4337 | na | na |
| | | HDHJ5 | 1.4337 | na | na |
| | | HDHJ6 | 1.4337 | na | na |
| | | HDHJ7 | 1.4337 | na | na |
| | | HDHJ8 | 1.4337 | na | na |
| C3F3S1 | Clinical=High,Functional=High,Service=Low | HDHK1 | 1.5147 | na | na |
| | | HDHK2 | 1.5147 | na | na |
| | | HDHK3 | 1.5147 | na | na |
| | | HDHK4 | 1.5147 | na | na |
| | | HDHK5 | 1.5147 | na | na |
| | | HDHK6 | 1.5147 | na | na |
| | | HDHK7 | 1.5147 | na | na |
| | | HDHK8 | 1.5147 | na | na |
| C3F3S2 | Clinical=High,Functional=High,Service=Mod | HDHL1 | 2.392 | HDHJ1 | 1.4337 |
| | | HDHL2 | 2.392 | HDHJ2 | 1.4337 |
| | | HDHL3 | 2.392 | HDHJ3 | 1.4337 |
| | | HDHL4 | 2.392 | HDHJ4 | 1.4337 |
| | | HDHL5 | 2.392 | HDHJ5 | 1.4337 |
| | | HDHL6 | 2.392 | HDHJ6 | 1.4337 |
| | | HDHL7 | 2.392 | HDHJ7 | 1.4337 |
| | | HDHL8 | 2.392 | HDHJ8 | 1.4337 |
| C3F3S3 | Clinical=High,Functional=High,Service=High | HDHM1 | 2.6437 | HDHK1 | 1.5147 |
| | | HDHM2 | 2.6437 | HDHK2 | 1.5147 |
| | | HDHM3 | 2.6437 | HDHK3 | 1.5147 |
| | | HDHM4 | 2.6437 | HDHK4 | 1.5147 |
| | | HDHM5 | 2.6437 | HDHK5 | 1.5147 |
| | | HDHM6 | 2.6437 | HDHK6 | 1.5147 |
| | | HDHM7 | 2.6437 | HDHK7 | 1.5147 |
| | | HDHM8 | 2.6437 | HDHK8 | 1.5147 |
| C3F4S0 | Clinical=High,Functional=Max,Service=Min | HDIJ1 | 1.6013 | na | na |
| | | HDIJ2 | 1.6013 | na | na |
| | | HDIJ3 | 1.6013 | na | na |
| | | HDIJ4 | 1.6013 | na | na |
| | | HDIJ5 | 1.6013 | na | na |
| | | HDIJ6 | 1.6013 | na | na |
| | | HDIJ7 | 1.6013 | na | na |
| | | HDIJ8 | 1.6013 | na | na |

| HHRG Description | HIPPS Table for Pricer Case Mix Description by Domains | HIPPS Code | Weight | Fallback HIPPS Code | Fallback code weight |
|---|---|---|---|---|---|
| C3F4S1 | Clinical=High,Functional=Max,Service=Low | HDIK1 | 1.6822 | na | na |
| | | HDIK2 | 1.6822 | na | na |
| | | HDIK3 | 1.6822 | na | na |
| | | HDIK4 | 1.6822 | na | na |
| | | HDIK5 | 1.6822 | na | na |
| | | HDIK6 | 1.6822 | na | na |
| | | HDIK7 | 1.6822 | na | na |
| | | HDIK8 | 1.6822 | na | na |
| C3F4S2 | Clinical=High,Functional=Max,Service=Mod | HDIL1 | 2.5596 | HDIJ1 | 1.6013 |
| | | HDIL2 | 2.5596 | HDIJ2 | 1.6013 |
| | | HDIL3 | 2.5596 | HDIJ3 | 1.6013 |
| | | HDIL4 | 2.5596 | HDIJ4 | 1.6013 |
| | | HDIL5 | 2.5596 | HDIJ5 | 1.6013 |
| | | HDIL6 | 2.5596 | HDIJ6 | 1.6013 |
| | | HDIL7 | 2.5596 | HDIJ7 | 1.6013 |
| | | HDIL8 | 2.5596 | HDIJ8 | 1.6013 |
| C3F4S3 | Clinical=High,Functional=Max,Service=High | HDIM1 | 2.8113 | HDIK1 | 1.6822 |
| | | HDIM2 | 2.8113 | HDIK2 | 1.6822 |
| | | HDIM3 | 2.8113 | HDIK3 | 1.6822 |
| | | HDIM4 | 2.8113 | HDIK4 | 1.6822 |
| | | HDIM5 | 2.8113 | HDIK5 | 1.6822 |
| | | HDIM6 | 2.8113 | HDIK6 | 1.6822 |
| | | HDIM7 | 2.8113 | HDIK7 | 1.6822 |
| | | HDIM8 | 2.8113 | HDIK8 | 1.6822 |

# Appendix 11B
# HHABN Service Flow Charts

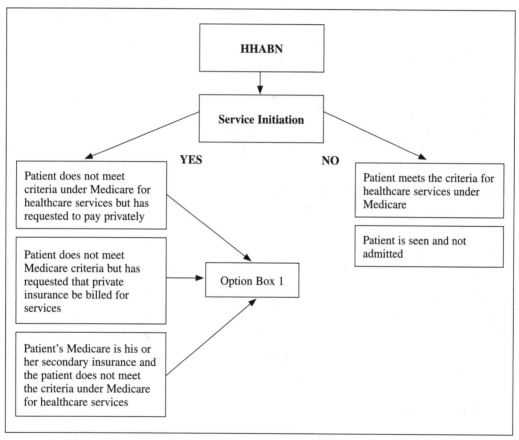

*If the patient refuses to sign the HHABN, the HHA must indicate that the patient refused to sign the HHABN itself and provide a copy of the annotated HHABN to the patient.

*If the patient is physically unable to sign but is fully capable of understanding the notice, the clinician can sign and date the notice under the direction of the patient (insert the patient's name as well as the clinician's name).

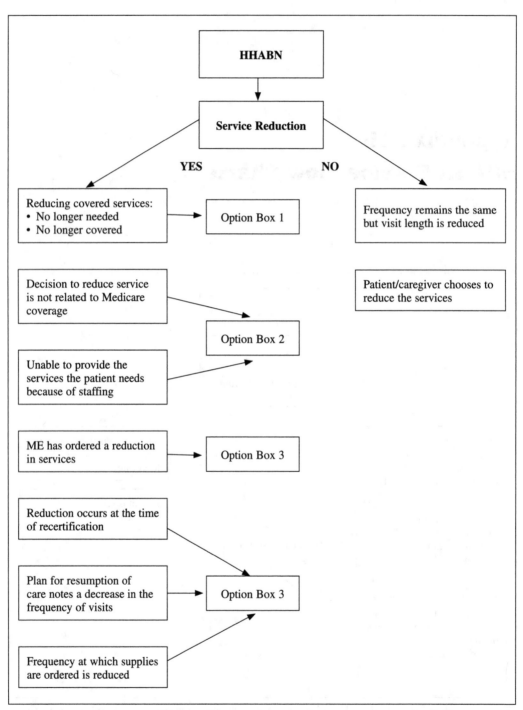

*If the patient refuses to sign the HHABN, the HHA must indicate that the patient refused to sign the HHABN itself and provide a copy of the annotated HHABN to the patient.

*If the patient is physically unable to sign but is fully capable of understanding the notice, the clinician can sign and date the notice under the direction of the patient (insert the patient's name as well as the clinician's name).

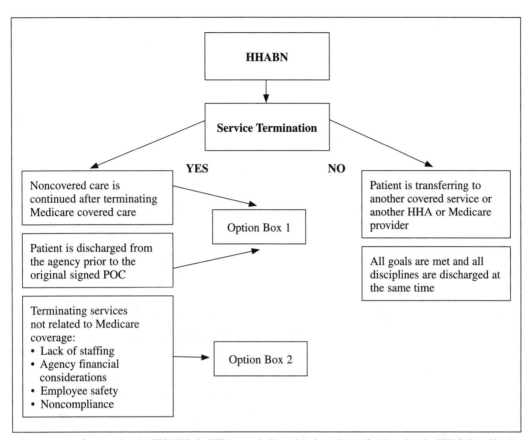

*If the patient refuses to sign the HHABN, the HHA must indicate that the patient refused to sign the HHABN itself and provide a copy of the annotated HHABN to the patient.

*If the patient is physically unable to sign but is fully capable of understanding the notice, the clinician can sign and date the notice under the direction of the patient (insert the patient's name as well as the clinician's name).

**REMEMBER:** The generic Expedited Determination Notice must be issued 48 hours prior to discharging the patient who is covered by Medicare.

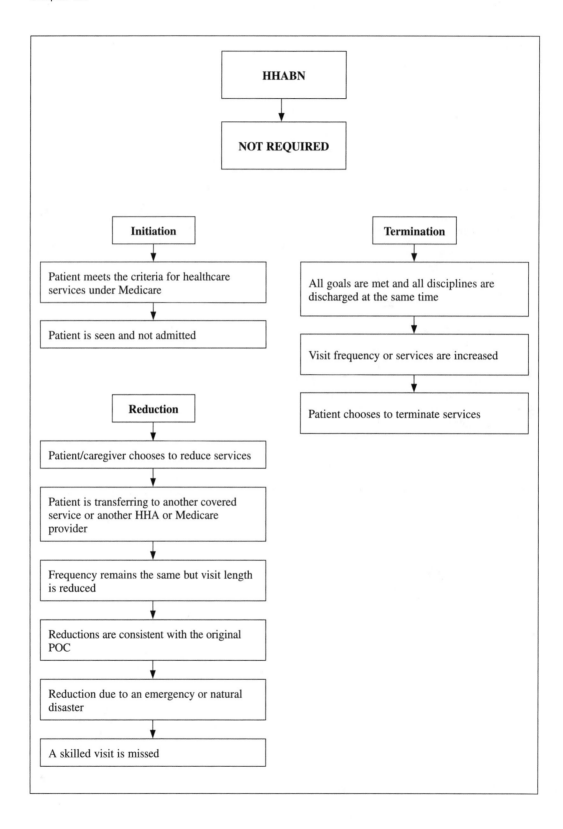

# Chapter 12
# Long-Term Acute Care Hospitals

*Ella James, RHIT*

Medicare defines long-term acute care hospitals (LTCHs) as hospitals that have an average inpatient length of stay greater than 25 days and typically provide extended medical and rehabilitative care for patients who are clinically complex and suffer from multiple acute or chronic conditions. LTCHs that are subject to the requirements of the LTCH PPS meet all of the following criteria:

- They are certified under Medicare as short-term acute care hospitals which have been excluded from the inpatient short-term acute care hospital prospective payment system (IPPS).

- They meet state licensure requirements for short-term acute care hospitals under section 1886(d)(B)(iv) of the Social Security Act.

- They are not excluded LTCH units in a facility, although they can be a satellite and/or hospital within a hospital, colocated within another facility. A hospital within a hospital is a hospital located in or on the campus of an acute care or host hospital. The Centers for Medicare and Medicaid Services (CMS) require an LTCH to have a separate governing body, medical staff, chief medical officer, and chief executive officer. "In addition, the hospital must perform basic functions independently from the host hospital, incur no more than 15 percent of its total inpatient operating costs for items and services supplied by the hospital in which it is located, and have an inpatient load of which at least 75 percent of patients are admitted from sources other than the host hospital" (CMS 2002a).

- LTCHs are identified by the last four digits of the Medicare provider number, which range between 2000 and 2299.

- Each LTCH has a provider agreement with Medicare in order to receive Medicare payment (CMS 2005).

- LTCHS are required to have Physician Acknowledgement Statements signed and dated from the attending physician just as do short-term acute care hospitals.

- LTCHs must have an agreement with a Quality Improvement Organization (QIO) for review that includes the following:

  —The medical necessity, reasonableness, and appropriateness of hospital admission and discharges

  —Inpatient hospital care for which outlier payments are sought

  —Validity of the hospital's diagnostic and procedural information

  —Completeness, adequacy, and quality of the services furnished in the hospital

  —Medical or other practices with respect to beneficiaries or billing for services furnished to the beneficiaries

The Medicare reimbursement for LTCHs is under a PPS based on the Medicare diagnosis-related groups (DRG) system used by short-term acute care hospitals and referred to as LTC-DRGs. The same short-term acute care DRGs are used, but "have been weighted to reflect the resources required to treat the medically complex patients treated at LTCHs" (Elements of the LTCH PPS are available at http://www.cms.hhs.gov). Each LTC-DRG includes an established Average Length of Stay (ALOS) for a patient assigned to the LTC-DRG. LTC-DRGs are paid according to the federal payment rate, including adjustments.

The annual changes to the short-term hospital DRGs also affect the LTCH PPS patient classification system. Because the patient classification system used under the LTCH PPS is based directly on the DRGs used under the IPPS for short-term acute care hospitals, the annual update of the LTC/DRG classifications and relative weights remains linked to the annual reclassification and recalibration of the CMS DRGs used under the IPPS. The update to the LTCH PPS rates—including the federal rate, outlier threshold, wage index and budget neutrality factor, and other policy changes to be effective for discharges occurring on or after July 1 through June 30 each year—is published annually in the *Federal Register* LTCH PPS "rate year proposed and final rules." The update to the LTC-DRG classifications and relative weights to be effective for discharges occurring on or after October 1 through September 30 each year is published in the annual IPPS fiscal year proposed and final rules.

"Relative weights (RW) for the LTC-DRGs are a primary element to account for the variation in cost per discharge because they reflect resource utilization for each diagnosis" (Elements of LTCH PPS). Relative weights for the LTC-DRGs, as in the short-term acute care hospitals, are a key factor that describes the difference in cost per discharge because they reflect resources used for each diagnosis. The different RWs try to account for the variation in cost by reflecting the resources used for each diagnosis. The LTC-DRG relative weights are updated annually using the most recently available claims data. Under the LTCH PPS, payment for a Medicare patient is made at a set, per discharge rate for each LTC-DRG. Adjustments are built into the LTCH PPS for short stay cases, interrupted stay cases, cases discharged and readmitted to colocated providers, and high-cost outlier cases. There are also adjustments for differences in area wages and a cost-of living adjustment (COLA) for LTCHs located in Alaska and Hawaii.

As in short-term acute care hospitals, LTCH DRG assignment is based on the following six elements:

1. Principal diagnosis

2. Up to eight additional diagnoses

3. Principal procedure

4. Patient's age

5. Patient's sex

6. Discharge status

LTCHs also are required to adhere to the Uniform Hospital Discharge Data Set (UHDDS) definitions of principal diagnosis, other diagnoses, and significant procedures.

LTCHs are expected to adhere to the *ICD-9-CM Official Guidelines for Coding and Reporting* and the coding advice provided in *Coding Clinic for ICD-9-CM*. In the LTCH PPS regulations, CMS has noted its concerns with the quality of coding and health record documentation in LTCHs, as was the case at the beginning of the short-term acute care hospital PPS. As in short-term acute care hospitals, inaccurate coding can result in inappropriate LTCH-DRG assignment and reimbursement. Inappropriate coding can adversely affect the uniformity of cases in each LTCH DRG and produce inappropriate weighting factors at calibration. CMS has urged LTCHs in the PPS regulations to focus on improved coding and physician documentation practices. It is imperative that LTCHs carefully analyze current coding and physician documentation practices, develop strategies for improvement, and monitor the effectiveness of these strategies. These are key components in an LTCH health information management (HIM) compliance program. Inappropriate coding and physician documentation practices can lead to fraud and abuse issues for an LTCH institution.

The Office of Inspector General (OIG) Work Plan for Fiscal Year 2007 includes recognized vulnerabilities of Department of Health and Human Services' (HHS) programs and activities. Within this 2007 plan, LTCH payments have been identified. The OIG will "review payments to long-term care hospitals under the prospective payment system to determine the extent to which these payments were made in accordance with Medicare laws and regulations. . . . [and] will review the appropriateness of early discharges to home, interrupted stays" (OIG 2007). This is a work in progress from the OIG 2006 Work Plan. Beginning in 2007, the OIG Work Plan "will determine whether hospitals currently reimbursed as LTCHs are in compliance with the average length of stay criteria" (OIG 2007). Additionally, the 2007 OIG Work Plan will "determine the extent to which LTCHs admit patients from a sole acute-care hospital, thus effectively functioning as units of those hospitals" (OIG 2007). This component is slated to begin in 2008.

The benefits of an HIM compliance program include those identified in short-term acute care hospitals, such as the following:

- Effective internal controls to ensure compliance with federal regulations, payment policies, and official coding rules and guidelines

- Identification of problematic coding and documentation practices and initiation of prompt and appropriate corrective action

- Improved health record documentation

- Improved education for organizational staff and physicians

- Improved coding accuracy

- Reduced claims denial

- Increased productivity due to better communication, more comprehensive policies and procedures, and more efficient operations

- Improved financial performance due to increased productivity and operational efficiency

- Improved collaboration and cooperation among healthcare practitioners and those processing and using health information

- Improved employee performance and morale

- Identification and reporting of unethical HIM practices

- Reduced exposure to civil and criminal penalties and sanctions in the event of a fraud investigation, and if wrongdoing is discovered by the government, a reduction in the severity of imposed penalties

The interrupted stay component of the LTCH PPS provides an additional concern for HIM from a compliance standpoint. "An interrupted stay occurs when a Long-Term Care Hospital (LTCH) patient is discharged from an LTCH and after a specific number of days away from the LTCH, is readmitted to the same LTCH for further medical treatment" (CMS 2004).

An interrupted stay may occur when a patient is discharged from an LTCH and is directly admitted to a specific type of Medicare provider such as an inpatient short-term acute care hospital, an inpatient rehabilitation facility (IRF), or skilled nursing facility (SNF)/swing bed, then returns to the original LTCH within a predetermined period of time. HIM compliance programs must include policies and procedures to ensure compliance with the interrupted stay rule. There are currently two different types of interrupted stays that must be considered, as follows:

- The 3-day-or-less interrupted stay

- The greater-than-3-day interrupted stay

If a stay falls within either designation, Medicare will pay only one LTC-DRG payment to the LTCH.

## The 3-day-or-less interrupted stay

This type of interrupted stay includes LTCH discharges and readmissions to the same LTCH within 3 days. During the 3-day interrupted stay, the patient may have received services in an outpatient or inpatient setting including tests, treatment, or care at a short-term acute care hospital, an IRF, or an SNF/swing bed, or "there may have been an intervening patient-stay at home for up to 3 days without the delivery of additional tests, treatment, or care. . . . The day count for purposes of determining the length of the stay away from the LTCH begins on the day that the patient is first discharged from the LTCH. Medicare payment for any test, procedure, or care provided to the patient on either an outpatient or inpatient basis during the 'interruption' would be the responsibility of the LTCH 'under arrangements'" (CMS 2004).

## The greater-than-3-day interrupted stay

The greater-than-3-day interrupted stay occurs when a patient who has been discharged from an LTCH and admitted to a short-term acute care hospital, an IRF, or an SNF/swing bed, is readmitted to the same LTCH after 3 days. This period of time varies depending on the type of facility that admits the patient from the LTCH: 9 days for a short-term acute care hospital, 27 days for an IRF, or 45 days for an SNF/swing bed. HIM compliance programs must address the appropriate monitoring of interrupted stays because the interrupted stay should not affect the LTC-DRG assignment.

To meet this definition of a greater than 3-day interrupted stay, the patient must meet the following criteria (CMS 2004):

> Discharged directly from the LTCH and admitted directly to an inpatient short-term acute care hospital, an IRF, or a SNF/swing bed.
>
> **AND**
>
> Discharged back to the original LTCH after a Length of Stay (LOS) less than or equal to the applicable fixed-day period.

If the patient is determined to have an interrupted stay at a short-term acute care hospital, an IRF, or an SNF/swing bed, when the patient is readmitted to the LTCH, the entire stay is considered an interrupted stay. The following is stated by CMS (2004):

> The day count to determine whether or not a patient has been away from the LTCH for purposes of the 'greater than 3-day interruption of stay' policy begins on the day of discharge and continues until the day of readmission, even though this policy governs beginning on the patient's fourth day away from the LTCH. A case may have multiple interrupted stays, but each stay must be evaluated separately to make certain that it meets the interrupted stay criteria.

Medicare offers examples of interrupted stays in its Long Term Care Hospital Interrupted Stay Fact Sheet available on its Web site to help LTCHs more clearly understand the interrupted stay rules (CMS 2004). It is imperative that the LTCH HIM compliance program includes processes to monitor this rule to avoid fraud and abuse issues.

Medicare makes one LTC-DRG payment for each patient whether it is a 3-day-or-less or a greater-than-3-day interrupted stay based on the initial admission. It is important to understand that the DRG assignment at the time of the initial admission to the LTCH cannot change due to an interrupted stay unless additional diagnoses or procedures affect the initial coding assignment. An example in which the DRG assignment would change would be a patient admitted to the LTCH with respiratory failure with no mechanical ventilation (DRG 087). After an interrupted stay, the patient is once again admitted with respiratory failure, but is now placed on mechanical ventilation (DRG 475). If the patient, however, is readmitted with respiratory failure and an additional diagnosis of late effect of a stroke, which will be treated, the LTCH DRG must remain as originally assigned, with the additional secondary diagnosis of the late effect of the stroke added to the patient's health records as a secondary diagnosis. The late effect of the stroke diagnosis cannot become the principal reason for admission because the patient has already been admitted and assigned the respiratory failure as the principal diagnosis. The interrupted stay rules are a key component in the LTCH compliance plan. The following has been stated by CMS (2004):

> If the patient's stay meets the interrupted stay criteria, the principal diagnosis should not be changed when the patient returns to the LTCH from the receiving facility. If other medical conditions are apparent upon the patient's return to the LTCH, the additional diagnosis codes should be noted on the claim.

If a patient is admitted **after** the period of time established in the interrupted stay rule, on day 10 or after for a short-term acute care hospital, day 28 or after for an IRF, or day 46 or after for an SNF/swing bed, the patient **does not** have an interrupted stay and HIM coding professionals may reevaluate the principal diagnosis and LTC-DRG assignment using Official Coding Guidance. Other instances when the patient does not have an interrupted stay include the following:

- "The patient is discharged to a type of facility other than the four types of facilities previously mentioned" (CMS 2004).

  Example: The patient is discharged to a psychiatric hospital.

- The patient is discharged to more than one facility.

  Example: The patient is discharged from the LTCH, is admitted to an SNF, and then is discharged from the SNF to a short-term acute care hospital.

- The patient is discharged home and readmitted to the LTCH after more than 3 days. CMS (2004) states the following:

  > If the patient is readmitted to the facility, the second admission begins a new stay. The LTCH would receive two LTC-DRG payments for two patient stays: one payment for the first stay and a separate payment for the stay after the readmission to the LTCH.

LTCH compliance components should contain the following considerations:

- ICD-9-CM coding must be accurate.
- ICD-9-CM coding systems that affect DRG assignment must be updated as changes occur. Changes become effective on April 1 and/or October 1 of each year.

- Annual short-term acute care DRG changes affect LTC-DRGs.

- Invalid diagnosis codes and invalid procedure codes should never be assigned. "Inappropriate coding of cases can adversely affect the uniformity of cases in each LTC-DRG and affect the facility's payment. The emphasis on the need for proper coding cannot be overstated" (CMS 2002b).

- "Each bill from an LTCH must contain the complete diagnosis and procedure coding for purposes of the Grouper software. The principal diagnosis must remain the same on every bill submitted for the LTCH stay" (CMS 2002b). An LTCH patient's hospital stay may have several interim bills for which the principal diagnosis must remain the same.

- If the patient is admitted to the LTCH from a short-term acute care hospital, the principal diagnosis at the LTCH may not be the same diagnosis for which the patient received services at the short-term acute care hospital.

- Diagnoses that are no longer being treated should not be coded in the LTCH setting.

- Procedures should be coded based on current ICD-9-CM coding guidance.

- Secondary or additional diagnoses should be coded as they develop and should never be removed from the patient's account or claims.

It is important for LTCHs to develop systems and processes to code patient records upon admission so that a working DRG can be established for financial tracking and trending and for admission case mix reporting. Although the working DRG may not accurately reflect the final DRG assignment, it provides the facility the ability to determine the average length of stay and projected reimbursement for each case. The working DRG can help the facility ensure that each patient is provided the correct level of care and that the LTCH admission is medically necessary. This process is also a good way to monitor interrupted stays.

Similarly, concurrent coding practices need to be developed to effectively capture all secondary diagnoses for which the patient is being treated. It is also important to concurrently code all procedures because these may affect the final DRG assignment. This practice will ensure that claims submissions are accurate. By establishing a working DRG at admission and concurrently coding the LTCH patient's diagnosis and procedures, final coding of the health record will be much more efficient and effective. Documentation practices can be monitored during admission, concurrently, and at final DRG assignment to improve compliance with proper documentation standards. Once firmly established, this methodology can improve patient placement, documentation and coding practices, DRG assignment, claims submission, and reimbursement.

Additional policies and procedures that are necessary for a thorough compliance plan are as follows:

- Audit controls such as DRG validation (See sample LTCH coding audit form and LTCH audit spreadsheet on the CD-ROM. These references are included to assist in HIM compliance programs for the LTCH organization.)

- Charge Description Master—the HIM role

- Coding competencies and qualifications

- Coding standards including coding timeliness, reference manuals or materials, and update requirements

- Documentation practices

- Education for coding staff not only for proper coding practices, but also compliance issues

- Physician query process: AHIMA provides excellent physician query guidelines in its Practice brief: Developing a physician query process (Prophet 2001). (See full text of this practice brief in appendix D on pp. 293–323.)

## References and Resources

Centers for Medicare and Medicaid Services. 2005 (Dec. 14). Elements of LTCH PPS. Available online from http://www.cms.hhs.gov.

Centers for Medicare and Medicaid Services. 2004 (June). Long-term care hospital interrupted stay fact sheet. Available online from http://www.cms.hhs.gov/LongTermCareHospitalPPS/Downloads/interrupted_stay_fs.pdf.

Centers for Medicare and Medicaid Services. 2002a . (Aug. 30). Medicare program: Prospective payment system for long-term care hospitals, final rule. 42 CFR, Parts 412, 413, and 476. *Federal Register* 67(169):55954–56001. Available online from http://www.cms.hhs.gov/LongTermCareHospitalPPS/downloads/55954-56002.pdf.

Centers for Medicare and Medicaid Services. 2002b (November). LTCH PPS training guide. Available online from http://www.cms.hhs.gov.

Office of Inspector General. 2006. Work plan, fiscal year 2006. Available online from http://oig.hhs.gov/publications/docs/workplan/2007/Work%20Plan%202007.pdf.

Prophet, S. 2001 (October). Practice brief: Developing a physician query process. *Journal of American Health Information Management Association* 72(9):88I–M.

# Chapter 13
# Compliance Considerations in Behavioral Health Facilities

*Linda Martins, RHIA, and Ruby Nicholson, RHIT*

Behavioral healthcare organizations have some of the same compliance challenges as acute care facilities, which require auditing, monitoring, education, and communication. However, following are additional challenges faced by behavioral health providers:

- The Emergency Medical Treatment and Labor Act (EMTALA)

- Prospective payment systems

- A diagnosis classification system (DSM-IV-TR) that requires a crosswalk to reimbursement coding (ICD-9-CM)

- Services that do not fit Current Procedural Terminology (CPT) definitions

- Justification of less-visible signs and symptoms determining medical necessity

- Documentation by and qualifications of paraprofessionals involved in service delivery

## EMTALA in Behavioral Care

Interpretative guidelines have not resolved confusion regarding specific definitions for behavioral health facilities given the unique nature of psychiatric patients and treatments. EMTALA regulations require that patients be treated for an emergency medical condition and be stabilized, but it does not define a psychiatric emergency condition. When EMTALA was implemented, the mental healthcare system was quite different. With the changes throughout the years, understanding how this law should apply to individuals with psychiatric conditions has been confusing. The EMTALA Technical Advisory Group (TAG) helps establish specific interpretative guidelines for psychiatric care and facilities. Some of the issues that affect behavioral healthcare systems regarding EMTALA are emergency medical condition and stabilization, clinically appropriate setting for the patient, financial burden, and conflicting legislation.

## Prospective Payment Systems

Communicating with third party payers the complexity of clinical situations and describing the heterogeneity of individuals presenting with the same diagnosis is another huge challenge. The newest challenge for inpatient psychiatric hospitals is the inpatient psychiatric facility prospective payment system (IPF PPS)—basically, diagnostic related group (DRG) designations used for payment groups for psychiatric hospitals. Each challenge necessitates a well-structured compliance program with auditing, monitoring, and education as its primary components. Although there are some differences between the inpatient and outpatient facilities, the issues with coding, justification, and documentation pose the same problem for HIM professionals regardless of the behavioral health setting.

One major difficulty in coding is that diagnostic formulation occurs in the multiaxial system found in the *Diagnostic and Statistical Manual of Mental Disorders, Fourth Edition, Text Revision* (DSM-IV-TR) (APA 2000). This system provides the clinician the ability to formulate a comprehensive assessment of clinical disorders, the patient's mental capacity, behaviors, general medical conditions, psychosocial and environmental factors, and overall functioning. (See figure 13.1)

**Figure 13.1.   Multiaxial assessment**

| | | |
|---|---|---|
| Axis I: | Clinical Disorders | |
| | Other Conditions That May be a Focus of Clinical Attention | |
| | Diagnosis Code | DSM IV Name |
| Axis II: | Personality Disorders | |
| | Mental Retardation | |
| | Diagnosis Code | DSM IV Name |
| Axis III: | General Medical Conditions | |
| | Diagnosis Code | ICD 9-CM Name |
| Axis IV: | Check those that apply | |
| | ___ Problems with primary support group | |
| | ___ Problems related to the social environment | |
| | ___ Educational problems | |
| | ___ Occupational problems | |
| | ___ Housing problems | |
| | ___ Economic problems | |
| | ___ Problems with access to healthcare services | |
| | ___ Problems related to interaction with the legal system/crime | |
| | ___ Other psychosocial and environmental problems | |
| Axis V: | Global Assessment of Functioning (GAF) Score_____ | |

Source: APA 2000.

# Crosswalk of Diagnostic to Reimbursement Coding

Since clinical staff completing the assessment and formulating a diagnosis are not trained in coding procedures, there are frequent errors due to the lack of specificity and sequencing of diagnoses. DSM-IV-TR diagnoses must be translated, or crosswalked, into *International Classification of Diseases,* Ninth Revision, Clinical Modification (ICD-9-CM) codes for reimbursement. Recently, the ICD-9-CM coordination and maintenance committee made changes to the mental health section (chapter 5). Although some of these changes to language made it easier to correlate the ICD-9-CM with the DSM-IV-TR, this only occurs when the descriptors are equivalent. The big issue that remains is manifestation codes. Manifestation codes are considered a primary Axis I (clinical disorders) principal diagnosis in psychiatry. However, for reimbursement purposes manifestation codes cannot be a principal diagnosis and the underlying physical condition needs to be coded first. Physical conditions are coded on Axis III (general medical conditions) in psychiatry and are not considered the primary principal diagnosis.

Hospitals have qualified coding professionals who are well-versed in medical conditions but additional training is necessary for psychiatric illnesses and criteria for assigning a psychiatric diagnosis. Assignment of a primary diagnosis for a patient with multiple psychiatric illnesses can be difficult because patients often are being treated for more than one diagnosis. That is, a patient may be treated for major depression and alcohol abuse simultaneously, or major depression and posttraumatic stress disorder (PTSD). The patient could be seen by a psychiatrist and prescribed treatment for depression while a counselor provides therapy for PTSD or alcohol abuse.

Assigning a primary diagnosis along with less specificity in some DSM-IV-TR codes creates additional coding problems for reimbursement. Training staff in the importance of crosswalks to ICD-9-CM codes and understanding the specificity and sequencing needed for billing is essential. Staff needs prompts and ongoing training for behavioral health diagnostic criteria and psychiatric diagnoses in the DSM-IV-TR that do not provide the same specificity found in the ICD-9-CM. In many ambulatory outpatient settings, establishing the knowledge base can be a huge task when there are usually no trained coding professionals employed by the organization. Unfortunately, in these settings coding validation is often left to billing staff, who are not versed in coding protocols. Validation of this problem was evident in a recent Office of Inspector General (OIG) report on outpatient mental health services in which a 34 percent claim error rate was reported (OIG 2001). Regardless of the setting or staff qualifications, training cannot be a one-time occurrence, instead it must be done regularly with clinical and nonclinical staff. A brief overview of topics addressed in compliance training is outlined in figure 13.2.

Additional attention has been given to coding since the recent changes Medicare has established for inpatient psychiatric facilities, making the quality of coding and understanding of behavioral health diagnostic criteria a significant factor.

The most recent change for inpatient psychiatric facilities is the IPF PPS published in the *Federal Register* (CMS 2004), which changed the way psychiatric hospitals would be reimbursed. Psychiatric hospitals were reimbursed on a per diem rate but now facilities have adjustment factors in order to establish the reimbursement rate for IPF PPS

**Figure 13.2.   Compliance training outline**

- What are compliance, fraud, and abuse
- Why have a compliance program
- Components of a compliance program
- Organization's code of conduct or code of ethics
- Monitoring and auditing procedures of organization
- Monitoring trends (organization and OIG audit reports)
- High-risk areas
- Assignment of diagnosis codes (DSM-IV-TR)
- Documentation of medical necessity and for justification of continued services
- Documentation of services and progress of treatment
- Crosswalk from DSM-IV-TR to ICD-9-CM
- CPT codes and DRGs
- Timely and accurate coding and billing of services
- Individual staff's role in compliance activities

under the DRG. These are the same DRGs currently used in the acute care hospital settings. All cases have a federal per diem base rate that is adjusted for patient, facility, and other factors. The facility level adjusters are wage index, rural hospital, cost of living for Alaska and Hawaii, and teaching and emergency department adjustment factors. Patient-related adjusters are principal diagnosis, comorbidity, age, variable per diem determined by the length of stay, and electroconvulsive therapy (ECT) rate for any patient who receives this treatment. Another important factor is the interrupted stay provision in the rule, which states any readmission to any IPF within three days of discharge counts as part of the same stay.

There are 15 psychiatric DRGs based on ICD-9-CM codes with adjustment factors for the specific principal diagnosis of the patient. This is a major change in the behavioral health setting because prior to January 2005, PPS was not a factor for psychiatric hospitals with an effective date of January 2005. Psychiatric hospitals adopted changes at the beginning of their first fiscal year post-January 2005. Table 13.1 lists the DRGs and their adjustment factors, and appendix 13A (pp. 245–252) contains a conversion chart of DRG categories to DSM IV diagnoses.

Another patient adjustment factor is comorbidity, which is classified as specific patient conditions that are secondary to the principal diagnosis and coexist at the time of admission, developed subsequently, or affect the resources received or the length of stay, or both. Comorbidities are clinically evaluated, therapeutically treated, require increased monitoring or nursing care, and can extend the length of stay. There are 17 comorbidity categories with specific diagnoses in each area. The diagnoses in these categories are the ones that have been identified previously by the Centers for Medicare and Medicaid Services as additional adjustment factors (CMS 2004). Table 13.2 contains a list of comorbidity adjustment factors.

**Table 13.1.   Psychiatric DRG adjustments**

| DRG | Diagnosis | Adjustment Factor |
|-----|-----------|-------------------|
| 012 | Degenerative Nervous System Disorder | 1.05 |
| 023 | Nontraumatic Stupor & Coma | 1.07 |
| 424 | O.R. Procedure w/ Principal Diagnosis of Mental Illness | 1.22 |
| 425 | Acute Adjustment Reaction & Psychosocial Dysfunction | 1.05 |
| 426 | Depressive Neuroses | 0.99 |
| 427 | Neuroses except Depressive | 1.02 |
| 428 | Disorders of Personality & Impulse Control | 1.02 |
| 429 | Organic Disturbances & Mental Retardation | 1.03 |
| 430 | Psychoses | 1.00 |
| 431 | Childhood Mental Disorders | 0.99 |
| 432 | Other Mental Disorder Diagnoses | 0.92 |
| 433 | Alcohol/Drug Abuse or Dependence Left AMA | 0.97 |
| 521 | Alcohol/Drug Abuse or Dependence W CC | 1.02 |
| 522 | Alcohol/Drug Abuse or Dependence w/ Rehab Therapy w/o CC | 0.98 |
| 523 | Alcohol/Drug Abuse or Dependence w/o Rehabilitation | 0.88 |

Source: CMS 2004 66938.

Another patient payment adjustment factor is age. The adjustment factor depends on the age of the patient, and applies to all patients older than age 45. The older the patient is the higher the adjustment factor due to the complications in treating the elderly population. See table 13.3 for age adjustments.

The final patient adjustment factor is the variable per diem rate, which changes on a day-by-day basis depending on the patient's length of stay in an inpatient psychiatric facility. CMS has recognized that higher cost incurs at the beginning of an inpatient hospitalization. (See table 13.4.)

Figure 13.3 contains a list of issues to review when monitoring for compliance with the IPF PPS.

**Table 13.2.   Comorbidity adjustments**

| Diagnosis* | Adjustment Factor |
|---|---|
| Developmental Disabilities | 1.04 |
| Coagulation Factor Deficit | 1.13 |
| Tracheostomy | 1.06 |
| Eating and Conduct Disorders | 1.12 |
| Infectious Diseases | 1.07 |
| Renal Failure, Acute | 1.11 |
| Renal Failure, Chronic | 1.11 |
| Oncology Treatment | 1.07 |
| Uncontrolled Type I Diabetes Mellitus | 1.05 |
| Severe Protein Malnutrition | 1.13 |
| Drug/Alcohol Induced Mental Disorders | 1.03 |
| Cardiac Conditions | 1.11 |
| Gangrene | 1.10 |
| Chronic Obstructive Pulmonary Disease | 1.12 |
| Artificial Openings—Digestive & Urinary | 1.08 |
| Musculoskeletal & Connective Tissue Diseases | 1.09 |
| Poisoning | 1.11 |

*See appendix 13B (p. 253) for specific diagnoses in each category.
Source: CMS 2004 66984.

**Table 13.3.   Age adjustments**

| Age | Adjustment Factor | Age | Adjustment Factor |
|---|---|---|---|
| Younger than 45 | 1.00 | 65 and younger than 70 | 1.10 |
| 45 and younger than 50 | 1.01 | 70 and younger than 75 | 1.13 |
| 50 and younger than 55 | 1.02 | 75 and younger than 80 | 1.15 |
| 55 and younger than 60 | 1.04 | 80 and older | 1.17 |
| 60 and younger than 65 | 1.07 | | |

Source: CMS 2004 66983.

**Table 13.4.   Variable IPF per diem adjustments**

| Day | Adjustment Factor |
|---|---|
| Day 1—Facility without a full-service emergency department | 1.19 |
| Day 1—Facility with a full-service emergency department | 1.31 |
| Day 2 | 1.12 |
| Day 3 | 1.08 |
| Day 4 | 1.05 |
| Day 5 | 1.04 |
| Day 6 | 1.02 |
| Day 7 | 1.01 |
| Day 8 | 1.01 |
| Day 9 | 1.00 |
| Day 10 | 1.00 |
| Day 11 | 0.99 |
| Day 12 | 0.99 |
| Day 13 | 0.99 |
| Day 14 | 0.99 |
| Day 15 | 0.98 |
| Day 16 | 0.97 |
| Day 17 | 0.97 |
| Day 18 | 0.96 |
| Day 19 | 0.95 |
| Day 20 | 0.95 |
| Day 21 | 0.95 |
| GT 21 Days | 0.92 |

Source: CMS 2004 66983–84.

**Figure 13.3.   IPF PPS compliance issues**

- Is the mix of your patients greater for mental illness or chemical dependence?
- What is your facility's Medicare average length of stay?
- Have you recently examined the staffing for psychiatric services?
- Does your facility use a case mix or resource sensitive method to staff or evaluate staffing?
- Have you recently or are you planning a capital replacement or expansion of your psychiatric facility?
- Does your facility monitor length of stay throughout the stay, after a specific threshold, at all?
- Does your facility have a psychiatric teaching program?
- Is your facility located in a rural area?
- What is your facility's average wage index?
- What is the proportion of Medicare days that fall into DRG 430 (Psychosis)?
- Does your facility's information system capture case complexity variables, such as DRG assignment, diabetes, ESRD, COPD, etc.?
- What is the case mix index for your psychiatric unit/hospital cases using the psychiatric DRGs?
- What is the proportion of your Medicare psychiatric days for patients who are 70 years of age and older?

## Crosswalk of Services to CPT Codes

Billing policies and procedures must be routinely reviewed as well as crosswalks used with CPT codes. Many organizations have service codes that align with state reimbursement definitions that must be correctly crosswalked or linked to the appropriate CPT code. There are a number of services reimbursed in a "bundled rate," particularly in children services or for mobile treatment teams, which also need to be reviewed with CPT coding and reporting rules. Strict procedures for emergency department billing, per diem billing, partial hospitalizations, psychosocial rehabilitation, case management, and other outpatient services must be implemented and audited routinely. According to OIG audits, 34 percent of outpatient individual therapy sessions in mental health services are billed inappropriately. Some types of billing errors are as follows:

- Incorrect place of service (facility type) on the claim form
- Incomplete listing of diagnoses on the claim form
- Incorrect principal diagnosis on the claim
- Incorrect clinician listed as the provider

Clinical documentation is the basis for treatment of the patient. Documentation on behavioral healthcare services contributes to continuity of care and treatment planning for the patient. Documentation is also the basis for selecting the correct procedural code and provides some protection against audit liability by providing factual information to support coding and charges. Also, clinical documentation supports medical decision making and provides the necessary information for claims review.

Documentation for evaluation and management (E&M) services are complex, and the American Medical Association (AMA) and CMS are exploring ways to revise the current guidelines, which are being reviewed for restructuring to make documentation more clinically relevant.

Several fiscal intermediaries (FIs) have published local coverage determination policies addressing documentation requirements for psychotherapy codes. This was done because there is no accepted universal standard for documenting psychotherapy services for E&M. Documentation requirements vary from carrier to carrier, but including the following information should satisfy most third party payers:

- Date of service

- Total time spent face-to-face with the patient

- Type of therapeutic intervention (insight oriented, supportive, behavior modification, interactive)

- Target symptoms

- Progress toward treatment goals

- E&M service provided

- Diagnoses

- Legible signature

Another important factor is the setting in which the service occurred, such as inpatient or outpatient. Refer to the current CPT codebook for specific psychiatric therapeutic codes that reflect the treatment setting provided to the patient.

## Justification of Medical Necessity

One of the most cited reasons for inappropriateness in the OIG audit was services that were not found medically necessary. The greatest challenge is getting clinical staff to clearly document the medical necessity for services. Signs and symptoms linking to the diagnosis and then justification for the need for services is frequently missing. Dealing with feelings, emotions, and one's individual self are not always physically visible and are difficult to describe in terms of medical need. Individuals providing outpatient services must ask questions such as the following:

- What am I or another behavioral health professional providing that a friend or family member cannot provide?

- Why is this service needed and how does the patient's signs, symptoms, and diagnosis warrant treatment?

- What are the functional deficits resulting from the mental illness that require professional intervention or case management services?

Another related compliance issue for inpatient psychiatric hospitals is determining if the patient not only requires care that is medically necessary but whether it can or cannot reasonably be delivered at a less intensive level of care. Medical necessity is an important factor for services rendered to any patient at any level of care. The need for services must be consistent with the symptoms or diagnosis of the illness or injury under treatment and consistent with generally accepted professional medical standards. Physician leadership and clinical involvement must be evident throughout the episode of care. A comprehensive individualized treatment plan should exist for each patient, based on professional assessment that offers an array and intensity of services that reflects a hospital level of care. Adequate numbers of appropriately qualified professionals should be available to evaluate each patient and formulate and deliver this individualized active treatment program. Medicare requires that upon admission to an inpatient psychiatric hospital, a physician certify that inpatient hospitalization is necessary for the patient to receive appropriate care. Recertification is required on day 18 by the attending physician. This requirement was changed in the proposed rule for IPF PPS on January 23, 2006 (CMS 2006c). Medical Necessity for psychiatric inpatient hospitalization was included on the OIG Work Plan for 2005. In 2006, the OIG reviewed psychiatric hospitals reimbursed under the IPF PPS to determine if they were in compliance with the Medicare laws and regulations. For 2007, the OIG expanded its review of behavioral health organizations and is focusing on the following areas:

- Reviewing IPF PPS claims for outliers

- Part B Mental Health Services

- Psychiatric services provided in an inpatient setting

Figure 13.4 lists some of the elements to review regarding medical necessity for inpatient behavioral facility hospitalization.

It is not surprising that the OIG reports that 65 percent of the problems for their findings in outpatient mental health services are due to poor documentation. In addition to documenting medical necessity, providers must be sure that documentation justifies the duration or frequency of services and validates the need for continued services. The symptoms exhibited, goals of treatment, client's capacity to participate in treatment, and progress as it relates to the interventions prescribed on the treatment plan must all be documented. An individualized treatment plan must state all services being provided and progress notes must reflect progress of treatment interventions. Services provided that are not identified on the treatment plan are disallowed. In the outpatient setting, providers must monitor documentation to ensure individual therapy sessions are truly psychotherapy and not case management services. Case management documentation often focuses on social service supports rather than on signs, symptoms, and functional deficits as a result of a diagnosis that impairs the patient from completing daily routine tasks. Training for clinical staff on service definitions and the interpretation of basic service elements is essential. Close attention should be given to documentation of case management, psychosocial rehabilitation, and recreational activities; many of these are delivered by paraprofessionals who are not trained in documenting signs and symptoms as they relate to a specific diagnosis and justify the activities provided.

**Figure 13.4. Elements to review for inpatient behavioral facility hospitalization**

- Any evidence of self-injurious behavior?
- Any evidence of threatening behavior?
- Any evidence of disorganized behavior?
- Any evidence of disordered thinking?
- Description of mood and affect?
- Is patient compliant with treatment plan?
- Is patient eating? How much?
- Is patient sleeping adequately? How many hours?
- Is patient attending to ADLs appropriately?
- Is patient compliant with medication? Is medication education provided?
- Use of PRNs and response
- Documentation of severity of symptoms, whether they have increased or decreased or different symptoms have emerged
- Does patient require 24-hour professional observation?
- Is there documentation of why passes are needed and the patient's response to a pass?
- At what level does the patient attend and participate in groups?
- Is the patient able and willing to participate in discharge planning?
- Is the family/significant other participating in the patient's treatment?
- If the patient has substance misuse or abuse issues, is the patient willing to address this in treatment?

# Paraprofessionals in Service Delivery

Another challenge is making sure paraprofessionals are providing services they are qualified to render and that documentation for these services meet the required standards.

Often documentation by paraprofessionals is vague. Many payers require the involvement of a licensed professional on treatment plans. Establishing quality checks of treatment plans can help reduce the risk of disallowed services due to poor documentation.

Depending on the setting and requirements of an organization, auditing and monitoring could be a random sample of each provider's records over a given period of time or auditing of each record prior to billing. Either method requires corrective action plans that ensure remediation, routine reviews of any trends, and protocols to ensure organizational value results. Auditors should review for both the existence of documentation and complete, comprehensive documents that identify signs, symptoms, the need for services, and progress of outcomes.

Questions for those conducting behavioral compliance documentation audits should include those listed in Figure 13.5.

**Figure 13.5.   Questions to consider in behavioral compliance documentation audits**

- Is there documentation of medical necessity, in other words, does documentation indicate why services are necessary?
- Does the diagnosis warrant the particular treatment being offered?
- Are correct diagnostic codes being used?
- Does the patient have the cognitive or communication skills necessary to benefit from treatment?
- Could services be provided by someone other than a mental health professional?
- Is there documentation of symptoms, goals, and client's capacity to participate in treatment?
- Do progress notes relate to the interventions prescribed on the treatment plan?
- Do progress notes document all services being prescribed on the treatment plan?
- Does documentation justify the duration or frequency of services?
- Does documentation justify any extension of services?
- Are services being provided by a qualified professional?
- Is documentation timely, legible, and signed?
- Is billing timely and accurate?
- Are services provided within the standard payer definitions and do these align with correct CPT codes?

The OIG Work Plan for 2007 identified the following areas in behavioral health services as areas they will audit to determine whether these services were appropriate:

- Part B mental health services to determine whether services provided in physician's offices were medically necessary and billed in accordance with Medicare requirements. Physician's office setting accounted for nearly 55 percent of the $1.3 billion in Medicare Part B mental health services in 2002. Prior audit reports indicated Medicare allowed for $185 million of inappropriate mental health services in an outpatient setting.
- Community mental health centers to determine if Medicaid payments were made in accordance with applicable federal and state regulation and guidance. Prior reviews for Medicare payments identified problems, including payments for noncovered services and payment for services to beneficiaries who did not meet eligibility requirements.
- Medicaid outpatient mental health services to identify improper payments and potential cost savings for Medicaid outpatient services. Based on the Medicare study, one-third of outpatient mental health services provided were medically unnecessary, billed incorrectly, rendered by unqualified providers, undocumented, or poorly documented. This study will determine if the issues are the same for Medicaid.

Additional areas of focus for 2007 are as follows:

- Medicaid for persons with mental disabilities
- Rehabilitation services for persons with mental illnesses
- Medicaid supplemental mental health payments to prepaid inpatient health plans
- Nursing home residents with mental illness and mental retardation
- Restraint and seclusion in children's psychiatric residential treatment facilities

- Medicaid/State Children's Health Insurance Programs (SCHIP)

- Adult rehabilitative services

- Outpatient alcoholism and substance abuse services

- Freestanding inpatient alcohol treatment providers

The Deficit Reduction Act of 2006 is also paying particular attention to case management and has targeted case management in adult and children outpatient mental health services.

For more information, see the OIG 2007 Work Plan (OIG 2007).

## References and Resources

American Medical Association. 2006. *Current Procedural Terminology.* Chicago: AMA.

American Medical Association. 2006. *International Classfication of Diseases, Ninth Revision, Clinical Modification (ICD-9-CM).* Chicago: AMA.

American Psychiatric Association. 2000. *Diagnostic and Statistical Manual of Mental Disorders, Fourth Edition, Text Revision.* Arlington, VA: American Psychiatric Publishing.

Centers for Medicare and Medicaid Services. 2006a (April 25). IPF PPS overview. Available online from http://www.cms.hhs.gov/InpatientPsychFacilPPS/.

Centers for Medicare and Medicaid Services. 2006b (May 3). IPF PPS tools and worksheets. Available online from http://www.cms.hhs.gov/InpatientPsychFacilPPS/04_tools.asp.

Centers for Medicare and Medicaid Services. 2006c (Jan. 23). Medicare Program: Inpatient Psychiatric Facilities Prospective Payment System Payment Update for Rate Year Beginning July 1, 2006 (RY 2007), Proposed Rule. 42 CFR Parts 412 and 424. *Federal Register* 71(14):3616–3752. Available online from http://a257.g.akamaitech.net/7/257/2422/01jan20061800/edocket.access.gpo.gov/2006/pdf/06-488.pdf.

Centers for Medicare and Medicaid Services. 2004 (Nov. 15). Medicare Program: Prospective Payment System for Inpatient Psychiatric Facilities, Final Rule. 42 CFR Parts 412 and 413. *Federal Register* 69(219):(66922–67015). Available online from http://a257.g.akamaitech.net/7/257/2422/15nov20040800/edocket.access.gpo.gov/2004/pdf/04-24787.pdf.

Office of Inspector General. 2006. Work Plan, fiscal year 2007. Available online from http://www.oig.hhs.gov/publications/docs/workplan/2007/Work%20Plan%202007.pdf.

Office of Inspector General. 2005. Work Plan, fiscal year 2006. Available online from http://oig.hhs.gov/publications/docs/workplan/2006/WorkPlanFY2006.pdf.

Office of Inspector General. 2001 (May). Outpatient mental health audit. Washington, DC: HHS.

# Appendix 13A
# ICD-9-CM-based DRGs Converted to DSM-IV

## DRG 12 Degenerative Nervous System Disorder (294.10 and 294.11 fall in this category)

*Adjustment Factor 1.05*

| **DSM-4 Codes** | 331.0 | Disease, Alzheimer's |
|---|---|---|
| | 331.1 | Disease, Pick's |
| | 331.2 | Degeneration brain senile |
| | 331.7 | Degeneration brain classified elsewhere |
| | 331.9 | Degeneration brain unspecified |
| | 332.0 | Disease Parkinson's |
| | 332.1 | Neuroleptic-Induced Parkinsonism |
| | 333.4 | Chorea Huntington's |
| | 333.7 | Dystonia, torsion symptomatic |
| | 333.90 | Medication Induced Movement Disorder NOS |
| | 333.99 | Neuroleptic-Induced Acute Akathisia |

## DRG 23 Nontraumatic Stupor or Coma

*Adjustment Factor 1.07*

**DSM-4 Code**    780.09    Delirium NOS

## DRG 424 O.R. Procedure with Principal Diagnosis of Mental Illness

*Adjustment Factor 1.22*

---

Sources: APA 2000, AMA 2006.

## DRG 425 Acute Adjustment Reactions and Psychosocial Dysfunction

*Adjustment Factor 1.05*

**DSM-4 Codes**

| | |
|---|---|
| 293.0 | Delirium due to General Medical Condition |
| 293.9 | Mental Disorder NOS |
| 300.00 | Anxiety Disorder NOS |
| 300.01 | Panic Disorder without Agoraphobia |
| 300.02 | Generalized Anxiety Disorder |
| 300.11 | Conversion Disorder |
| 300.12 | Dissociative Amnesia |
| 300.13 | Dissociative Fugue |
| 300.15 | Dissociative Disorder NOS |
| 300.16 | Factitious Disorder with Predominantly Psychological Signs and Symptoms |
| 300.19 | Factitious Disorder NOS |
| 300.9 | Unspecified Mental Disorder |
| 308.3 | Acute Stress Disorder |
| V71.01 | Adult Antisocial Behavior |
| V71.02 | Child or Adolescent Antisocial Behavior |

## DRG 426 Depressive Neuroses

*Adjustment Factor .99*

**DSM-4 Codes**

| | |
|---|---|
| 300.4 | Dysthymic Disorder |
| 309.0 | Adjustment Disorder with Depressed Mood |
| 311 | Depressive Disorder NOS |

## DRG 427 Neuroses Except Depressive

*Adjustment Factor 1.02*

**DSM-4 Codes**

| | |
|---|---|
| 300.2 | PHOBIA, UNSPECIFIED |
| 300.21 | Panic Disorder with Agoraphobia |
| 300.22 | Agoraphobia without history of Panic Disorder |
| 300.23 | Social Phobia |
| 300.29 | Specific Phobia |
| 300.3 | Obsessive-Compulsive Disorder |
| 300.6 | Depersonalization Disorder |
| 300.7 | Body Dysmorphic Disorder |
| 300.81 | Somatization Disorder |

| | |
|---|---|
| 300.82 | Somatoform Disorder NOS |
| 300.82 | Undifferentiated Somatoform Disorder |
| 307.53 | Rumination Disorder |
| 307.80 | Pain Disorder Associated with Psychological Factors |
| 307.89 | Pain Disorder Associated with Both Psychological Factors and a General Medical Condition |
| 309.21 | Separation Anxiety Disorder |
| 309.24 | Adjustment Disorder with Anxiety |
| 309.28 | Adjustment Disorder with Depressed Mood and Anxiety |
| 309.3 | Adjustment Disorder with Disturbance of Conduct |
| 309.4 | Adjustment Disorder with Mixed Disturbance of Emotions and Conduct |
| 309.81 | Posttraumatic Stress Disorder |
| 309.9 | Adjustment Disorder Unspecified |

## DRG 428 Disorders of Personality and Impulse Control

*Adjustment Factor 1.02*

**DSM-4 Codes**

| | |
|---|---|
| 300.14 | Dissociative Identity Disorder |
| 301.0 | Paranoid Personality Disorder |
| 301.13 | Cyclothymic Disorder |
| 301.20 | Schizoid Personality Disorder |
| 301.22 | Schizotypal Personality Disorder |
| 301.4 | Obsessive-Compulsive Personality Disorder |
| 301.50 | Histrionic Personality Disorder |
| 301.6 | Dependent Personality Disorder |
| 301.7 | Antisocial Personality Disorder |
| 301.81 | Narcissistic Personality Disorder |
| 301.82 | Avoidant Personality Disorder |
| 301.83 | Borderline Personality Disorder |
| 301.9 | Personality Disorder NOS |
| 307.1 | Anorexia Nervosa |
| 312.31 | Pathological Gambling |
| 312.32 | Kleptomania |
| 312.34 | Intermittent Explosive Disorder |
| 312.39 | Trichotillomania |

## DRG 429 Organic Disturbances and Mental Retardation

*Adjustment Factor 1.03*

**DSM-4 Codes**

| | |
|---|---|
| 290.40 | Vascular Dementia Uncomplicated |
| 290.41 | Vascular Dementia with Delirium |
| 290.42 | Vascular Dementia with Delusions |
| 290.43 | Vascular Dementia with Depressed Mood |
| 293.81 | Psychotic Disorder due to General Medical Condition with Delusions |
| 293.82 | Psychotic Disorder due to General Medical Condition with Hallucinations |
| 293.83 | Mood Disorder due to General Medical Condition |
| 293.84 | Anxiety Disorder due to General Medical Condition |
| 293.89 | Catatonic Disorder due to General Medical Condition |
| 294.0 | Amnestic Disorder due to General Medical Condition |
| 294.10 | Dementia in Conditions Classified Elsewhere without Behavioral Disturbance |
| 294.11 | Dementia in Conditions Classified Elsewhere with Behavioral Disturbance |
| 294.8 | Dementia NOS |
| 294.8 | Amnestic Disorder NOS |
| 294.9 | Cognitive Disorder NOS |
| 299.00 | Autistic Disorder |
| 299.10 | Childhood Disintegrative Disorder |
| 307.9 | Communication Disorder NOS |
| 310.1 | Personality Change due to General Medical Condition |
| 316 | Psychological factor affecting General Medical Condition |
| 317 | Mild Mental Retardation |
| 318.0 | Moderate Mental Retardation |
| 318.1 | Severe Mental Retardation |
| 318.2 | Profound Mental Retardation |
| 319 | Mental Retardation Severity Unspecified |

## DRG 430 Psychosis (denotes all specifity for the diagnosis)

*Adjustment Factor 1.00*

**DSM-4 Codes**

| | |
|---|---|
| 295.1 | Schizophrenia Disorganized Type |
| 295.2 | Schizophrenia Catatonic Type |
| 295.3 | Schizophrenia Paranoid Type |
| 295.4 | Schizophreniform Type |
| 295.6 | Schizophrenia Residual Type |
| 295.7 | Schizoaffective Disorder |
| 295.9 | Schizophrenia Undifferentiated Type |
| 296.0 | Bipolar I Disorder Single Manic Episode |

| | | |
|---|---|---|
| 296.2 | Major Depression Single Episode |
| 296.3 | Major Depression Recurrent Episode |
| 296.4 | Bipolar I Disorder Most Recent Episode Manic |
| 296.5 | Bipolar I Disorder Most Recent Episode Depressed |
| 296.6 | Bipolar I Disorder Most Recent Episode Mixed |
| 296.7 | Bipolar I Disorder Most Recent Episode Unspecified |
| 296.80 | Bipolar Disorder NOS |
| 296.89 | Bipolar II Disorder |
| 296.90 | Mood Disorder NOS |
| 297.1 | Delusional Disorder |
| 297.3 | Shared Psychotic Disorder |
| 298.8 | Brief Psychotic Disorder |
| 298.9 | Psychotic Disorder NOS |
| 299.8 | Aspergers/Pervasive Developmental/Retts Disorder |

## DRG 431 Childhood Mental Disorder

*Adjustment Factor .99*

**DSM-4 Codes**

| | | |
|---|---|---|
| 307.52 | Pica |
| 307.6 | Enuresis Not due to Medical Condition |
| 307.7 | Encopresis without Constipation and Overflow Incontinence |
| 312.30 | Impulse-Control Disorder NOS |
| 312.33 | Pyromania |
| 312.81 | Conduct Disorder Childhood Onset Type |
| 312.82 | Conduct Disorder Adolescent Onset Type |
| 312.89 | Conduct Disorder Unspecified Onset Type |
| 312.9 | Disruptive Behavior Disorder NOS |
| 313.23 | Selective Mutism |
| 313.81 | Oppositional Defiant Disorder |
| 313.82 | Identity Problem |
| 313.89 | Reactive Attachment Disorder of Infancy or Early Childhood |
| 313.9 | Disorder of Infancy, Childhood or Adolescence NOS |
| 314.00 | Attention Deficit Hyperactivity Disorder Predominantly Inattentive Type |
| 314.01 | Attention Deficit Hyperactivity Disorder Combined/ Hyperactive/Impulsive Type |
| 314.9 | Attention-Deficit/Hyperactivity Disorder NOS |
| 315.00 | Reading Disorder |
| 315.1 | Mathematics Disorder |
| 315.2 | Disorder of Written Expression |
| 315.31 | Expressive Language Disorder |
| 315.32 | Mixed Receptive-Expressive Language Disorder |
| 315.4 | Developmental Coordination Disorder |
| 315.9 | Learning Disorder NOS |

## DRG 432 Other Mental Disorder Diagnoses

*Adjustment Factor .92*

**DSM-4 Codes**

| | |
|---|---|
| 302.2 | Pedophilia |
| 302.3 | Transvestic Fetishism |
| 302.4 | Exhibitionism |
| 302.6 | Gender Identity Disorder NOS |
| 302.70 | Sexual Dysfunction NOS |
| 302.71 | Hypoactive Sexual Desire Disorder |
| 302.72 | Female Sexual Arousal Disorder/Male Erectile Disorder |
| 302.73 | Female Orgasmic Disorder |
| 302.74 | Male Orgasmic Disorder |
| 302.75 | Premature Ejaculation |
| 302.76 | Dyspareunia Not due to General Medical Condition |
| 302.79 | Sexual Aversion Disorder |
| 302.81 | Fetishism |
| 302.82 | Voyeurism |
| 302.83 | Sexual Masochism |
| 302.84 | Sexual Sadism |
| 302.85 | Gender Identity Disorder in Adolescents or Adults |
| 302.89 | Frotteurism |
| 302.9 | Paraphilia NOS/Sexual Disorder NOS |
| 307.0 | Stuttering |
| 307.3 | Stereotypic Movement Disorder |
| 307.42 | Insomnia Related to Axis I or II Disorder/Primary Insomnia |
| 307.44 | Hypersomnia Related to Axis I or II Disorder/Primary Hypersomnia |
| 307.45 | Circadian Rhythm Sleep Disorder |
| 307.46 | Sleep Terror Disorder/Sleepwalking Disorder |
| 307.47 | Dyssomnia NOS/Nightmare Disorder/Parasomnia NOS |
| 307.50 | Eating Disorder NOS |
| 307.51 | Bulimia Nervosa |
| 307.59 | Feeding Disorder of Infancy or Early Childhood |
| 780.52 | Sleep Disorder Due to General Medical Condition, Insomnia Type |
| 780.54 | Sleep Disorder Due to General Medical Condition, Hypersomnia Type |
| 780.59 | Breathing Related Sleep Disorder/Sleep Disorder due to General Medical Condition, Mixed or Parasomnia Type |
| V71.09 | No Diagnosis on Axis I or II |

## DRG 433 Alcohol/Drug Abuse or Dependence (AMA)

*Adjustment Factor .97*

[Note: Discharge status must be AMA]

## DRG 521 Alcohol/Drug Abuse or Dependence with CC

*Adjustment Factor 1.02*

| **DSM-4 Codes** | 291.0 | Alcohol Intoxication/Withdrawal Delirium |
|---|---|---|
| | 291.1 | Alcohol-Induced Persisting Amnestic Disorder |
| | 291.2 | Alcohol-Induced Persisting Dementia |
| | 291.3 | Alcohol-Induced Psychotic Disorder with Hallucinations |
| | 291.5 | Alcohol-Induced Psychotic Disorder with Delusions |
| | 291.81 | Alcohol Withdrawal |
| | 291.89 | Alcohol-Induced Anxiety/Mood/Sexual/Sleep Disorder or Dysfunction |
| | 291.9 | Alcohol-Related Disorder NOS |
| | 292.0 | Amphetamine/Cocaine/Nicotine/Opioid/Other Substance Withdrawal |
| | 292.11 | Amphetamine/Cocaine/Nicotine/Opioid/Cannabis/Phencyclidine Induced Psychotic Disorder with Delusions |
| | 292.12 | Amphetamine/Cocaine/Nicotine/Opioid/Cannabis/Phencyclidine Induced Psychotic Disorder with Hallucinations |
| | 292.81 | Amphetamine/Cocaine/Nicotine/Opioid/Cannabis/Phencyclidine Intoxification Delirium |
| | 292.82 | Inhalant/Other/Sedative/Hypnotic or Anxiolytic Persisting Dementia |
| | 292.83 | Other/Sedative/Hypnotic or Anxiolytic Induced Persisting Amnestic Disorder |
| | 292.84 | Amphetamine/Cocaine/Nicotine/Opioid/Cannabis/Phencyclidine/Sedative/Hypnotic/Anxiolytic Induced Mood Disorder |
| | 292.89 | Amphetamine Induced Anxiety/Sexual/Sleep Disorder/Intoxication |
| | 292.89 | Caffeine Induced Anxiety/Sleep Disorder |
| | 292.89 | Cannabis Induced Anxiety/Sleep Disorder/Intoxication |
| | 292.89 | Cocaine Induced Anxiety/Sexual/Sleep Disorder/Intoxication |
| | 292.89 | Hallucinogen Induced Anxiety/Intoxication/Perception Disorder |
| | 292.89 | Inhalant Induced Anxiety/Intoxication Disorder |
| | 292.89 | Opioid Induced Sexual/Sleep Disorder/Intoxication |
| | 292.89 | Other Substance Induced Anxiety/Sexual/Sleep/Intoxication Disorder |

| | | |
|---|---|---|
| 292.89 | Phencyclidine Induced Anxiety/Intoxication Disorder |
| 292.89 | Sedative/Hypnotic or Anxiolytic Induced Anxiety/Sexual/ Sleep/Intoxication Disorder |
| 292.9 | Amphetamine/Caffeine/Cannabis/Cocaine/Hallucinogen/ Inhalant/Nicotine/Opioid/Other Substance/Phencyclidine/ Sedative/Hypnotic/Anxiolytic Related Disorder NOS |
| 303.00 | Alcohol Intoxication |
| 303.90 | Alcohol Dependence |
| 304.00 | Opioid Dependence |
| 304.10 | Sedative Hypnotic or Anxiolytic Dependence |
| 304.20 | Cocaine Dependence |
| 304.30 | Cannabis Dependence |
| 304.40 | Amphetamine Dependence |
| 304.50 | Hallucinogen Dependence |
| 304.60 | Inhalant/Phencyclidine Dependence |
| 304.80 | Polysubstance Dependence |
| 304.90 | Other Unknown Substance Dependence |
| 305.00 | Alcohol Abuse |
| 305.20 | Cannabis Abuse |
| 305.30 | Hallucinogen Abuse |
| 305.40 | Sedative/Hypnotic or Anxiolytic Abuse |
| 305.50 | Opioid Abuse |
| 305.60 | Cocaine Abuse |
| 305.70 | Amphetamine Abuse |
| 305.90 | Caffeine Intoxication/Inhalant/Phencyclidine/Other Substance |

## DRG 522 Alcohol/Drug Abuse or Dependence with Rehab without CC

*Adjustment Factor .98*

**Same Codes as DRG 521 in conjunction with the following procedure**

| | |
|---|---|
| 94.61 | Rehabilitation Alcohol |
| 94.63 | Rehabilitation/Detoxification Alcohol |
| 94.64 | Rehabilitation Drug |
| 94.66 | Rehabilitation/Detoxification Drug |
| 94.67 | Rehabilitation Combined Alcohol and Drug |
| 94.69 | Rehabilitation/Detoxification Alcohol and Drug combined |

## DRG 523 Alcohol/Drug Abuse or Dependence without Rehabilitation Therapy without CC

*Adjustment Factor .88*

**Same Codes as DRG 521**

# Appendix 13B
# Comorbidity Descriptions and Adjustment Factors

| Description of Comorbidity | ICD-9-CM Code | Adjustment Factor |
|---|---|---|
| Developmental Disabilities | 317, 3180, 3181, 3182, and 319 | 1.04 |
| Coagulation Factor Deficits | 2860 through 2864 | 1.13 |
| Tracheotomy | 51900 through 51909 and V440 | 1.06 |
| Renal Failure, Acute | 5845 through 5849, 63630, 63631, 63632, 63730, 63731, 63732, 6383, 6393, 66932, 66934, 9585 | 1.11 |
| Renal Failure, Chronic | 40301, 40311, 40391, 40402, 40403, 40412, 40413, 40492, 40493, 585, 586, V451, V560, V561, and V562 | 1.11 |
| Oncology Treatment | 1400 through 2399 with a radiation therapy code 92.21–92.29 or chemotherapy code 99.25 | 1.07 |
| Uncontrolled Diabetes-Mellitus with or without Complications | 25002, 25003, 25012, 25013, 25022, 25023, 25032, 25033, 25042, 25043, 25052, 25053, 25062, 25063, 25072, 25073, 25082, 25083, 25092, and 25093 | 1.05 |
| Severe Protein Calorie Malnutrition | 260 through 262 | 1.13 |
| Eating and Conduct Disorders | 3071, 30750, 31203, 31233, and 31234 | 1.12 |
| Infectious Disease | 01000 through 04110, 042, 04500 through 05319, 05440 through 05449, 0550 through 0770, 0782 through 07889, and 07950 through 07959 | 1.07 |
| Drug and/or Alcohol Induced Mental Disorders | 2910, 2920, 29212, 2922, 30300, and 30400 | 1.03 |
| Cardiac Conditions | 3910, 3911, 3912, 40201, 40403, 4160, 4210, 4211, and 4219 | 1.11 |
| Gangrene | 44024 and 7854 | 1.10 |
| Chronic Obstructive Pulmonary Disease | 49121, 4941, 5100, 51883, 51884, V4611 and V4612 | 1.12 |
| Artificial Openings—Digestive and Urinary | 56960 through 56969, 9975, and V441 through V446 | 1.08 |
| Severe Musculoskeletal and Connective Tissue Diseases | 6960, 7100, 73000 through 73009, 73010 through 73019, and 73020 through 73029 | 1.09 |
| Poisoning | 96500 through 96509, 9654, 9670 through 9699, 9770, 9800 through 9809, 9830 through 9839, 986, 9890 through 9897 | 1.11 |

# References

Abraham, Prinny Rose, and Reesa Gottschalk. 2004. *ICD-9-CM Diagnostic Coding for Long-Term Care and Home Care.* Chicago: American Health Information Management Association.

Abraham, Prinny Rose. 2001. Trends to watch in home health compliance. *Journal of the American Health Information Management Association* 72(5): 47.

Amatayakul, Margret, Mary Brandt, and Michelle Dougherty. 2003. Cut, Copy, Paste: EHR Guidelines. *Journal of the American Health Information Management Association* 72(9): 72, 74.

American Health Information Management Association. 2004 (Nov-Dec). AHIMA Practice Brief: Delving into Computer-Assisted Coding. Available online from www.ahima.org.

American Health Information Management Association. 2005 (Nov-Dec). AHIMA Practice Brief: Update: Maintaining a Legally Sound Health Record—Paper and Electronic. Available online from www.ahima.org.

American Health Information Management Association. 2005 (July). FORE Report: Automated Coding Software: Development and Use to Enhance Anti-Fraud Activities. Available online from www.ahima.org.

American Health Information Management Association. 2005 (September). FORE Report: Use of Health Information Technology to Enhance and Expand Health Care Anti-Fraud Activities. Available online from www.ahima.org.

American Health Information Management Association. 2001 (February). AHIMA Position Statement: Privacy official. Available online from www.ahima.org.

American Health Information Management Association. Help wanted: Privacy officer. 2001. *Journal of the American Health Information Management Association* 72(6): 37–39.

Centers for Medicare and Medicaid Services. *Medicare Program Integrity Manual.* Available online from www.cms.hhs.gov.

Centers for Medicare and Medicaid Services. 2003 (November 7). Medicare Program: Review of national coverage determinations and local coverage determinations, Final Rule. *Federal Register* 68(216): 63693. Available online from www.access.gpo.gov/su_docs/fedreg/a031107c.html.

Centers for Medicare and Medicaid Services. *Medicare Coverage Issues Manual.* Available online from www.cms.hhs.gov.

Centers for Medicare and Medicaid Services. 2001 (September 26). Program Memorandum, Intermediaries/ Carriers: ICD-9-CM coding for diagnostic tests. Transmittal AB-01-144. Available under "CMS Program Memoranda" at www.cms.hhs.gov/transmittals.

Drach, Maureen, Althea Davis, and Carmen Sagrati. 2001. Ten steps to successful chargemaster reviews. *Journal of the American Health Information Management Association* 72(1): 42–48.

Dunn, Rose T. 2003 (November). ABNs: Always been neglected. *Journal of the American Health Information Management Association.* Available online from www.ahima.org.

Estrella, Renato. 2003. What happened to PEPP? QIOs plan for hospital payment monitoring program. *Journal of the American Health Information Management Association* 74(7): 43–48.

General Accounting Office. 2001 (June). Health Care: Consultants' billing advice may lead to improperly paid insurance claims. GAO-01-818. Available online from www.gao.gov/new.items/d01818.pdf.

General Accounting Office. 1999 (April). Medicare: Early evidence of compliance effectiveness is inconclusive. GAO/HEHS-99-59. Available online from www.gao.gov/archive/1999/he99059.pdf.

Glondys, Barbara. 2003. AHIMA Practice Brief: Ensuring legibility of patient records. *Journal of the American Health Information Management Association* 74(5): 64A–D.

Hammen, Cheryl. 2001. Choosing consultants without compromising compliance. *Journal of the American Health Information Management Association* 72(9): 26, 28, 30.

Hanna, Joette. 2002. Constructing a coding compliance plan. *Journal of the American Health Information Management Association* 73(7): 48–56.

Health Care Compliance Association. 2003. *Evaluating and Improving a Compliance Program: A Resource for Health Care Board Members, Health Care Executives, and Compliance Officers.* Minneapolis: HCCA. Available online from http://www.hcca-info.org/content/navigationmenu/compliance_resources/ evaluation_improvement/evaluation_improvement.htm.

HPMP Compliance Workbook, 2005, page 8.

Hull, Susan. 2003. Long-term care hospital PPS creates opportunity for coders: Proposed rule addresses related coding issues. *Journal of the American Health Information Management Association* 74(6): 58–60.

Jones, Lolita. 2001. *Reimbursement Methodologies for Healthcare Services.* Chicago: American Health Information Management Association.

Neville, Deborah, and Francine Katz. 2001. Six steps to compliance for small practices. *Journal of the American Health Information Management Association* 72(5): 40–44.

Office of Inspector General. 2001 (June). Special Advisory Bulletin: Practices of business consultants. Available online from http://oig.hhs.gov/fraud/docs/alertsandbulletins/consultants.pdf.

Office of Inspector General. 2000 (October 5). OIG Compliance Program Guidance for Individual and Small Group Physician Practices. *Federal Register* 65(194): 59434–52. Available online from http://oig.hhs.gov/ authorities/docs/physician.pdf.

Office of Inspector General. 1998 (February 23). OIG Compliance Program Guidance for Hospitals. *Federal Register* 63(35): 8987–98. Available online from http://oig.hhs.gov/authorities/docs/cpghosp.pdf.

Office of Inspector General. 2005 (January 31). OIG Supplemental Compliance Program Guidance for Hospitals. *Federal Register* 70(19): 4858–76. Available online from http://oig.hhs.gov/fraud/docs/ complianceguidance/012705HospSupplementalGuidance.pdf.

Ortquist, Steve, and Sheryl Vacca. 2004. Evaluating compliance program effectiveness. *Journal of the American Health Information Management Association* 75(1): 74–75.

Prophet-Bowman, Sue. 2003. Observation services present compliance challenges: Know these complex, changing requirements to avoid risk. *Journal of the American Health Information Management Association* 74(3): 60–65.

Russo, Ruthann. 1998. *Seven Steps to HIM Compliance.* Marblehead, Mass.: Opus Communications.

Scichilone, Rita. 2002. Best practices for medical necessity validation. *Journal of the American Health Information Management Association* 73(2): 48, 50.

Skurka, Margaret A. 2001. Navigating the physician services maze. *Journal of the American Health Information Management Association* 72(7): 51–58.

Stanfill, Mary. 2003 (October). Strategies for effective auditing of physician evaluation and management services. Proceedings of the AHIMA 2003 National Convention, San Francisco.

Stewart, Margaret Morgan. 2001. *Coding and Reimbursement under the Outpatient Prospective Payment System.* Chicago: American Health Information Management Association.

Texas Medical Foundation Health Quality Institute. 2005 (December). Hospital Payment Monitoring Program Compliance Workbook. Available online from http://www.tmf.org/hpmp/tools/workbook/index.htm.

Green-Shook, Sheila. 2004 (October). IFHRO Congress and AHIMA Convention Proceedings.

AHIMA Workgroup on Electronic Health Records Management. "The Strategic Importance of Electronic Health Records Management. Appendix A: Issues in Electronic Health Records Management." *Journal of AHIMA* 75, no. 9 (October 2004): Web extra.

Tegan, Anne, et al. 2005 (May). The EHR's Impact on HIM Functions. *Journal of the American Health Information Management Association* 76 (5): 56C–H.

Williams, Adrian. 2006 (February). Design for Better Data: How Software and Users Interact Onscreen Matters to Data Quality. *Journal of AHIMA* 77 (2): 56–60.

Micheletti, Julie A. and Thomas J. Shlala. 2006 (February). Documentation Rx: Strategies for Improving Physician Contribution to Hospital Records. *Journal of the American Health Information Management Association* 77 (2): 66–68.

Rollins, Gina. "Following the Digital Trail: Weak Auditing Functions Spell Trouble for an Electronic Record." *Journal of the American Health Information Management Association* 77, no.3 (March 2006): 38–41.

Hanson, Susan P. and Bonnie S. Cassidy. "Fraud Control: New Tools, New Potential." *Journal of the American Health Information Management Association* 77, no.3 (March 2006): 24–27,30.

Hornung Garvin, Jennifer, Sohrab Moeini, and Valerie Watzlaf, PhD, RHIA, FAHIMA; and Sohrab Moeini, BSIS. " Fighting Fraud, Automatically: How Coding Automation Can Prevent Healthcare Fraud." *Journal of the American Health Information Management Association* 77, no.3 (March 2006).

# Appendices

# Appendix A
# Health Information Management Skills Fundamental to Effective Compliance

The background of health information management (HIM) professionals is invaluable to the process of achieving effective compliance and reducing the risk of future fraudulent or abusive practices. HIM professionals have specialized education, training, and certification in the management of health information, and they are responsible for the achievement and maintenance of data of the highest quality. They are specialists in collecting, analyzing, processing, integrating, storing, and securing healthcare data. Their education includes extensive training in the classification and coding of healthcare information for reimbursement, statistical, and research purposes. Finally, they are responsible for translating clinical information into coded data and then evaluating, analyzing, and maintaining its accuracy, validity, and meaningfulness.

HIM professionals are employed in a variety of healthcare settings, including hospitals, clinics, mental health facilities, nursing homes, and physicians' offices, as well as payers, managed care organizations, government agencies, law firms, accounting firms, consulting firms, vendors of healthcare products and services, health data organizations, and educational institutions. They possess many skills that are critical to an effective compliance program, including the following:

- A strong knowledge base in complete and accurate clinical documentation in all healthcare settings and for all healthcare disciplines

- A strong knowledge base and experience in appropriate coding and billing practices

- Knowledge of the conventions, rules, and guidelines for multiple classification systems

- Knowledge of multiple reimbursement systems

- Knowledge of multiple regulations, standards, policies, and requirements pertaining to clinical documentation, coding, and billing

- Knowledge of multiple third-party payer requirements
- The ability to accurately interpret and implement regulatory standards
- The ability to interpret legal requirements
- An established rapport with physicians and other healthcare practitioners
- Strong managerial, leadership, and interpersonal skills
- Strong communication and presentation skills
- Strong analytical skills

The HIM profession has a long history of deep-rooted commitment to honesty, integrity, and professional ethics.

# Appendix B
# High-Risk Areas for Fraud and Abuse Enforcement

## Risk Areas Targeted by the HHS Office of Inspector General

The following are risk areas identified in the Office of Inspector General (OIG) 2007 Work Plan that would be of particular interest to HIM professionals. This is not an all-inclusive list. As new annual OIG Work Plans are released, review them carefully to identify new focus areas impacting HIM functions. For information on the process the OIG uses during a government audit, see the OIG document titled *The Audit Process* (information on accessing this document can be found in appendix F).

### Short-term, Acute Care Hospitals

**Payments for Observation Services versus Inpatient Admissions for Dialysis Services:** The objective of this audit will be to determine whether payments were made for inpatient admissions for dialysis services when the physicians' orders stated the level of care as admission to observation status.

**Inpatient Hospital Payments for New Technologies:** The OIG will review payments made to hospitals for new services and technologies and will examine the costs associated with the new devices and technologies to determine if the reimbursement was appropriate.

**Outpatient Department Payments:** The OIG will review payments to hospital outpatient departments under the outpatient hospital prospective payment system (PPS) to determine the extent to which they were made in accordance with Medicare laws and regulations. The appropriateness of payments made for multiple procedures, repeat procedures, and global surgeries will be reviewed.

**Unbundling of Hospital Outpatient Services:** The OIG will determine the extent to which hospitals and other providers are submitting claims for services that should be bundled into outpatient services.

**"Inpatient Only" Services Performed in an Outpatient Setting:** The OIG will determine if Medicare payments are appropriately denied for "inpatient only" and related services performed in an outpatient setting and assess the extent to which Medicare beneficiaries are held liable for denied inpatient claims for these services.

**Medical Appropriateness and Coding of Diagnosis Related Group Services:** The OIG will analyze inpatient hospital claims to identify providers who exhibit high or unusual patterns for selected DRGs. They will then determine the medical necessity, the appropriate level of coding, and reimbursement for a sample of services billed by these providers. In earlier work, the OIG found the DRG system vulnerable to abuse by providers who wish to increase reimbursement inappropriately through upcoding.

## Inpatient Rehabilitation Facilities

**Inpatient Rehabilitation Facility Classification Criteria:** The OIG will review the extent to which admissions to inpatient rehabilitation facilities (IRFs) met specific regulatory requirements and whether the facilities billed for services in compliance with Medicare regulations. The Deficit Reduction Act modified the compliance threshold criteria, that is, the percentage criterion that must be met to be classified as a rehabilitation hospital under the Medicare program.

**Inpatient Rehabilitation Facility Compliance with Medicare Requirements:** The OIG will continue to review payments to IRFs under the PPS to determine the extent to which they were made in accordance with Medicare requirements. For example, they will determine the extent to which admissions to IRFs met Medicare requirements and whether a claim paid as a discharge should have been paid as a transfer. They will also review outlier claims.

**Inpatient Rehabilitation Payments—Late Assessments:** The OIG will determine the accuracy of Medicare payments for inpatient rehabilitation stays when patient assessments are entered late.

## Inpatient Psychiatric Hospitals

**Inpatient Psychiatric Hospitals:** The OIG will review payments to psychiatric hospitals under the inpatient psychiatric facility PPS to determine the extent to which they were made in accordance with Medicare laws and regulations. Outlier payments and payments for interrupted stays will be reviewed.

## Long-Term Care Hospitals

**Long-Term Care Hospital Payments:** The OIG will review payments to long-term care hospitals under the PPS to determine the extent to which these payments were made in accordance with Medicare laws and regulations. They will review the appropriateness of early discharges to home and interrupted stays.

**Long-Term Care Hospital Admissions:** The OIG will determine the extent to which long-term care hospitals admit patients from a sole acute-care hospital.

## Home Health

**Enhanced Payments for Home Health Therapy:** The OIG will determine whether home health agencies' therapy services met the threshold for higher payments in compliance with Medicare regulations. They will analyze the number and the duration of therapy visits provided per episode period.

**Accurately Coding Claims for Medicare Home Health Resource Groups:** This review will determine the extent to which Medicare home health agencies accurately code the home health resource group in the Outcome and Assessment Information Set. The OIG will also determine the extent to which providers improperly code home health resource groups and the level of inappropriate payments made as a result of any miscoding.

**Home Health Rehabilitation Therapy Services:** This review will determine the extent to which rehabilitation therapy services provided by home health agencies were provided by appropriate staff and were medically necessary. The OIG will determine the extent to which patients' plans of care identified the need for the amount and level of therapy they received. They will also determine the amount of reimbursement that providers received due to medically unnecessary home health agency therapy.

## Nursing Homes

**Skilled Nursing Facility Rehabilitation and Infusion Therapy Services:** Through medical review, the OIG will analyze whether rehabilitation and infusion therapy services provided to Medicare beneficiaries in skilled nursing facilities (SNF) were medically necessary, adequately supported, and actually provided as ordered.

**Skilled Nursing Facilities' Involvement in Consecutive Inpatient Stays:** The OIG will determine whether SNF care provided to Medicare beneficiaries with consecutive inpatient stays was medically reasonable and necessary. This study will focus on beneficiaries who experience three or more consecutive stays, including at least one SNF facility stay.

**Skilled Nursing Facility Consolidated Billing:** The OIG will determine whether controls are in place to preclude duplicate billings under Medicare Part B for services covered under the SNF PPS and assess the effectiveness of the Common Working File edits established in 2002 to prevent and detect improper payments.

**Nursing Home Residents Minimum Data Set Assessments and Care Planning:** The type, frequency, and severity of nursing home deficiencies related to Minimum Data Set assessments and care planning will be examined. The OIG will also examine methods the state survey agencies use in identifying assessments and care plans that do not address individualized needs of residents.

**Imaging and Laboratory Services in Nursing Homes:** The OIG will determine the extent and nature of any medically unnecessary or excessive billing for imaging and laboratory services provided to nursing home residents.

## Physicians and Other Health Professionals

**Billing Service Companies:** The OIG will identify and review the relationships between billing companies and the physicians and other Medicare providers who use their services. They will also identify the types of arrangements physicians and other Medicare providers have with billing services and determine the impact of these arrangements on physicians' billings.

**Physician Pathology Services:** The OIG will focus on pathology services performed in physicians' offices. They will determine if the billings for pathology laboratory services comply with Medicare Part B requirements. The relationships between physicians who furnish pathology services in their offices and outside pathology companies will be identified and reviewed.

**Cardiography and Echocardiography Services:** Medicare payments for cardiography and echocardiography services will be reviewed to determine whether physicians billed appropriately for the professional and technical components of the services.

**Physical and Occupational Therapy Services:** Medicare claims for therapy services provided by physical and occupational therapists will be reviewed to determine whether the services were reasonable and medically necessary, adequately documented, and certified by physician certification statements.

**Payments to Providers of Care for Initial Preventive Physical Examination:** The impact of Medicare coverage for an initial preventive physical examination on Medicare payments and physician billing practices will be evaluated.

**Medicare Part B Mental Health Services:** The OIG will determine whether Medicare Part B mental health services provided in physicians' offices were medically necessary and billed in accordance with Medicare requirements.

**Wound Care Services:** The OIG will determine whether claims for wound care services were medically necessary and billed in accordance with Medicare requirements. The adequacy of controls to prevent inappropriate payments for wound care services will also be examined.

**Evaluation of "Incident to" Services:** The purpose of this study is to evaluate the appropriateness of Medicare services performed "incident to" the professional services of physicians. The OIG will identify services performed "incident to" physicians' professional services and will determine the extent to which the services met Medicare standards for medical necessity, documentation, and quality of care.

**Potential Duplicate Physical Therapy Claims:** The OIG will assess whether the Centers for Medicare and Medicaid Services' (CMS) systems are able to identify and prevent payment for potential duplicate claims for physical therapy submitted by providers.

**Review of Evaluation and Management Services During Global Surgery Periods:** The OIG will determine whether (1) physicians received separate payments for evaluation and management (E&M) services provided during the global surgery period and (2) industry practices related to the number of E&M services provided during the global surgery period have changed since the global surgery fee concept was initially developed in 1992.

## Other Medicare Services

**Therapy Services Provided by Comprehensive Outpatient Rehabilitation Facilities:** The OIG will determine whether comprehensive outpatient rehabilitation facilities (CORF) provided and billed physical therapy, speech language pathology, and occupational therapy services in accordance with Medicare eligibility and reimbursement requirements.

**Separately Billable Laboratory Services under the End-Stage Renal Disease Program:** Providers' compliance with the Medicare payment policies for automated multichannel chemistry tests furnished to end-stage renal disease beneficiaries will be reviewed.

## Non-Medicare Services

**Preadmission Screening and Resident Review for Younger Nursing Facility Residents with Serious Mental Illness and Mental Retardation:** The OIG will assess the Preadmission Screening and Resident Review (PASRR) program for Medicaid nursing facility residents aged 22 to 64 with serious mental illness or mental retardation. This review will evaluate CMS' oversight of States' PASRR programs, State Medicaid agencies' oversight of the process, and the extent to which nursing facilities comply with the PASRR requirements.

**Medicaid Physical and Occupational Therapy Services—Appropriateness of Payments:** Improper payments and potential cost savings for Medicaid physical and occupational therapy services will be identified. In past Medicaid studies, the OIG found that physical and occupational therapy services provided were medically unnecessary, billed incorrectly, or rendered by unqualified providers.

## Information Systems Controls

**Smart Card Technology:** The OIG will assess the use of "smart card" technology in Medicare demonstrations as a means of creating portable, electronic patient medical records. Their review will focus on information security, data privacy, and program integrity concerns.

**Quality Concerns Identified Through Quality Improvement Organizations' Medical Record Reviews:** The OIG will determine the extent to which the quality improvement organizations identify quality of care concerns through medical record reviews and what interventions they take in response to confirmed concerns.

## Investigations

**Healthcare Fraud:** The OIG's Office of Investigations will investigate individuals, facilities, or entities that bill Medicare and/or Medicaid for services not rendered, claims that manipulate payment codes in an effort to inflate reimbursement amounts, claims for care not provided to nursing home residents, and other false claims submitted to obtain program funds. They will also investigate business arrangements that may violate the Federal healthcare antikickback statute. Investigations of potential violations of the Medicare Part D drug benefit, including enrollment and marketing schemes and prescription shorting, are being undertaken.

The following risk areas have been identified in the OIG's Supplemental Program Guidance for Hospitals:

1) Outpatient Procedure Coding
   a) Billing on an outpatient basis for "inpatient-only" procedures
   b) Submitting claims for medically unnecessary services by failing to follow the fiscal intermediaries' (FI) local policies
   c) Submitting duplicate claims or otherwise not following the NCCI guidelines
   d) Submitting incorrect claims for ancillary services because of outdated Charge Description Masters
   e) Circumventing the multiple procedure discounting rules
   f) Improper evaluation and management code selection
   g) Improperly billing for observation services

2) Admissions and Discharges
    a) Failure to follow the "same-day rule"
    b) Abuse of partial hospitalization payments
    c) Same-day discharges and readmissions
    d) Violation of Medicare's postacute transfer policy
    e) Improper churning of patients by long-term care hospitals colocated in acute care hospitals

# Additional High-Risk Areas

## Billing for Items or Services Not Actually Rendered

This practice involves submitting a claim representing that the provider performed a service, all or part of which was not performed.

## Billing for Items or Services Not Actually Documented

This involves submitting a claim that cannot be substantiated in the documentation.

## Providing Medically Unnecessary Services

By law, no payment may be made under Medicare Part A or Part B for any expenses incurred for items or services that are not reasonable and necessary for the diagnosis or treatment of illness or injury, or to improve the functioning of the malformed body member. A claim requesting payment for medically unnecessary services intentionally seeks reimbursement for a service that is not warranted by the patient's current and documented medical condition.

## Local Coverage Determinations

An area of concern relating to determinations of reasonable and necessary services is the variation in Local Coverage Determinations (LCDs) among carriers. Federal health programs should only be billed for items and services that are covered. In order to determine if an item or service is covered for Medicare, providers must be knowledgeable of the LCDs applicable to them. When the LCD indicates that an item or service may not be covered by Medicare, the provider is responsible for conveying this information to the patient so that the patient can make an informed decision concerning the healthcare services he or she may want to receive. This information is conveyed through advance beneficiary notices (ABNs).

## Advance Beneficiary Notices

The use of ABNs is an area where physician practices and other providers experience numerous difficulties. Problems in this area can be reduced through physician education on the correct use of ABNs, obtaining guidance from the Medicare contractor regarding their interpretation of whether an ABN is necessary where the service is not covered, developing a standard form for all diagnostic tests, and developing a process for handling patients who refuse to sign ABNs.

## Billing for Noncovered Services as if Covered

Claims are sometimes submitted for services in order to receive a denial from the carrier, thereby enabling the patient to submit the denied claim for payment to a secondary payer. In instances in which a claim is being submitted to Medicare for this purpose, the provider should indicate on the claim that it is being submitted for the purpose of receiving a denial in order to bill a secondary payer. This step should assist Medicare contractors and prevent inadvertent payments to which the provider is not entitled. In some instances, however, Medicare pays the claim even though the service is noncovered and the provider did not intend for payment to be made. When this occurs, the provider has a responsibility to refund the amount paid and indicate that the service is not covered.

## Duplicate Billing

This occurs when more than one claim is submitted for the same service or the bill is submitted to more than one primary payer at the same time. The OIG acknowledged that duplicate billing could occur as a result of simple errors, but that known duplicate billing, which is sometimes evidenced by systematic or repeated double billing, can create liability under criminal, civil, or administrative law, particularly if any overpayment is not promptly refunded.

## Upcoding

Upcoding is the practice of using a code that provides a higher payment rate than the code that actually reflects the service furnished to the patient.

## DRG Creep

DRG creep is the practice of billing using a DRG that provides a higher payment rate than the DRG that accurately reflects the service furnished to the patient.

## Unbundling

Unbundling is the practice of submitting bills piecemeal or in fragmented fashion to maximize reimbursement for various tests or procedures that are required to be billed together and thus at a reduced cost.

## Failure to Properly Use Modifiers

Because the use of CPT modifiers can determine whether a service is reimbursed or whether additional reimbursement is warranted, improper use of modifiers can result in inappropriate reimbursement.

## Internal Coding Practices

The OIG noted that internal coding practices, including software edits, should be reviewed periodically to determine consistency with all applicable federal, state, and private payer healthcare program requirements.

## Assumption Coding

This refers to the coding of a diagnosis or procedure without supporting clinical documentation.

## Clustering

This refers to the practice of coding one or two middle levels of E/M codes exclusively, under the philosophy that some will be higher and some will be lower, and it will average out over time (in reality, this method overcharges some patients while undercharging others).

## Coding Without Proper Documentation of All Physician and Other Professional Services

The OIG noted that although proper documentation is the responsibility of the healthcare provider, the coding professional should be aware of proper documentation requirements and should encourage providers to document their services appropriately.

## Lack of Integrity in Computer Systems

This involves the failure to have systems and processes in place to ensure the integrity of health information and records that can be easily located and accessed.

## Resource Utilization Groups (RUG) Creep

This is a risk created by the nursing facility PPS in which there is an incentive to over-assess residents in order to achieve higher payment rates.

## Third-Party Billing Services

Physicians should remember that they remain responsible to the Medicare program for bills sent in the physician's name or containing the physician's signature, even if the physician had no actual knowledge of a billing impropriety. It is no defense for the physician if the physician's billing service improperly bills Medicare. One of the most common risk areas involving billing services deals with physician practices contracting with billing services on a percentage basis. Although percentage-based billing arrangements are not illegal per se, the OIG has a long-standing concern that such arrangements may increase the risk of intentional upcoding and similar abusive billing practices, such as the following:

- Alteration of documentation
- Unavailability of all necessary documentation at the time of coding
- Failure to maintain the confidentiality of information or records
- Computer software programs that encourage billing personnel to enter data in fields indicating services were rendered although not actually performed or documented

- Overutilization (furnishing more services than medically necessary) and under-utilization (knowingly denying needed care in order to keep costs low)

- False dating of amendments to nursing notes

- Falsified plans of care

- Untimely and/or forged physician certification on plans of care

- Falsifying information on the claim form, certificate of medical necessity, and/or accompanying documentation

- Providing misleading information about a resident's medical condition on the minimum data set (MDS) or otherwise providing inaccurate information used to determine the RUG assigned to the resident

- Failure to comply with applicable requirements for verbal orders for hospice services

- **One-day hospital admissions:** One-day inpatient stays raise the question of medical necessity and whether the patient could have been treated as an out-patient instead of an inpatient.

- **Same-day readmissions:** Readmissions on the same day as discharge could be an indication of a premature discharge from the first admission and possibly result in a claims denial for the second admission under the premise that the care should have been provided during the first admission and, therefore, only the DRG payment for the first admission should be paid. Patterns of premature discharges raise red flags regarding quality of care and potential fraudulent practices of attempting to maximize Medicare reimbursement at the expense of patient care.

- **Three-day payment window:** Were diagnostic services provided within 3 days prior to a Medicare inpatient admission combined with the inpatient admission, or were they incorrectly billed separately from the inpatient admission? Were therapeutic services provided within 3 days prior to a Medicare inpatient admission that were related to the reason for the inpatient admission, combined with the inpatient admission?

- **Modifiers 25 and 59:** Are these modifiers being applied correctly? Do they seem to be overutilized? How does your organization or practice's use of these modifiers compare to regional and national benchmarks?

## Transfers between Inpatient PPS Hospitals

CMS' definition of a transfer under the hospital inpatient PPS includes any patient who is admitted to another inpatient PPS hospital on the same day that the patient is discharged from an inpatient PPS hospital, unless the first hospital can demonstrate that the patient's treatment was completed at the time of discharge from that hospital. Therefore, unless the same-day readmission at the second hospital is to treat a condition that is unrelated to the condition treated during the first admission, an admission to a second hospital on the same day as a discharge from another hospital would be considered a transfer from the first hospital. This means that if a patient signs out of the first hospital against medical advice and is subsequently admitted to another hospital later that day, without the knowledge of the first hospital, CMS still considers it a transfer from the hospital and the discharge status code should reflect a transfer. CMS acknowledges that there may be situations in which the first hospital could not have known the patient was admitted to another hospital on the day of discharge from the first hospital. In those instances, the Medicare contractor will notify the first hospital of the need to submit an adjustment claim reflecting the discharge status code for a transfer to another acute care PPS hospital.

If the first hospital can present documentation showing that the patient's care was completed before discharge, it is not required that the first hospital report the discharge as a transfer. The documentation requirement is expected to be similar to the type of documentation necessary to demonstrate to the Medicare contractor and quality improvement organizations (QIOs) that a patient was not prematurely discharged.

## Transfers from an Inpatient PPS Hospital to Postacute Care

The Medicare postacute care transfer policy has been expanded significantly beyond the original 10 DRGs (a total of 182 DRGs for fiscal year 2006). This policy requires discharges to one of the following postacute settings to be paid as transfers when they are classified to select DRGs:

- Psychiatric hospitals and units
- Rehabilitation hospitals and units
- Children's hospitals
- Long-term care hospitals
- Cancer treatment hospitals
- Skilled nursing facilities
- Home health services provided by a home health agency, if the services relate to the condition or diagnosis for which the individual received inpatient hospital services and if the home health services are provided within 3 days after the date of discharge

Postacute transfer was identified as a compliance risk in the OIG's Supplemental Compliance Guidance for Hospitals. The OIG has conducted reviews of hospitals' compliance with the Medicare postacute transfer policy and identified problems with hospitals miscoding a postacute transfer as a discharge to home. They noted that this miscoding occurred because some hospitals did not have the necessary controls to ensure the accuracy of discharge status.

It is important for hospitals to implement processes to ensure discharges meet the qualifying criteria for a transfer to be billed with the appropriate discharge status code for a transfer. It also is important to monitor discharges to these postacute settings, as well as cases in which the patient left against medical advice, to ensure the correct discharge status code is being reported. The OIG has identified problems with claims being coded as discharges to home rather than transfers to postacute care. Discharges to home health are particularly challenging because the medical record documentation may not clearly indicate plans for home health services following discharge or the hospital may not be aware that these services were not initiated within three days after discharge.

## Consecutive Medicare Inpatient Stays

Same-day discharges and readmissions were identified as a compliance risk in the OIG's Supplemental Compliance Guidance for Hospitals. The OIG examined services to Medicare beneficiaries who had three or more inpatient stays, each within one day of discharge from the last facility. Although the OIG found that most such consecutive inpatient stays were appropriate, for 20% of the stays, medical record reviews showed that Medicare inpatient stays were associated with quality of care problems and/or unnecessary fragmentation of healthcare services across multiple inpatient stays. Ten percent of individual stays within consecutive inpatient stay sequences were associated with poor quality of patient care.

## High-Risk DRGs

The common reasons or contributing factors given for misclassification to these DRGs are not intended to be all-inclusive.

- **Complication/comorbidity pairs:** When a DRG is split based on the presence or absence of a complication/comorbidity (CC), miscoding of CCs can result in inappropriate DRG assignment.

- **Major Cardiovascular Conditions:** For those cardiovascular DRGs split on the basis of the presence or absence of a major cardiovascular condition, miscoding of the principal or secondary diagnoses can result in incorrect DRG assignment.

- **DRG 14, Intracranial hemorrhage or cerebral infarction:** Some cases may be classified more appropriately to DRG 524 (Transient Ischemia) or DRG 15 (Nonspecific CVA and Precerebral Occlusion without Infarction). For example, the neurologic deficits may have been transient in nature. The physician documentation may be ambiguous as to whether the patient experienced a stroke or a transient ischemic attack (TIA). The coding professional may have coded a cerebrovascular accident (CVA) from a radiology report without supporting documentation from the attending physician. There also are variable interpretations as to the meaning of the fifth digits for categories 433 and 434, which may result in misclassification of some cases to DRG 14.

- **DRG 79, Respiratory infections and inflammations, age older than 17 with CC:** A specific type of pneumonia may be presumed, the causal organism may be picked up from culture reports without supporting documentation from the attending physician, or pneumonia documented as due to multiple specified organisms may be coded inappropriately as "mixed" bacterial pneumonia.

- **DRG 87, Pulmonary edema and respiratory failure:** Misapplication of coding guidelines for respiratory failure may result in incorrect classification of cases to this DRG. Clinical findings (such as arterial blood gases) may be used to justify reporting a principal diagnosis of respiratory failure without supporting documentation from the attending physician. Respiratory failure may be sequenced inappropriately as the principal diagnosis when another diagnosis, such as myocardial infarction, congestive heart failure, chronic obstructive pulmonary disease, or CVA, more appropriately meets the definition of principal diagnosis. Pulmonary edema may be inappropriately coded separately from congestive heart failure.

- **DRG 88, Chronic obstructive pulmonary disease:** If asthma and bronchitis are coded incorrectly as "chronic obstructive pulmonary disease," the case will be classified to this DRG instead of DRG 96 or 97.

- **DRG 89, Simple pneumonia and pleurisy, age older than 17 with CC:** Pneumonia may be reported as the principal diagnosis, but the medical record documentation only supports a diagnosis of bronchitis.

- **DRG 121, Circulatory disorders with acute myocardial infarction and major complications, discharged alive:** A major complication may be coded without supporting physician documentation. If there is no major complication, the case is classified to DRG 122. If an acute myocardial infarction is incorrectly coded, DRG misclassification also will occur.

- **DRG 124, Circulatory disorders except acute myocardial infarction with cardiac catheterization and complex diagnosis:** A complex diagnosis may be coded without supporting physician documentation. Cases without a complex diagnosis are classified to DRG 125.

- **DRG 127, Heart failure and shock:** Congestive heart failure may be sequenced inappropriately as the principal diagnosis instead of angina or another condition.

- **DRG 130, Peripheral vascular disorders with CC:** Thrombophlebitis of the lower extremities may be coded inappropriately as thrombophlebitis of the superficial vessels without supporting physician documentation. Thrombophlebitis of the superficial vessels of the lower extremities is classified to DRG 130, but unspecified thrombophlebitis or that of deep vessels is classified to DRG 128.

- **DRG 132, Atherosclerosis with CC:** Arteriosclerotic heart disease may be sequenced inappropriately as the principal diagnosis instead of angina. If the physician documents that the angina is due to arteriosclerotic heart disease, or links them, the arteriosclerotic heart disease should be sequenced first. However, if the physician does not link the two conditions, angina should be sequenced as the principal diagnosis.

- **DRG 138, Cardiac arrhythmia and conduction disorders with CC:** Cardiac arrhythmia may be sequenced inappropriately as the principal diagnosis instead of angina.

- **DRG 144, Other circulatory system diagnoses with CC:** A common problem resulting in misclassification to this DRG is determination of whether the appropriate principal diagnosis is a subsequent episode of care for a myocardial infarction (within the applicable 8-week time frame), arteriosclerotic heart disease, chest pain, or angina.

- **DRG 174, Gastrointestinal hemorrhage with CC:** Gastrointestinal disorders, such as diverticulitis or gastritis, may be coded inappropriately as that with hemorrhage instead of without hemorrhage. Physician documentation linking the patient's bleeding with the identified gastrointestinal disorder is necessary in order to assign the fifth digit for "with hemorrhage."

- **DRG 182, Esophagitis, gastroenteritis, and miscellaneous digestive disorders, age older than 17 with CC:** Some cases may be classified more appropriately to DRG 296, Nutritional and miscellaneous metabolic disorders, age older than 17 with CC. A key issue is whether the patient was admitted for dehydration or the underlying gastrointestinal disorder.

- **DRG 188, Other digestive system diagnoses, age older than 17 with CC:** Classification to the appropriate digestive system DRG depends on clear documentation of the digestive system symptom or definitive diagnosis necessitating admission. For example, abdominal pain is classified to DRG 182, whereas abdominal rigidity is classified to DRG 188. Diaphragmatic hernia is classified to DRG 182, whereas other types of hernia are classified to DRG 188. Toxic gastroenteritis and colitis and that due to radiation are classified to DRG 188, whereas other types of gastroenteritis and colitis are classified to DRG 182. Also, a digestive disorder classified to DRG 188 may be sequenced inappropriately as the principal diagnosis instead of gastrointestinal obstruction.

- **DRG 239, Pathological fractures and musculoskeletal and connective tissue malignancy:** Misclassification to this DRG can occur when pathologic fracture is sequenced inappropriately as the principal diagnosis, but the correct principal diagnosis is a traumatic fracture or osteoporosis.

- **DRG 320, Kidney and urinary tract infections, age older than 17 with CC:** In some cases, dehydration may be the more appropriate principal diagnosis.

- **DRG 416, Septicemia, age older than 17:** Some cases may be classified more appropriately to DRG 320 or 321. The key issue is whether the patient has septicemia or a urinary tract infection. The confusion typically results from physician documentation of the term urosepsis.

- **DRG 429, Organic disturbances and mental retardation:** When psychosis is coded inappropriately as a "senile" condition, it is classified to this DRG instead of DRG 430.

- **DRG 475, Respiratory system diagnosis with ventilator support:** A common reason for misclassification of cases to this DRG is inappropriate sequencing of a respiratory condition as the principal diagnosis. Patients with a respiratory principal diagnosis on mechanical ventilation are classified to DRG 475, but those with a nonrespiratory principal diagnosis are not classified to this DRG. Factors resulting in cases being misclassified to DRG 475 include the following:

—unclear physician documentation as to the reason for hospital admission

—incorrect coding of bilevel positive airway pressure (BPAP) or continuous positive airway pressure (CPAP) as continuous mechanical ventilation

—continuous mechanical ventilation was coded, but ventilator was only used during surgery

—miscoding respiratory failure resulting from sepsis as the principal diagnosis

- **DRG 559, Acute ischemic stroke with use of thrombolytic agent:** If use of a thrombolytic agent is coded when the patient did not receive a thrombolytic agent, DRG 559 will be incorrectly assigned. An admission for a stroke that did not involve the use of a thrombolytic agent is classified to DRG 14.

## CMS Initiatives to Reduce Medicare Payment Errors

### Improper Medicare Fee-for-Service Payments Report

Since 1996, HHS has annually determined the rate of improper payments for fee-for-service (FFS) claims paid by Medicare contractors. Until fiscal year 2003, the survey was conducted by the OIG on a relatively small sample of claims. For fiscal year 2003, CMS launched an expanded initiative to determine a national payment error rate. CMS established two programs for monitoring the accuracy of Medicare payments. The Comprehensive Error Rate (CERT) program monitors payment decisions made by carriers, durable medical equipment regional carriers (DMERCs), and FIs for claims submitted by physicians, diagnostic and laboratory facilities, durable medical equipment (DME) suppliers, non-PPS inpatient hospitals, hospital outpatient services, skilled nursing facilities, home health agencies, and hospices. The CERT program was designed to establish the Medicare fee-for-service payment error rate for all types of Medicare services other than acute care inpatient hospital services and to determine the underlying reasons for claim errors, and to develop appropriate action plans to improve compliance with payment, claims processing, and provider billing requirements. The Hospital Payment Monitoring Program (HPMP), discussed in more detail in the following paragraphs, monitors decisions made by FIs and QIOs for claims submitted by PPS acute care inpatient hospital services. CMS' new initiative for measuring the payment error rate provides CMS with contractor-specific error rates, error rates by provider type, and error rates by service type.

CMS calculates the Medicare FFS error rate and improper payment estimate using a methodology approved by the OIG. This methodology includes the following:

- Random sample selection of submitted claims

- Requesting medical records from the healthcare providers that submitted the claims in the sample

- Where medical records were submitted by the provider, reviewing the claims in the sample and the associated medical records to see if the claims complied with Medicare coverage, coding, and billing rules, and, if not, assigning errors to the claims

- Where medical records were not submitted by the provider, classifying the case as a no documentation claim and counting it as an error

- Sending providers overpayment letters/notices or making adjustments for claims that were overpaid or underpaid

For the reporting period covered by the November 2005 report (the most recent available report at the time this book was being developed), the Medicare paid claims error rate was estimated at 5.2 percent, which is a 4.9 percent decrease from the previous reporting period. For Medicare contractors, the report included claims submitted between 01/01/04 and 12/31/04. For QIOs, the report included inpatient PPS hospital discharges between 7/1/03 and 6/30/04.

One of the performance goals for CMS is the reduction of improper payments made under the FFS program to 7.9 percent or less by the November 2005 reporting period, 6.9 percent or less by the November 2006 reporting period, 5.4 percent or less by the November 2007 reporting period, and 4.7 percent by the 2008 reporting period. The findings in this November 2005 report indicate that CMS exceeded the November 2005 goal and is well on the way toward meeting the November 2008 goal.

Insufficient documentation accounted for 1.1 percent of the dollars improperly paid; medically unnecessary services accounted for 1.6 percent; incorrect coding accounted for 1.5 percent; no documentation accounted for 0.7 percent; and 0.2 percent of the improper payments was due to other reasons.

"No documentation" means the provider did not submit any documentation to support the services provided. "Insufficient documentation" means that the provider did not include pertinent patient facts in the medical record documentation submitted. "Nonresponse" also means that the provider did not submit any documentation to support the services provided. The "medically unnecessary" category includes situations in which the reviewers identified enough documentation in the medical record to make an informed decision that the services billed to Medicare were not medically necessary. The "other errors" category includes instances when providers' claims did not meet benefit category requirements or other billing requirements.

For most of the coding errors, the reviewers determined that providers submitted documentation that supported a lower-paying code than the code submitted (that is, the provider "upcoded" the claim). However, for some of the coding errors, it was determined that the documentation supported a higher code than the code submitted by the provider (that is, the provider "undercoded" the claim). There were significantly fewer instances of undercoding among claims submitted to FIs than among claims submitted to carriers. A common error involved upcoding or downcoding by one level on a scale of five code levels. Published studies suggest that under certain circumstances, experienced reviewers may disagree on the most appropriate code to describe a particular service. This could explain some of the identified coding errors. CMS is investigating procedures to minimize the occurrence of this type of error in the future.

The insufficient documentation rate improved significantly over the previous FFS payment error report. Among the corrective actions CMS has taken to reduce this rate is to encourage Medicare contractors to educate providers about the importance of submitting thorough and complete documentation.

The percentage of total dollars in errors attributed to medically unnecessary services remained steady for the November 2005 reporting period. CMS has undertaken the following actions to correct this problem:

- CMS has developed a tool that generates state-specific hospital billing reports to help QIOs analyze administrative claims data.

- CMS has developed projects with the QIOs that address problems identified in state-specific hospital billing reports.

- CMS will provide hospitals with training on using comparative data reports to help them prioritize auditing and monitoring efforts with the goal of preventing payment errors.

- CMS conducts an annual payment error cause analysis to discern sources of payment error. CMS will be developing and distributing QIO-specific payment error cause analyses.

- CMS is working to address possible issues with observation versus inpatient admission that could be contributing to inappropriate inpatient admissions.

- CMS has completed and distributed an extensive workbook designed to be a resource for hospitals in their compliance efforts and activities.

- CMS has tasked each Medicare contractor with developing an Error Rate Reduction Plan (ERRP) that targets medical necessity errors in their jurisdiction.

The percentage of sampled dollars found to be in error due to incorrect coding increased from 1.2 percent in November 2004 to 1.5 percent in the November 2005 reporting period. CMS will continue the following corrective actions:

- QIOs will continue to work with hospitals to reduce coding errors through educational efforts and the use of statewide and hospital specific reports from First Look Analysis Tool for Hospital Outlier Monitoring (FATHOM). FATHOM is designed to identify emerging problem areas through data analysis. FATHOM includes reports on DRG-based target areas such as the ratio of the count of discharges with DRG 0079 (respiratory infections and inflammations age older than 17 years with complications or comorbidity) to the count of discharges with DRGs 079, 080, 089, or 090 (lower paying pneumonia DRGs).

- CMS is considering a resolution passed by the American Medical Association (AMA), the owner of the CPT coding system, that recommends CMS defer to the billing physician's judgment in E/M cases where a reviewer and the billing physician disagree by only one coding level.

## Hospital Payment Monitoring Program

HPMP evolved from the Payment Error Prevention Program (PEPP) and was established by CMS to measure, monitor, and reduce the incidence of improper PPS acute care inpatient Medicare payments (including payments to both short-term, acute care inpatient hospitals, and long-term acute care hospitals). HPMP operates through the QIO program as QIOs have responsibility for ascertaining the accuracy of these payments through the physician peer review process. The purpose of HPMP is to measure, monitor, and reduce the incidence of improper FFS inpatient Medicare payments. This includes the provision of medically unnecessary services, the provision of services in inappropriate settings, errors in DRG assignment and/or coding, errors in billing, and errors in prepayment denials. The long-term goal of HPMP is to help inpatient PPS hospitals monitor payment patterns by analyzing data, conducting focused audits, and implementing system changes to prevent payment errors. HPMP ongoing process improvement activities should be integrated into the organization's compliance program.

The Program for Evaluating Payment Patterns Electronic Report (PEPPER) is an HPMP tool developed to help short-term, acute care hospitals prioritize auditing tasks. The PEPPER reports are made available to the hospitals by the QIOs. Additional information about the use of the PEPPER reports can be found in the Auditing and Monitoring section of chapter 5.

## Recovery Audit Contractors

CMS launched a demonstration project using recovery audit contractors (RACs) to search for improper Medicare payments that may have been made to healthcare providers and were not detected through existing program integrity efforts. The initial recovery audit contracts focused on Part A Medicare claims and excluded E/M services.

Because Medicare contractors will continue to review claims in the current fiscal year, each RAC will work on claims that are at least one year old. Using an audit plan developed especially for Medicare, the RACs analyze claims that have a tendency to be incorrect despite clear guidance from Medicare. If an overpayment is detected, the RAC will pursue payment and will be reimbursed a percentage of the recoveries. For underpayments, the RAC will provide the necessary documentation to the Medicare contractors for processing payment to the provider.

# Appendix C
# Sample Tools for Implementation of an HIM Compliance Program

## Sample Outlines for Internal Educational Programs

Following are suggested agenda items for educational programs on HIM compliance issues aimed at different target audiences. The programs may be presented by the HIM compliance specialist or another designated HIM representative. Each organization should customize its educational programs to meet its own needs. The specific information to be covered on each subject would be at the discretion of the presenter. Additional topics should be included, as appropriate. Pertinent elements of the organization's HIM compliance program should be covered in educational programs, as appropriate for the particular audience. It would be helpful to include a few examples or to provide case scenarios that fit the audience. Educational programs should be interactive in order to demonstrate the participants' understanding of the material presented.

### Admitting Department

- Background of fraud and abuse enforcement
- OIG target areas
- Accurate and complete diagnosis
- Relationship to HIM and coding
- Medical necessity issues
- Data quality (including overview of key coding rules and guidelines)
- New regulations and payment methodologies
- Pertinent review and audit results (positive and negative)
- Pertinent payer-specific policies
- HIM role in systemwide compliance (Where does HIM fit in?)

- Input from participants on process improvements (for example, suggestions from participants regarding ways to streamline operations or improve documentation to ensure compliance)

- Design of educational programs for admitting staff (that is, suggested topics for ongoing educational initiatives and areas that should be covered in new employee training)

## Ancillary Services (Nursing, Laboratory, Radiology, Dietary, Physical Medicine, and Other Departments)

- Background of fraud and abuse enforcement
- OIG target areas
- Accurate and complete documentation
- Relationship of documentation and coding
- Skills necessary for accurate coding
- Medical necessity issues
- Chargemaster maintenance
- Regulatory requirements pertaining to coding and documentation
- Pertinent payer-specific policies
- New coding requirements (for example, new ICD-9-CM or CPT codes affecting ancillary services)
- Data quality
- New regulations and payment methodologies
- Pertinent audit results (positive and negative)
- HIM role in systemwide compliance (Where does HIM fit in?)
- Input from participants on process improvements
- Design of educational programs for ancillary services (initial and ongoing)

## Business Office Services

- Background of fraud and abuse enforcement
- OIG target areas
- Relationship of documentation and coding
- Coding process
- Skills necessary for accurate coding

- Relationship between coding and billing functions
- Role of coding in resolution of claims rejections
- Medical necessity issues
- Chargemaster maintenance
- Coding and billing compliance
- Communication with payers (for example, documentation of payer advice)
- Communication of payer memos or bulletins to all affected departments
- Pertinent payer-specific policies
- Data quality
- New regulations and payment methodologies
- HIM role in systemwide compliance (Where does HIM fit in?)
- Input from participants on process improvements
- Design of educational programs for business office personnel (initial and ongoing)

## Administration

- Background of fraud and abuse enforcement
- OIG target areas
- Consequences of noncompliance
- Linkage of documentation and coding to compliance
- OIG model compliance programs
- Compliance and the medical staff
- HIM recommendations for process improvements (for example, suggestions based on risk assessment or audit results)
- New regulations payment methodologies
- HIM as a vital link to systemwide compliance (Where does HIM fit in?)

## Medical Staff

- Background of fraud and abuse enforcement
- OIG target areas
- Complete and accurate documentation practices
- Relationship of documentation and coding

- Pertinent payer-specific policies

- Medical necessity documentation requirements

- Data quality

- New regulations and payment methodologies

- Pertinent review and audit results (positive and negative)

- Design of review programs and audits for physician practices (prospective versus retrospective)

- HIM role in systemwide compliance (Where does HIM fit in?)

- Understanding of the physician's role in compliance

- Input from participants on process improvements

## Sample Communication Tools for Improving Physician Documentation

The following are sample forms to be used to provide guidance to physicians regarding appropriate documentation of history and physicals, discharge summaries, operative reports, and consultations. Each healthcare organization should design its own tool(s) to assist in communicating regulatory requirements on documentation (The Joint Commission, Centers for Medicare and Medicaid Services [CMS], and others) to physicians. Common documentation deficiencies identified by the organization may be incorporated.

## History and Physical Examinations

**Date:**

**To:**     *[Insert medical staff or specific physician name]*

**From:**   *[Insert HIM director name, title, and telephone number]*

**Re:**     Health Record Documentation Requirements

The following information is provided to assist and guide the physician in proper health record documentation compliance. Increasing scrutiny is being directed toward complete and accurate physician documentation.

All dictated reports *must* include:

- Patient name
- Health record number
- Date of admission, consult, operation, and so on
- List of physicians for sending copies
- Type of report

To determine medical necessity and ensure proper coding and billing, the following elements are recommended for history and physical examination reports:

- Chief complaint, admitting diagnosis
- Present illness
- Past history (including allergies, current medication, and conditions)
- Family and social histories
- Review of systems
- Physical examination (*must include* pelvic, breast, and rectal examinations *or reason why deferred*)
- Diabetic patient (fundoscopic eye examination and peripheral pulses)
- Treatment plan (plan of care)
- Impression

For preoperative history and physical examinations, a statement regarding the risks, benefits, options, and potential complications of the procedure, as well as blood transfusion, if applicable, should be included. This statement is required in some states.

**Discharge Summaries**

---

**Date:**

**To:**      *[Insert medical staff or specific physician name]*

**From:**    *[Insert HIM director name, title, and telephone number]*

**Re:**      Health Record Documentation Requirements

The following information is provided to assist and guide the physician in proper health record documentation compliance. Increasing scrutiny is being directed toward complete and accurate physician documentation.

All dictated reports must include:

- Patient name
- Health record number
- Date of admission, consult, operation, and so on
- List of physicians for sending copies
- Type of report

To determine medical necessity and ensure proper coding and billing, the following elements are recommended for discharge summaries:

- Date of admission/date of discharge
- Admitting diagnosis and history
- Significant findings
- Hospital course (including procedures performed and treatment rendered)
- Complications
- Discharge instructions (including activity, diet, and medications)
- Condition on discharge
- Disposition (if transferred, state what level of care the receiving facility will provide [such as rehabilitation or acute care])
- Principal diagnosis (condition found after study to be chiefly responsible for admission)
- Additional diagnoses (those conditions identified, evaluated, treated, or that required additional resources or extended the length of stay)
  —Comorbid conditions (such as chronic obstructive pulmonary disease, congestive heart failure, and diabetes)
  —Complications
- Plan for follow-up care

## Operative Reports

**Date:**

**To:**        *[Insert medical staff or specific physician name]*

**From:**     *[Insert HIM director name, title, and telephone number]*

**Re:**        Health Record Documentation Requirements

The following information is provided to assist and guide the physician in proper health record documentation compliance. Increasing scrutiny is being directed toward complete and accurate physician documentation.

All dictated reports must include:

- Patient name
- Health record number
- Date of admission, consult, operation, and so on
- List of physicians for sending copies
- Type of report

To determine medical necessity and ensure proper coding and billing, the following elements are recommended for operative reports:

- Preoperative diagnosis
- Postoperative diagnosis
- Operation(s)/procedure(s) performed (do not use abbreviations)
- Indications
- Surgeon
- Assistant surgeon
- Anesthesiologist
- Type of anesthesia
- Findings
- Description of procedure
- Specimens removed
- Sutures/drains
- Estimated blood loss
- Fluids replaced (for example, blood transfusions)
- Complications (describe)
- Disposition (condition at conclusion of procedure)

## Consultations

---

**Date:**

**To:**    *[Insert medical staff or specific physician name]*

**From:**    *[Insert HIM director name, title, and telephone number]*

**Re:**    Health Record Documentation Requirements

The following information is provided to assist and guide the physician in proper health record documentation compliance. Increasing scrutiny is being directed toward complete and accurate physician documentation.

All dictated reports must include:

- Patient name
- Health record number
- Date of admission, consult, operation, and so on
- List of physicians for sending copies
- Type of report

To determine medical necessity and ensure proper coding and billing, the following elements are recommended for consultation reports:

- Reason for consultation or evaluation
- Requesting physician
- Current history
- Past medical history
- Physical examination and review of systems (may be limited depending on circumstances)
- Pertinent laboratory/radiology findings and/or studies
- Treatment plan
- Impression/conclusion

---

# Sample Job Description for HIM Compliance Specialist

**Title:** HIM Compliance Specialist        **Reports to:** Corporate Compliance Officer

**Qualifications:**

- RHIA or RHIT
- CCS preferred (or CCS-P for professional services coding)
- Extensive knowledge of ICD-9-CM and CPT coding principles and guidelines
- Extensive knowledge of reimbursement systems
- Extensive knowledge of proper use of Healthcare Common Procedure Coding System codes
- Chargemaster experience
- Extensive knowledge of federal, state, and payer-specific regulations and policies pertaining to documentation, coding, and billing
- Understanding of relationship among coding, billing, and reimbursement
- Experience with reviewing and analyzing claims, denials, and rejections
- Five years of hospital coding experience (for ambulatory services, ambulatory coding experience)
- Strong managerial, leadership, and interpersonal skills
- Excellent written and oral communication skills
- Excellent analytical skills

**Responsibilities:**

- Oversees and monitors implementation of the HIM compliance program
- Develops and coordinates educational and training programs regarding elements of the HIM compliance program, such as appropriate documentation and accurate coding, to all appropriate personnel, including HIM coding staff, physicians, billing personnel, and ancillary departments
- Maintains attendance rosters and documentation (agenda, handouts, and so on) for HIM training programs
- Ensures that coding consultants and other contracted entities (for example, outsourced coding personnel) understand and agree to adhere to the organization's HIM compliance program
- Conducts regular audits and coordinates ongoing monitoring of coding accuracy and documentation adequacy
- Provides feedback and focused educational programs on the results of auditing and monitoring activities to affected staff and physicians
- Conducts trend analyses to identify patterns and variations in coding practices and case-mix index

- Compares coding and reimbursement profile with national and regional norms to identify variations requiring further investigation
- Reviews claim denials and rejections pertaining to coding and medical necessity issues and, when necessary, implements corrective action plan, such as educational programs, to prevent similar denials and rejections from recurring
- Conducts internal investigations of changes in coding practices or reports of other potential problems pertaining to coding
- Initiates corrective action to ensure resolution of problem areas identified during an internal investigation or auditing/monitoring activity
- Reports noncompliance issues detected through auditing and monitoring, nature of corrective action plans implemented in response to identified problems, and results of follow-up audits to the corporate compliance officer
- Receives and investigates reports of HIM compliance violations and communicates this information to the corporate compliance officer
- Recommends disciplinary action for violation of the compliance program, the organization's standards of conduct, or coding policies and procedures to the corporate compliance officer
- Ensures the appropriate dissemination and communication of all regulation, policy, and guideline changes to affected personnel
- Serves as a resource for department managers, staff, physicians, and administration to obtain information or clarification on accurate and ethical coding and documentation standards, guidelines, and regulatory requirements
- Monitors adherence to the HIM compliance program
- Revises the HIM compliance program in response to changing organizational needs or new or revised regulations, policies, and guidelines
- Serves on the compliance committee
- Recommends revisions to the corporate compliance program to improve its effectiveness

# HIM Compliance Checklist

☐ Has an HIM code of conduct been developed and signed by HIM staff?

☐ Has an individual been designated to oversee the HIM compliance program?

☐ Has an internal risk assessment been conducted?

☐ Have comprehensive coding and documentation policies and procedures been developed and/or revised?

☐ Have educational programs been designed to ensure that staff and physicians are receiving adequate training on the elements of the compliance program, with particular emphasis on coding and documentation requirements?

☐ Do job descriptions for coding positions accurately reflect the necessary qualifications for these positions?

☐ Have processes been established for reporting, investigating, correcting, and following up on compliance-related violations?

☐ Have mechanisms for reporting compliance-related issues been communicated to employees, physicians, and contractors?

☐ Has a mechanism been established for employees, physicians, and contractors to obtain clarification on a policy, procedure, or element of the compliance program (including answers to billing and coding questions)?

☐ Is there a centralized source and systematic process for disseminating statutory and regulatory information in a timely fashion?

☐ Have processes been put in place for regular auditing and monitoring of coding accuracy and for addressing any identified problems?

☐ Have processes been established to investigate variations or other problems identified through auditing and monitoring such that the cause, scope, and seriousness of the problem can reasonably be determined and appropriate corrective action initiated?

☐ Has an action plan for responding to state or federal investigations been developed and approved?

☐ Has compliance been incorporated into the staff performance evaluation process?

☐ Have the various levels of disciplinary action that may be imposed for failure to comply been communicated to all affected individuals?

# Appendix D
# AHIMA Resources

**Practice Brief: Developing a Physician Query Process**

**Practice Brief: Developing a Coding Compliance Policy Document**

**Position Statement: Consistency of Healthcare Diagnostic and Procedural Coding**

**Practice Brief: Managing and Improving Data Quality**

**Resolution: Advocating for Quality Documentation and Adherence to Official Coding Guidelines**

**Position Statement: Quality Healthcare Data and Information**

# AHIMA Practice Brief
# Developing a Physician Query Process

## Principles of Medical Record Documentation

Medical record documentation is used for a multitude of purposes, including:

- Serving as a means of communication between the physician and the other members of the healthcare team providing care to the patient

- Serving as a basis for evaluating the adequacy and appropriateness of patient care

- Providing data to support insurance claims

- Assisting in protecting the legal interests of patients, healthcare professionals, and healthcare facilities

- Providing clinical data for research and education

To support these various uses, it is imperative that medical record documentation be complete, accurate, and timely. Facilities are expected to comply with a number of standards regarding medical record completion and content promulgated by multiple regulatory agencies.

### Joint Commission on Accreditation of Healthcare Organizations

The Joint Commission's *2000 Hospital Accreditation Standards* state, "the medical record contains sufficient information to identify the patient, support the diagnosis, justify the treatment, document the course and results, and promote continuity among health care providers" (IM.7.2).[1] The Joint Commission's Standards also state, "medical record data and information are managed in a timely manner" (IM.7.6).

Reprinted from: Prophet, S. 2001 (October). Practice brief: Developing a physician query process. *Journal of American Health Information Management Association* 72(9):88I–M.

Timely entries are essential if a medical record is to be useful in a patient's care. A complete medical record is also important when a patient is discharged, because information in the record may be needed for clinical, legal, or performance improvement purposes. The Joint Commission requires hospitals to have policy and procedures on the timely entry of all significant clinical information into the patient's medical record, and they do not consider a medical record complete until all final diagnoses and complications are recorded without the use of symbols or abbreviations.

Joint Commission standards also require medical records to be reviewed on an ongoing basis for completeness of timeliness of information, and action is taken to improve the quality and timeliness of documentation that affects patient care (IM.7.10). This review must address the presence, timeliness, legibility, and authentication of the final diagnoses and conclusions at termination of hospitalization.

## Medicare

The Medicare Conditions of Participation require medical records to be accurately written, promptly completed, properly filed and retained, and accessible.[2] Records must document, as appropriate, complications, hospital-acquired infections, and unfavorable reactions to drugs and anesthesia. The conditions also stipulate that all records must document the final diagnosis with completion of medical records within 30 days following discharge.

# Relationship between Coding and Documentation

Complete and accurate diagnostic and procedural coded data must be available, in a timely manner, in order to:

- Improve the quality and effectiveness of patient care

- Ensure equitable healthcare reimbursement

- Expand the body of medical knowledge

- Make appropriate decisions regarding healthcare policies, delivery systems, funding, expansion, and education

- Monitor resource utilization

- Permit identification and resolution of medical errors

- Improve clinical decision making

- Facilitate tracking of fraud and abuse

- Permit valid clinical research, epidemiologic studies, outcomes and statistical analyses, and provider profiling

- Provide comparative data to consumers regarding costs and outcomes, average charges, and outcomes by procedure

Physician documentation is the cornerstone of accurate coding. Therefore, assuring the accuracy of coded data is a shared responsibility between coding professionals and physicians. Accurate diagnostic and procedural coded data originate from collaboration between physicians, who have a clinical background, and coding professionals, who have an understanding of classification systems.

## Expectations of Physicians

Physicians are expected to provide complete, accurate, timely, and legible documentation of pertinent facts and observations about an individual's health history, including past and present illnesses, tests, treatments, and outcomes. Medical record entries should be documented at the time service is provided. Medical record entries should be authenticated. If subsequent additions to documentation are needed, they should be identified as such and dated. (Often these expectations are included in the medical staff or house staff rules and regulations.) Medical record documentation should:

- Address the clinical significance of abnormal test results

- Support the intensity of patient evaluation and treatment and describe the thought processes and complexity of decision making

- Include all diagnostic and therapeutic procedures, treatments, and tests performed, in addition to their results

- Include any changes in the patient's condition, including psychosocial and physical symptoms

- Include all conditions that coexist at the time of admission, that subsequently develop, or that affect the treatment received and the length of stay. This encompasses all conditions that affect patient care in terms of requiring clinical evaluation, therapeutic treatment, diagnostic procedures, extended length of hospital stay, or increased nursing care and monitoring[3]

- Be updated as necessary to reflect all diagnoses relevant to the care or services provided

- Be consistent and discuss and reconcile any discrepancies (this reconciliation should be documented in the medical record)

- Be legible and written in ink, typewritten, or electronically signed, stored, and printed

## Expectations of Coding Professionals

AHIMA's Code of Ethics sets forth ethical principles for the HIM profession. HIM professionals are responsible for maintaining and promoting ethical practices. This Code of Ethics states, in part: "Health information management professionals promote high standards for health information management practice, education, and research."

Another standard in this code states, "Health information management professionals strive to provide accurate and timely information." Data accuracy and integrity are fundamental values of HIM that are advanced by:

- Using practices that produce complete, accurate, and timely information to meet the health and related needs of individuals

- Following the guidelines set forth in the organization's compliance plan for reporting improper preparation, alteration, or suppression of information or data by others

- Not participating in any improper preparation, alteration, or suppression of health record information or other organization data

A conscientious goal for coding and maintaining a quality database is accurate clinical and statistical data. AHIMA's Standards of Ethical Coding were developed to guide coding professionals in this process. As stated in the standards, coding professionals are expected to support the importance of accurate, complete, and consistent coding practices for the production of quality healthcare data. These standards also indicate that coding professionals should only assign and report codes that are clearly and consistently supported by physician documentation in the medical record. It is the responsibility of coding professionals to assess physician documentation to assure that it supports the diagnosis and procedure codes reported on claims.

Dialogue between coding professionals and clinicians is encouraged, because it improves coding professionals' clinical knowledge and educates the physicians on documentation practice issues. AHIMA's Standards of Ethical Coding state that coding professionals are expected to consult physicians for clarification and additional documentation prior to code assignment when there is conflicting or ambiguous data in the health record. Coding professionals should also assist and educate physicians by advocating proper documentation practices, further specificity, and resequencing or inclusion of diagnoses or procedures when needed to more accurately reflect the acuity, severity, and the occurrence of events. It is recommended that coding be performed by credentialed HIM professionals.[4]

It is inappropriate for coding professionals to misrepresent the patient's clinical picture through incorrect coding or add diagnoses or procedures unsupported by the documentation to maximize reimbursement or meet insurance policy coverage requirements. Coding professionals should not change codes or the narratives of codes on the billing abstract so that meanings are misrepresented. Diagnoses or procedures should not be inappropriately included or excluded, because payment or insurance policy coverage requirements will be affected. When individual payer policies conflict with official coding rules and guidelines, these policies should be obtained in writing whenever possible. Reasonable efforts should be made to educate the payer on proper coding practices in order to influence a change in the payer's policy.

## Proper Use of Physician Queries

The process of querying physicians is an effective and, in the current healthcare environment, necessary mechanism for improving the quality of coding and medical record documentation and capturing complete clinical data. Query forms have become an accepted tool for communicating with physicians on documentation issues influencing proper code assignment. Query forms should be used in a judicious and appropriate manner. They must be used as a communication tool to improve the accuracy of code assignment and the quality of physician documentation, not to inappropriately maximize reimbursement. The query process should be guided by AHIMA's Standards of Ethical Coding and the official coding guidelines. An inappropriate query—such as a form that is poorly constructed or asks leading questions—or overuse of the query process can result in quality-of-care, legal, and ethical concerns.

## The Query Process

The goal of the query process should be to improve physician documentation and coding professionals' understanding of the unique clinical situation, not to improve reimbursement. Each facility should establish a policy and procedure for obtaining physician clarification of documentation that affects code assignment. The process of querying physicians must be a patient-specific process, not a general process. Asking "blanket" questions is not appropriate. Policies regarding the circumstances when physicians will be queried should be designed to promote timely, complete, and accurate coding and documentation.

Physicians should not be asked to provide clarification of their medical record documentation without the opportunity to access the patient's medical record.

Each facility also needs to determine if physicians will be queried concurrently (during the patient's hospitalization) or after discharge. Both methods are acceptable. Querying physicians concurrently allows the documentation deficiency to be corrected while the patient is still in-house and can positively influence patient care.

The policy and procedure should stipulate who is authorized to contact the physician for clarifications regarding a coding issue. Coding professionals should be allowed to contact physicians directly for clarification, rather than limiting this responsibility to supervisory personnel or a designated individual.

The facility may wish to use a designated physician liaison to resolve conflicts between physicians and coding professionals. The appropriate use of the physician liaison should be described in the facility's policy and procedures.

### Query Format

Each facility should develop a standard format for the query form. Post-it notes or scratch paper should not be allowed. Each facility should develop a standard design and format for physician queries to ensure clear, consistent, appropriate queries.

The query form should:

- Be clearly and concisely written

- Contain precise language

- Present the facts from the medical record and identify why clarification is needed

- Present the scenario and state a question that asks the physician to make a clinical interpretation of a given diagnosis or condition based on treatment, evaluation, monitoring, and/or services provided. "Open-ended" questions that allow the physician to document the specific diagnosis are preferable to multiple-choice questions or questions requiring only a "yes" or "no" response. Queries that appear to lead the physician to provide a particular response could lead to allegations of inappropriate upcoding.

- Be phrased such that the physician is allowed to specify the correct diagnosis. It should not indicate the financial impact of the response to the query.

- Include:

  —Patient name

  —Admission date

  —Medical record number

  —Name and contact information (phone number and e-mail address) of the coding professional

  —Specific question and rationale (that is, relevant documentation or clinical findings)

  —Place for the physician to document his or her response

  —Place for the physician to sign and date his or her response

The query forms should not:

- "Lead" the physician

- Sound presumptive, directing, prodding, probing, or as though the physician is being led to make an assumption

- Ask questions that can be responded to in a "yes" or "no" fashion

- Indicate the financial impact of the response to the query

- Be designed so that all that is required is a physician signature

## When Is a Query Appropriate?

Physicians should be queried whenever there is conflicting, ambiguous, or incomplete information in the medical record regarding any significant reportable condition or procedure. Querying the physician only when reimbursement is affected will skew national healthcare data and might lead to allegations of upcoding.

Every discrepancy or issue not addressed in the physician documentation should not necessarily result in the physician being queried. Each facility needs to develop policies and procedures regarding the clinical conditions and documentation situations warranting a request for physician clarification. For example, insignificant or irrelevant findings may not warrant querying the physician regarding the assignment of an additional diagnosis code. Also, if the maximum number of codes that can be entered in the hospital information system has already been assigned, the facility may decide that it is not necessary to query the physician regarding an additional code. Facilities need to balance the value of marginal data being collected against the administrative burden of obtaining the additional documentation.

Members of the medical staff in consultation with coding professionals should develop the specific clinical criteria for a valid query. The specific clinical documentation that must be present in the patient's record to generate a query should be described. For example, anemia, septicemia, and respiratory failure are conditions that often require physician clarification. The medical staff can assist the coding staff in determining when it would be appropriate to query a physician regarding the reporting of these conditions by describing the specific clinical indications in the medical record documentation that raise the possibility that the condition in question may be present.

## When Is a Query Not Necessary?

Queries are not necessary if a physician involved in the care and treatment of the patient, including consulting physicians, has documented a diagnosis and there is no conflicting documentation from another physician. Medical record documentation from any physician involved in the care and treatment of the patient, including documentation by consulting physicians, is appropriate for the basis of code assignment. If there is conflicting documentation between different physicians, clarification should be sought from the attending physician, who is ultimately responsible for the final diagnosis.

Queries are also not necessary when a physician has documented a final diagnosis, and clinical indicators—such as test results—do not appear to support this diagnosis. Although coding professionals are expected to advocate complete and accurate physician documentation and to collaborate with physicians to realize this goal, they are not expected to challenge the physician's medical judgment in establishing the patient's diagnosis. However, because a discrepancy between clinical findings and a final diagnosis is a clinical issue, a facility may choose to establish a policy that the physician will be queried in these instances.

## Documentation of Query Response

The physician's response to the query must be documented in the patient's medical record. Each facility must develop a policy regarding the specific process for incorporating this additional documentation in the medical record. For example, this policy might stipulate that the physician is required to add the additional information to the body of the medical record. As an alternative, a form, such as a medical record "progress note" form, might be attached to the query form and the attachment is then filed in the medical record. However, another alternative is to file the query form itself in the permanent medical record. Any documentation obtained after discharge must be included in the discharge summary or identified as a late entry or addendum.

Any decision to file this form in the medical record should involve the advice of the facility's corporate compliance officer and legal counsel, due to potential compliance and legal risks related to incorporating the actual query form into the permanent medical record (such as its potential use as evidence of poor documentation in an audit, investigation, or malpractice suit, risks related to naming a nonclinician in the medical record, or quality of care concerns if the physician response on a query form is not clearly supported by the rest of the medical record documentation).

If the query form will serve as the only documentation of the physician's clarification, the use of open-ended questions (those that require the physician to specifically document the additional information) are preferable to multiple-choice questions or the use of questions requiring only a "yes" or "no" answer. The query form would need to be approved by the medical staff/medical records committee before implementation of a policy allowing this form to be maintained in the medical record. Also, the Joint Commission hospital accreditation standards stipulate that only authorized individuals may make entries in medical records (IM.7.1.1). Therefore, the facility needs to consider modifying the medical staff bylaws to specify coding professionals as individuals authorized to make medical record entries prior to allowing query forms to become a permanent part of the medical record.

## Auditing, Monitoring, and Corrective Action

Ideally, complete and accurate physician documentation should occur at the time care is rendered. The need for a query form results from incomplete, conflicting, or ambiguous documentation, which is an indication of poor documentation. Therefore, query form usage should be the exception rather than the norm. If physicians are being queried frequently, facility management or an appropriate medical staff committee should investigate the reasons why.

A periodic review of the query practice should include a determination of what percentage of the query forms are eliciting negative and positive responses from the physicians. A high negative response rate may be an indication that the coding staff are not using the query process judiciously and are being overzealous.

A high positive response rate may indicate that there are widespread poor documentation habits that need to be addressed. It may also indicate that the absence of certain reports (for example, discharge summary, operative report) at the time of coding is forcing the coding staff to query the physicians to obtain the information they need for proper coding.

If this is the case, the facility may wish to reconsider its policy regarding the availability of certain reports prior to coding. Waiting for these reports may make more sense in terms of turnaround time and productivity rather than finding it necessary to frequently query the physicians. The question of why final diagnoses are not available at the time of discharge may arise at the time of an audit, review by the peer review organization, or investigation.

The use of query forms should also be monitored for patterns, and any identified patterns should be used to educate physicians on improving their documentation at the point of care. If a pattern is identified, such as a particular physician or diagnosis, appropriate steps should be taken to correct the problem so the necessary documentation is present prior to coding in the future and the need to query this physician, or to query physicians regarding a particular diagnosis, is reduced. Corrective action might include targeted education for one physician or education for the entire medical staff on the proper documentation necessary for accurate code assignment.

Patterns of poor documentation that have not been addressed through education or other corrective action are signs of an ineffective compliance program. The Department of Health and Human Services Office of Inspector General has noted in its *Compliance Program Guidance for Hospitals* that "accurate coding depends upon the quality of completeness of the physician's documentation" and "active staff physician participation in educational programs focusing on coding and documentation should be emphasized by the hospital."[5]

The format of the queries should also be monitored on a regular basis to ensure that they are not inappropriately leading the physician to provide a particular response. Inappropriately written queries should be used to educate the coding staff on a properly written query. Patterns of inappropriately written queries should be referred to the corporate compliance officer.

## Prepared by

Sue Prophet, RHIA, CCS

## Acknowledgments

AHIMA Advocacy and Policy Task Force

AHIMA's Coding Practice Team

AHIMA Coding Policy and Strategy Committee

AHIMA Society for Clinical Coding

Dan Rode, MBA, FHFMA

## Notes

1. Joint Commission on Accreditation of Healthcare Organizations. *Comprehensive Accreditation Manual for Hospitals: The Official Handbook.* Oakbrook Terrace, IL: Joint Commission, 2000.

2. Health Care Financing Administration, Department of Health and Human Services. "Conditions of Participation for Hospitals." *Code of Federal Regulations,* 2000. 42 CFR, Chapter IV, Part 482.

3. Official ICD-9-CM Guidelines for Coding and Reporting developed and approved by the American Hospital Association, American Health Information Management Association, Health Care Financing Administration, and the National Center for Health Statistics.

4. AHIMA is the professional organization responsible for issuing several credentials in health information management: Registered Health Information Administrator (RHIA), Registered Health Information Technician (RHIT), Certified Coding Specialist (CCS), and Certified Coding Specialist—Physician-based (CCS-P).

5. Office of Inspector General, Department of Health and Human Services. "Compliance Program Guidance for Hospitals." Washington, DC: Office of Inspector General, 1998.

## References

AHIMA Code of Ethics, 1998.

AHIMA Standards of Ethical Coding, 1999.

AHIMA Coding Policy and Strategy Committee. "Practice Brief: Data Quality." *Journal of AHIMA* 67, no. 2 (1996).

# AHIMA Practice Brief: Developing a Coding Compliance Policy Document

Organizations using diagnosis and procedure codes for reporting healthcare services must have formal policies and corresponding procedures in place that provide instruction on the entire process—from the point of service to the billing statement or claim form. Coding compliance policies serve as a guide to performing coding and billing functions and provide documentation of the organization's intent to correctly report services. The policies should include facility-specific documentation requirements, payer regulations and policies, and contractual arrangements for coding consultants and outsourcing services. This information may be covered in payer/provider contracts or found in Medicare and Medicaid manuals and bulletins.

Following are selected tenets that address the process of code selection and reporting. These tenets may be referred to as coding protocols, a coding compliance program, organizational coding guidelines, or a similar name. These tenets are an important part of any organization's compliance plan and the key to preventing coding errors and resulting reimbursement problems. Examples are taken from both outpatient and inpatient coding processes for illustration purposes only. This document cannot serve as a complete coding compliance plan, but will be useful as a guide for creating a more comprehensive resource to meet individual organizational needs.

A coding compliance plan should include the following components:

- **A general policy statement about the commitment of the organization to correctly assign and report codes.**

  **Example:** Memorial Medical Center is committed to establishing and maintaining clinical coding and insurance claims processing procedures to ensure that reported codes reflect actual services provided, through accurate information system entries.

Reprinted from: AHIMA Coding Practice Team. 2001 (August). Practice brief: Developing a coding compliance policy document. *Journal of American Health Information Management Association* 72(7) 88A–C.

- **The source of the official coding guidelines used to direct code selection.**

  **Example:** ICD-9-CM code selection follows the Official Guidelines for Coding and Reporting, developed by the cooperating parties and documented in *Coding Clinic for ICD-9-CM*, published by the American Hospital Association.

  **Example:** CPT code selection follows the guidelines set forth in the CPT manual and in *CPT Assistant,* published by the American Medical Association.

- **The parties responsible for code assignment. The ultimate responsibility for code assignment lies with the physician (provider). However, policies and procedures may document instances where codes may be selected or modified by authorized individuals.**

  **Example:** For inpatient records, medical record analyst I staff are responsible for analysis of records and assignment of the correct ICD-9-CM codes based on documentation by the attending physician.

  **Example:** Emergency department evaluation and management levels for physician services will be selected by the physician and validated by outpatient record analysts using the HCFA/AMA documentation guidelines. When a variance occurs, the following steps are taken for resolution: (The actual document should follow with procedure details.)

- **The procedure to follow when the clinical information is not clear enough to assign the correct code.**

  **Example:** When the documentation used to assign codes is ambiguous or incomplete, the physician must be contacted to clarify the information and complete/amend the record, if necessary. (The actual document should follow with details of how the medical staff would like this to occur, for example, by phone call or by note on the record). Standard protocols for adding documentation to a record must be followed, in accordance with the applicable laws and regulations.

- **Specify the policies and procedures that apply to specific locations and care settings. Official coding guidelines for inpatient reporting and outpatient/physician reporting are different. This means that if you are developing a facility-specific coding guideline for emergency department services, designate that the coding rules or guidelines only apply in this setting.**

  **Example:** When reporting an injection of a drug provided in the emergency department to a Medicare beneficiary, the appropriate CPT code for the administration of the injection is reported in addition to the evaluation and management service code and drug code. CPT codes are reported whether a physician provides the injection personally or a nurse is carrying out a physician's order. This instruction does not always apply for reporting of professional services in the clinics, because administration of medication is considered bundled with the corresponding evaluation and management service for Medicare patients.

**Example:** Diagnoses that are documented as "probable," "suspected," "questionable," "rule-out," or "working diagnosis" are not to have a code assigned as a confirmed diagnosis. Instead, the code for the condition established at the close of the encounter should be assigned, such as a symptom, sign, abnormal test result, or clinical finding. This guideline applies only to outpatient services.

- **Applicable reporting requirements required by specific agencies. The document should include where instructions on payer-specific requirements may be accessed.**

  **Example:** For patients with XYZ care plan, report code S0800 for patients having a LASIK procedure rather than an unlisted CPT code.

  **Example:** For Medicare patients receiving a wound closure by tissue adhesive only, report HCPCS Level II code G0168 rather than a CPT code.

  Many of these procedures will be put into software databases and would not be written as a specific policy. This is true with most billing software, whether for physician services or through the charge description master used by many hospitals.

- **Procedures for correction of inaccurate code assignments in the clinical database and to the agencies where the codes have been reported.**

  **Example:** When an error in code assignment is discovered after bill release and the claim has already been submitted, this is the process required to update and correct the information system and facilitate claim amendment or correction. (The actual document should follow with appropriate details.)

- **Areas of risk that have been identified through audits or monitoring. Each organization should have a defined audit plan for code accuracy and consistency review and corrective actions should be outlined for problems that are identified.**

  **Example:** A hospital might identify that acute respiratory failure is being assigned as the principal diagnosis with congestive heart failure as a secondary diagnosis. The specific reference to *Coding Clinic* could be listed with instructions about correct coding of these conditions and the process to be used to correct the deficiency.

- **Identification of essential coding resources available to and used by the coding professionals.**

  **Example:** Updated ICD-9-CM, CPT, and HCPCS Level II code books are used by all coding professionals. Even if the hospital uses automated encoding software, at least one printed copy of the coding manuals should be available for reference.

  **Example:** Updated encoder software, including the appropriate version of the NCCI edits and DRG and APC grouper software, is available to the appropriate personnel.

**Example:** *Coding Clinic* and *CPT Assistant* are available to all coding professionals.

- **A process for coding new procedures or unusual diagnoses.**

**Example:** When the coding professional encounters an unusual diagnosis, the coding supervisor or the attending physician is consulted. If, after research, a code cannot be identified, the documentation is submitted to the American Hospital Association for clarification.

- **A procedure to identify any optional codes gathered for statistical purposes by the facility and clarification of the appropriate use of E codes.**

**Example:** All ICD-9-CM procedure codes in the surgical range (ICD-9-CM Volume III codes 01.01-86.99) shall be reported for inpatients. In addition, codes reported from the nonsurgical section include the following: (Completed document should list the actual codes to be reported.)

**Example:** All appropriate E codes for adverse effects of drugs must be reported. In addition, this facility reports all E codes, including the place of injury for poisonings, all cases of abuse, and all accidents on the initial visit for both inpatient and outpatient services.

- **Appropriate methods for resolving coding or documentation disputes with physicians.**

**Example:** When the physician disagrees with official coding guidelines, the case is referred to the medical records committee following review by the designated physician liaison from that group.

- **A procedure for processing claim rejections.**

**Example:** All rejected claims pertaining to diagnosis and procedure codes should be returned to coding staff for review or correction. Any chargemaster issues should be forwarded to appropriate departmental staff for corrections. All clinical codes, including modifiers, must never be changed or added without review by coding staff with access to the appropriate documentation.

**Example:** If a claim is rejected due to the codes provided in the medical record abstract, the billing department notifies the supervisor of coding for a review rather than changing the code to a payable code and resubmitting the claim.

- **A statement clarifying that codes will not be assigned, modified, or excluded solely for the purpose of maximizing reimbursement. Clinical codes will not be changed or amended merely due to either physicians' or patients' request to have the service in question covered by insurance. If the initial code assignment did not reflect the actual services, codes may be revised based on supporting documentation. Disputes with either physicians or patients are handled only by the coding supervisor and are appropriately logged for review.**

**Example:** A patient calls the business office saying that her insurance carrier did not pay for her mammogram. After investigating, the HIM coding staff discover that the coding was appropriate for a screening mammogram and that this is a noncovered service with the insurance provider. The code is not changed and the matter is referred back to the business office for explanation to the patient that she should contact her insurance provider with any dispute over coverage of service.

**Example:** Part of a payment is denied and after review, the supervisor discovers that a modifier should have been appended to the CPT code to denote a separately identifiable service. Modifier 25 is added to the code set and the corrected claim is resubmitted.

**Example:** A physician approaches the coding supervisor with a request to change the diagnosis codes for his patient because she currently has a pre-existing condition that is not covered by her current health plan. The coding supervisor must explain to the physician that falsification of insurance claims is illegal. If the physician insists, the physician liaison for the medical record committee is contacted and the matter is turned over to that committee for resolution if necessary.

- **The use of and reliance on encoders within the organization. Coding staff cannot rely solely on computerized encoders. Current coding manuals must be readily accessible and the staff must be educated appropriately to detect inappropriate logic or errors in encoding software. When errors in logic or code crosswalks are discovered, they are reported to the vendor immediately by the coding supervisor.**

**Example:** During the coding process, an error is identified in the crosswalk between the ICD-9-CM Volume III code and the CPT code. This error is reported to the software vendor, with proper documentation and notification of all staff using the encoder to not rely on the encoder for code selection.

- **Medical records are analyzed and codes selected only with complete and appropriate documentation by the physician available. According to coding guidelines, codes are not assigned without physician documentation. If records are coded without the discharge summary or final diagnostic statements available, processes are in place for review after the summary is added to the record.**

**Example:** When records are coded without a discharge summary, they are flagged in the computer system. When the summaries are added to the record, the record is returned to the coding professional for review of codes. If there are any inconsistencies, appropriate steps are taken for review of the changes.

## Additional Elements

A coding compliance document should include a reference to AHIMA's Standards of Ethical Coding, which can be downloaded from AHIMA's Web site at www.ahima.org. Reference to the data quality assessment procedures must be included in a coding compliance plan to establish the mechanism for determining areas of risk. Reviews will identify the need for further education and increased monitoring for those areas where either coding variances or documentation deficiencies are identified.

Specific and detailed coding guidelines that cover the reporting of typical services provided by a facility or organization create tools for data consistency and reliability by ensuring that all coding professionals interpret clinical documentation and apply coding principles in the same manner. The appropriate medical staff committee should give final approval of any coding guidelines that involve clinical criteria to assure appropriateness and physician consensus on the process.

The format is most useful when organized by patient or service type and easily referenced by using a table of contents. If the facility-specific guidelines are maintained electronically, they should be searchable by key terms. Placing the coding guidelines on a facility Intranet or internal computer network is an efficient way to ensure their use and it also enables timely and efficient updating and distribution. Inclusion of references to live links should be provided to supporting documents such as Uniform Hospital Discharge Data Sets or other regulatory requirements outlining reporting procedures or code assignments.

### Prepared by

AHIMA's Coding Practice Team and reviewed by the Coding Policy and Strategy Committee and the Society for Clinical Coding Data Quality Committee

# AHIMA Position Statement on Consistency of Healthcare Diagnostic and Procedural Coding

## AHIMA's Position

AHIMA believes the collection of accurate and complete coded data is critical to healthcare delivery, research and analysis, reimbursement, and policymaking. The integrity of coded data and the ability to turn it into functional information requires that all users consistently apply the same official coding rules, conventions, guidelines, and definitions (the basis of coding standards). Use of uniform coding standards reduces administrative costs, enhances data quality and integrity, and improves decision-making—all factors that lead to quality healthcare delivery and information.

For the United States to have and maintain quality data and information, coding standards must be required and promoted for uniform application and use, and not violated to meet parochial or short-term requirements. In order for the nation to obtain, store, and use quality information, coding standards must be uniformly applied across sites of service and developed and maintained to meet the national and international needs of healthcare delivery, research, policy making, and the interpretation of healthcare data for the benefit of humankind. AHIMA's coding professionals are educated and certified to ethically apply and use national uniform coding standards to support these data quality, analysis, and maintenance functions.

## Current Situation

Coded clinical data are used by healthcare providers, payers, researchers, government agencies, and others for the following reasons:

- Measuring the quality, safety, and efficacy of care

- Managing care and disease processes

Approved by the AHIMA Board of Directors, May 18, 2002.

- Tracking public health and risks

- Providing data to consumers regarding costs and outcomes of treatment options

- Payment system design and processing of claims for reimbursement

- Research, epidemiologic studies, and clinical trials

- Designing healthcare delivery systems and monitoring resource utilization

- Identifying fraudulent practices

- Setting health policy

The coding of clinical diagnostic and procedure data involves the translation of clinical information collected during healthcare encounters into diagnostic and procedural codes that accurately reflect the patients' medical conditions and services provided. A medical code set is an established system for encoding specific data elements pertaining to the provision of healthcare services, such as medical conditions, signs and symptoms, diagnostic and therapeutic procedures, devices, and supplies. A code set includes the codes and code descriptions and, potentially, the rules, conventions, and guidelines for proper use of the codes.

Currently, many coding practices are driven by health plan or payer reimbursement contracts or policies requiring providers to add, modify, or omit selected medical codes to reflect the plan or payer's coverages, policies, or government regulations, contrary to standards for proper use of the code sets. Payers do not uniformly abide by such standards for proper application of the medical code sets. Code sets are not revised on the same date, and often payers require the continued use of deleted or invalid codes. Individual health plans, and even different contractors for the same plan (including Medicare and other government contractors), develop their own rules and definitions for the reporting of given codes. These variable requirements, which affect all the medical code sets currently required for reimbursement claims submission to third-party payers, undermine the integrity and comparability of healthcare data.

New uses of healthcare data are constantly evolving, further demanding that careful attention be paid to accurate and consistent application and reporting of coded data. Code sets must be sufficiently flexible to meet these changing needs, while maintaining stability and continuity over time to ensure data comparability. Those responsible for coding clinical data must be educated and trained to apply coding standards correctly and uniformly. The current situation, resulting in inconsistent coding practices, leads to potentially bad healthcare decisions now and in the future.

## Consistency of Healthcare Diagnostic and Procedure Coding

Consistency of healthcare diagnostic and procedure coding will be achieved when:

- All healthcare entities agree to:

    —Use only valid versions of the medical code sets and coding standards, and

    —Refrain from establishing or accepting rules (for example, reimbursement rules), regulations, or contracts that force healthcare entities to violate coding standards.

- Certified coding professionals assign and validate codes and assist in the development of policies that affect or depend on coding accuracy.

- Medical Code Set Maintenance Organizations:

  —Provide fully public processes for input to the update and maintenance of the code set standard;

  —Include representation by all groups of stakeholders in decisions regarding code set revisions; and

  —Publish and implement code set revisions and standards on a scheduled basis for clarity of implementation requirements, due dates, and timely publishing of education materials by others outside the organization.

- Medical Code Sets are:

  —Flexible to accommodate changes in healthcare that affect diagnoses, changes in medical and clinical practices, and so forth;

  —Maintained to ensure stability and comparability of coded data over time;

  —Maintained and updated on a timely basis to accommodate advances in medicine;

  —Unique, so that users do not have to choose between or among different code sets;

  —Capable of uniform use across different sites of service when the service is the same;

  —Subject to a national central coordinating authority; and

  —Serve to facilitate a national healthcare information in infrastructure.

# AHIMA Practice Brief:
# Managing and Improving Data Quality

Complete and accurate diagnostic and procedural coded data is necessary for research, epidemiology, outcomes and statistical analyses, financial and strategic planning, reimbursement, evaluation of quality of care, and communication to support the patient's treatment.

Consistency of coding has been a major AHIMA initiative in the quest to improve data quality management in healthcare service reporting. AHIMA has also taken a stand on the quality of healthcare data and information.[1]

## Data Quality Mandates

Adherence to industry standards and approved coding principles that generate coded data of the highest quality and consistency remains critical to the healthcare industry and the maintenance of information integrity throughout healthcare systems. HIM professionals must continue to meet the challenges of maintaining an accurate and meaningful database reflective of patient mix and resource use. As long as diagnostic and procedural codes serve as the basis for payment methodologies, the ethics of clinical coding professionals and healthcare organization billing processes will be challenged.

Ensuring accuracy of coded data is a shared responsibility between HIM professionals, clinicians, business services staff, and information systems integrity professionals. The HIM professional has the unique responsibility of administration, oversight, analysis, and/or coding clinical data in all healthcare organizations. Care must be taken in organizational structures to ensure that oversight of the coding and data management process falls within the HIM department's responsibility area so data quality mandates are upheld and appropriate HIM principles are applied to business practices.

Reprinted from: AHIMA Coding Products and Services Team. 2003 (July/August). Practice brief: Managing and improving data quality (Updated)." *Journal of American Health Information Management Association* 74(7):64A–C.

## Clinical Collaboration

The Joint Commission and the Medicare Conditions of Participation as well as other accreditation agencies require final diagnoses and procedures to be recorded in the medical record and authenticated by the responsible practitioner. State laws also provide guidelines concerning the content of the health record as a legal document.

Clinical documentation primarily created by physicians is the cornerstone of accurate coding, supplemented by appropriate policies and procedures developed by facilities to meet patient care requirements. Coded data originates from the collaboration between clinicians and HIM professionals with clinical terminology, classification system, nomenclature, data analysis, and compliance policy expertise.

Thus, the need for collaboration, cooperation, and communication between clinicians and support personnel continues to grow as information gathering and storage embrace new technology. Movement of the coding process into the business processing side of a healthcare organization must not preclude access to and regular communication with clinicians.

## Clinical Database Evaluation

Regulatory agencies are beginning to apply data analysis tools to monitor data quality and reliability for reimbursement appropriateness and to identify unusual claims data patterns that may indicate payment errors or health insurance fraud. Examples include the Hospital Payment Monitoring Program tool First Look Analysis Tool for Hospital Outlier Monitoring (FATHOM), used by Quality Improvement Organizations, and the comprehensive error rate testing (CERT) process to be used by Centers for Medicare and Medicaid Services carriers to produce national, contractor, provider type, and benefit category-specific paid claims error rates.

Ongoing evaluation of the clinical database by health information managers facilitates ethical reporting of clinical information and early identification of data accuracy problems for timely and appropriate resolution. Pattern analysis of codes is a useful tool for prevention of compliance problems by identifying and correcting clinical coding errors.

Coding errors have multiple causes, some within the control of HIM processes and others that occur outside the scope of HIM due to inadequacy of the source document or the lack of information integrity resulting from inappropriate computer programming routines or software logic.

## Data Quality Management and Improvement Initiatives

The following actions are required in any successful program:

- Evaluation and trending of diagnosis and procedure code selections, the appropriateness of reimbursement group assignment, and other coded data elements such as discharge status are required. This action ensures that clinical concept validity, appropriate code sequencing, specific code use requirements, and clinical pertinence are reflected in the codes reported.

- Reporting data quality review results to organizational leadership, compliance staff, and the medical staff. This stresses accountability for data quality to everyone involved and allows the root causes of inconsistency or lack of reliability of data validity to be addressed. If the source for code assignment is inadequate or invalid, the results may reflect correct coding by the coding professional, but still represent a data quality problem because the code assigned does not reflect the actual concept or event as it occurred.

- Following up on and monitoring identified problems. HIM professionals must resist the temptation to overlook inadequate documentation and report codes without appropriate clinical foundation within the record just to speed up claims processing, meet a business requirement, or obtain additional reimbursement. There is an ethical duty as members of the healthcare team to educate physicians on appropriate documentation practices and maintain high standards for health information practice. Organizational structures must support these efforts by the enforcement of medical staff rules and regulations and continuous monitoring of clinical pertinence of documentation to meet both business and patient care requirements.

HIM clinical data specialists who understand data quality management concepts and the relationship of clinical code assignments to reimbursement and decision support for healthcare will have important roles to play in the healthcare organizations of the future. Continuing education and career-boosting specialty advancement programs are expected to be the key to job security and professional growth as automation continues to change healthcare delivery, claims processing, and compliance activities.[2]

## Data Quality Recommendations

HIM coding professionals and the organizations that employ them are accountable for data quality that requires the following behaviors.

HIM professionals should:

- Adopt best practices made known in professional resources and follow the code of ethics for the profession or their specific compliance programs.[3] This guidance applies to all settings and all health plans.

- Use the entire health record as part of the coding process in order to assign and report the appropriate clinical codes for the standard transactions and codes sets required for external reporting and meeting internal abstracting requirements.

- Adhere to all official coding guidelines published in the HIPAA standard transactions and code sets regulation. ICD-9-CM guidelines are available for downloading at www.cdc.gov/nchs/data/icd9/icdguide.pdf. Additional official coding advice is published in the quarterly publication AHA *Coding Clinic for ICD-9-CM*. CPT guidelines are located within the CPT code books and additional information and coding advice is provided in the AMA monthly publication *CPT Assistant.* Modifications to the initial HIPAA standards for electronic transactions or adoption of additional standards are submitted first to the designated standard maintenance organization. For more information, go to http://aspe.os.dhhs.gov/admnsimp/final/dsmo.htm and www.hipaa-dsmo.org/.

- Develop appropriate facility or practice-specific guidelines when available coding guidelines do not address interpretation of the source document or guide code selection in specific circumstances. Facility practice guidelines should not conflict with official coding guidelines.

- Maintain a working relationship with clinicians through ongoing communication and documentation improvement programs.

- Report root causes of data quality concerns when identified. Problematic issues that arise from individual physicians or groups of clinicians should be referred to medical staff leadership or the compliance office for investigation and resolution.

- Query when necessary. Best practices and coding guidelines suggest that when coding professionals encounter conflicting or ambiguous documentation in a source document, the physician must be queried to confirm the appropriate code selection.[4]

- Consistently seek out innovative methods to capture pertinent information required for clinical code assignment to minimize unnecessary clinician inquiries. Alternative methods of accessing information necessary for code assignment may prevent the need to wait for completion of the health record, such as electronic access to clinical reports.

- Ensure that clinical code sets reported to outside agencies are fully supported by documentation within the health record and clearly reflected in diagnostic statements and procedure reports provided by a physician.

- Provide the physician the opportunity to review reported diagnoses and procedures on preclaim or postclaim or postbill submission, via mechanisms such as:

  —providing a copy (via mail, fax, or electronic transmission) of the sequenced codes and their narrative descriptions, taking appropriate care to protect patient privacy and security of the information.

  —placing the diagnostic and procedural listing within the record and bringing it to the physician's attention within the appropriate time frame for correction when warranted.

- Create a documentation improvement program or offer educational programs concerning the relationship of health record entries and health record management to data quality, information integrity, patient outcomes, and business success of the organization.

- Conduct a periodic or ongoing review of any automated billing software (charge-masters, service description masters, practice management systems, claims scrubbers, medical necessity software) used to ensure code appropriateness and validity of clinical codes.

- Require a periodic or ongoing review of encounter forms or other resource tools that involve clinical code assignment to ensure validity and appropriateness.

- Complete appropriate continuing education and training to keep abreast of clinical advancements in diagnosis and treatment, billing and compliance issues, regulatory requirements, and coding guideline changes, and to maintain professional credentials.

HIM coding professionals and the organizations that employ them have the responsibility to not engage in, promote, or tolerate the following behaviors that adversely affect data quality.

HIM professionals should not:

- Make assumptions requiring clinical judgment concerning the etiology or context of the condition under consideration for code reporting.

- Misrepresent the patient's clinical picture through code assignment for diagnoses/procedures unsupported by the documentation in order to maximize reimbursement, affect insurance policy coverage, or because of other third-party payer requirements. This includes falsification of conditions to meet medical necessity requirements when the patient's condition does not support health plan coverage for the service in question or using a specific code requested by a payer when, according to official coding guidelines, a different code is mandatory.

- Omit the reporting of clinical codes that represent actual clinical conditions or services but negatively affect a facility's data profile, negate health plan coverage, or lower the reimbursement potential.

- Allow changing of clinical code assignments under any circumstances without consultation with the coding professional involved and the clinician whose services are being reported. Changes are allowed only with subsequent validation of the documentation supporting the need for code revision.

- Fail to use the physician query process outlined by professional practice standards or required by quality improvement organizations under contract for federal and state agencies that reimburse for healthcare services.

- Assign codes to an incomplete record without organizational policies in place to ensure the codes are reviewed after the records are complete. Failure to confirm the accuracy and completeness of the codes submitted for a reimbursement claim upon completion of the medical record can increase both data quality and compliance risks.[5]

- Promote or tolerate the falsification of clinical documentation or misrepresentation of clinical conditions or service provided.

## Prepared by

AHIMA's Coding Products and Services team:
Kathy Brouch, RHIA, CCS
Susan Hull, MPH, RHIA, CCS
Karen Kostick, RHIT, CCS, CCS-P
Rita Scichilone, MHSA, RHIA, CCS, CCS-P
Mary Stanfill, RHIA, CCS, CCS-P
Ann Zeisset, RHIT, CCS, CCS-P

## Acknowledgments

AHIMA Coding (SCC) Community of Practice

AHIMA Coding Policy and Strategy Committee

Sue Prophet-Bowman, RHIA, CCS

## Notes

1. For details, see AHIMA's Position Statements on Consistency of Healthcare Diagnostic and Procedural Coding and on the Quality of Healthcare Data and Information at www.ahima.org/dc/positions.

2. For more information on AHIMA's specialty advancement programs, go to http://campus.ahima.org.

3. AHIMA's Standards of Ethical Coding are available at www.ahima.org/infocenter/guidelines.

4. Prophet, Sue. "Practice Brief: Developing a Physician Query Process." *Journal of AHIMA* 72, no. 9 (2001): 88I–M.

5. More guidelines for HIM policy and procedure development are available in *Health Information Management Compliance: A Model Program for Healthcare Organizations* by Sue Prophet, AHIMA, 2002. Coding from incomplete records is also discussed in the AHIMA Practice Brief "Developing a Coding Compliance Document" in the July/August 2001 *Journal of AHIMA* (vol. 72, no. 7, prepared by AHIMA's Coding Practice Team).

# AHIMA Resolution:
# Advocating for Quality Documentation and Adherence to Official Coding Guidelines

## Background Information

In August 1996, the Health Insurance Portability and Accountability Act (HIPAA) [Public Law 104-191] established the infrastructure and funding for federal fraud and abuse efforts. This legislation authorizes the appropriation of $104 million in 1997, with increases in 15 percent increments until 2003, to defray the costs of the Department of Health and Human Services (HHS) Office of Inspector General's (OIG's) and the Federal Bureau of Investigation's enforcement activities. Section 201(b) establishes the Health Care Fraud and Abuse Control Account within the Medicare Trust Fund. Under the legislation, this account will receive proceeds from: (1) criminal fines from "federal health care offenses"; (2) civil money penalties from cases involving Medicare and Medicaid or the peer review provisions; (3) forfeitures of property arising from federal healthcare offenses; and (4) penalties and damages obtained from health-related False Claims Act actions.

Section 201 of HIPAA also creates the Fraud and Abuse Control Program through which Congress grants the OIG and the U.S. Attorney General joint authority to coordinate federal, state, and local law enforcement programs to control all healthcare fraud and abuse. Section 203 mandates the creation of a program to encourage individuals to report suspected fraud and abuse violations. The Secretary of HHS is directed to establish a program for encouraging individuals to report persons who are, or have been, engaged in any activity that constitutes fraud and abuse against Medicare.

Sections 241 through 250 of HIPAA revise the federal criminal law to provide for a federal healthcare offense relating to a healthcare benefit program. The definition of healthcare benefit program includes federal healthcare programs and "any public or private plan or contract, affecting commerce, under which any medical benefit, item, or service is provided to any individual, and includes any individual or entity who is providing a medical benefit, item, or service for which payment may be made under the plan or contract."

Reprinted from: AHIMA. 1998 (January). Advocating for Quality Documentation and Adherence to Official Coding Guidelines. Journal of American Health Information Management Association 69(1):insert before p.49.

HIPAA establishes new criminal provisions covering a wide range of activities: healthcare fraud, theft, or embezzlement in connection with healthcare; false statements relating to healthcare matters; obstruction of criminal investigations of healthcare offenses; and laundering of monetary instruments related to a federal healthcare offense.

Section 231 of HIPAA increases the intent standard that the government must meet for civil monetary penalties. To establish liability, the government must demonstrate that the defendant "knowingly" submitted false claims. Knowingly is defined so that one may be liable if a false claim or statement is made: (1) with actual knowledge that it is false; (2) in deliberate ignorance of the truth or falsity of the information; or (3) in reckless disregard of the truth or falsity of the information.

In the regulatory arena, OIG expects to complete more than 100 reviews of various healthcare providers, including hospitals, physicians, home health care agencies, clinical labs, and managed care plans to detect whether they are correctly billing the Medicare and Medicaid program for services. The healthcare fraud and abuse initiative, Operation Restore Trust, will add twelve mores states to the five already targeted by the two-year-old program. The program focuses on home health providers, nursing homes, and durable medical equipment suppliers.

During the past several months, the federal government has instituted the second half of its enforcement activities concerning billing under Medicare Part B for physician services performed at teaching hospitals. In 1996, the Healthcare Financing Administration (HCFA) [renamed as Centers for Medicare & Medicaid Services (CMS) in 2001] adopted a variety of standards that teaching hospitals must now meet to bill for physician services under Medicare Part B. More recently, OIG announced that it will conduct audits nationwide to evaluate compliance of teaching hospitals in past years with regulatory requirements.

The healthcare field is highly regulated by a complex statutory and regulatory scheme. HIM professionals, at the crossroads of healthcare and information management, are profoundly impacted by the interpretation and implementation of government policy for reimbursement of institutional and provider claims. HIM professionals are uniquely qualified to provide leadership in healthcare organizations to ensure that the documentation in the health record is accurate and appropriate to support the diagnoses and procedures selected for reimbursement.

## Resolution

**Topic:**          Advocating for Quality Documentation and Adherence to Official Coding Guidelines

**Intent:**          Promote the quality of documentation to support the appropriate use of codes for institutional and provider reimbursement

**Addressed to:** All HIM professionals and AHIMA's strategic partners

**Approved by:** 1997 House of Delegates

**Date:**          October 19, 1997

Whereas, detection of healthcare fraud and abuse is a major activity at the federal, state, and local areas of government;

Whereas, ever-changing guidelines for reimbursement impact the ability of healthcare organizations to submit appropriate claims;

Whereas, insurers and payers do not uniformly adhere to official coding guidelines;

Whereas, AHIMA and its component organizations encourage healthcare providers, organizations, insurers, and other appropriate parties to adhere to official coding guidelines in submitting institutional and provider claims for reimbursement;

Whereas, AHIMA members promote accurate and ethical coding; therefore, be it

Resolved, That AHIMA members promote accurate and complete documentation that reflects the level of services provided to the patient and ensure that the HIM profession continues to play a pivotal role in addressing fraud and abuse; and

Resolved, That AHIMA and its component organizations advocate that the federal government and insurers adopt nationwide official coding standards and guidelines used in the development and interpretation of policy for institutional reimbursement and provider claims.

# AHIMA Position Statement on Quality Healthcare Data and Information

## AHIMA's Position

Healthcare data and its transformation into meaningful information should be a central concern for consumers, healthcare providers, the healthcare industry, and the government. Standards, technologies, education, and research are required to capture, use, and maintain accurate healthcare data and facilitate the transition from paper to electronic systems.

## AHIMA Calls for the Following Actions:

- Develop and implement standards for data content, data mapping, and documentation within the healthcare industry.

- Implement continuous quality improvement strategies to support quality data and information.

- Research issues surrounding data variability to quantify their impact and identify solutions.

- Design application technology that supports collection of high-quality data at the point of care, data aggregation, exchange, and retrieval.

- Educate consumers regarding their role in ensuring the quality of healthcare data.

## Rationale

Improving the quality of data, information, and knowledge in the U.S. healthcare system is paramount as we transition from paper to electronic health records. Many errors and adverse incidents in healthcare occur as a result of poor data and information.[1] In addition to threatening patient safety, poor data quality increases healthcare costs and inhibits health information exchange, research, and performance measurement initiatives.[2,3]

---

Revised and Adopted by the AHIMA Board of Directors, October 7, 2006.

Everyone involved with documenting or using health information is responsible for its quality. According to AHIMA's Data Quality Management Model,[4] there are four key processes for data:

- Application—The purpose for which the data are collected

- Collection—The processes by which data elements are accumulated

- Warehousing—The processes and systems used to store and maintain data and data journals

- Analysis—The process of translating data into information utilized for an application

These processes are evaluated with regard to 10 different data characteristics:

- Accuracy—Ensure data are the correct values, valid, and attached to the correct patient record.

- Accessibility—Data items should be easily obtainable and legal to access with strong protections and controls built into the process.

- Comprehensiveness—All required data items are included. Ensure that the entire scope of the data is collected and document intentional limitations.

- Consistency—The value of the data should be reliable and the same across applications.

- Currency—The data should be up to date.

- Definition—Clear definitions should be provided so that current and future data users will know what the data mean. Each data element should have clear meaning and acceptable values.

- Granularity—The attributes and values of data should be defined at the correct level of detail.

- Precision—Data values should be just large enough to support the application or process.

- Relevancy—The data are meaningful to the performance of the process or application for which they are collected.

- Timeliness—Timeliness is determined by how the data are being used and their context.

Unfortunately, the quality of data within an individual organization is essential, but not sufficient. Healthcare enterprises are tasked with integrating multiple systems which may operate according to this data quality model; however, they do not have the ability to share data between applications within the enterprise. Enterprise integration requires a metadata approach with specified enterprise data standards. In addition, the healthcare industry is now facing data interoperability issues between enterprises, requiring universally accepted data standards, such as those being developed by a variety of standards development organizations (e.g., HL7, ASTM, etc.).

Healthcare quality and safety require that the right information be available at the right time to support patient care and health system management decisions. Gaining consensus on essential data content and documentation standards is a necessary prerequisite for high-quality data in the interconnected healthcare system of the future. Further, continuous quality management of data standards and content is key to ensuring that information is useable and actionable.

## Notes

1. Institute of Medicine. To Err is Human: Building a Safer Health System. Washington, DC: National Academy Press, 2000.

2. AHIMA e-HIM Workgroup on EHR Data Content. "Data Standard Time: Data Content Standardization and the HIM Role." Journal of AHIMA 77, no. 1 (2006): 26–32.

3. Crerand, William J., et al. "Building Data Quality into Clinical Trials." Journal of AHIMA 73, no. 10 (2002): 44ff.

4. AHIMA Data Quality Management Task Force. "Practice Brief: Data Quality Management Model." *Journal of AHIMA* 69, no. 6 (1998): p. 2-7 of insert before p. 73.

# Appendix E
# AHIMA Code of Ethics

The following ethical principles are based on the core values of the American Health Information Management Association and apply to all health information management professionals.

Health information management professionals:

I. Advocate, uphold, and defend the individual's right to privacy and the doctrine of confidentiality in the use and disclosure of information.

II. Put service and the health and welfare of persons before self-interest and conduct themselves in the practice of the profession so as to bring honor to themselves, their peers, and to the health information management profession.

III. Preserve, protect, and secure personal health information in any form or medium and hold in the highest regard the contents of the records and other information of a confidential nature, taking into account the applicable statutes and regulations.

IV. Refuse to participate in or conceal unethical practices or procedures.

V. Advance health information management knowledge and practice through continuing education, research, publications, and presentations.

VI. Recruit and mentor students, peers and colleagues to develop and strengthen professional workforce.

VII. Represent the profession accurately to the public.

VIII. Perform honorably health information management association responsibilities, either appointed or elected, and preserve the confidentiality of any privileged information made known in any official capacity.

IX. State truthfully and accurately their credentials, professional education, and experiences.

X. Facilitate interdisciplinary collaboration in situations supporting health information practice.

XI. Respect the inherent dignity and worth of every person.

Revised July 2004.

# AHIMA Standards of Ethical Coding

In this era of payment based on diagnostic and procedural coding, the professional ethics of health information coding professionals continue to be challenged. A conscientious goal for coding and maintaining a quality database is accurate clinical and statistical data. The following standards of ethical coding, developed by the AHIMA Coding Policy and Strategy Committee and approved by the AHIMA Board of Directors, are offered to guide coding professionals in this process.

1. Coding professionals are expected to support the importance of accurate, complete, and consistent coding practices for the production of quality healthcare data.

2. Coding professionals in all healthcare settings should adhere to the ICD-9-CM *(International Classification of Diseases, Ninth Revision, Clinical Modification)* coding conventions, official coding guidelines approved by the Cooperating Parties,* the CPT *(Current Procedural Terminology)* rules established by the American Medical Association, and any other official coding rules and guidelines established for use with mandated standard code sets. Selection and sequencing of diagnoses and procedures must meet the definitions of required data sets for applicable healthcare settings.

3. Coding professionals should use their skills, their knowledge of the currently mandated coding and classification systems, and official resources to select the appropriate diagnostic and procedural codes.

4. Coding professionals should only assign and report codes that are clearly and consistently supported by physician documentation in the health record.

*The Cooperating Parties are the American Health Information Management Association, American Hospital Association, Health Care Financing Administration, and National Center for Health Statistics. All rights reserved. Reprint and quote only with proper reference to AHIMA's authorship.

Reprinted from: AHIMA. 2000 (March). Standards of ethical coding. *Journal of American Health Information Management Association* 71(3): insert after p.8.

5. Coding professionals should consult physicians for clarification and additional documentation prior to code assignment when there is conflicting or ambiguous data in the health record.

6. Coding professionals should not change codes or the narratives of codes on the billing abstract so that the meanings are misrepresented. Diagnoses or procedures should not be inappropriately included or excluded because the payment or insurance policy coverage requirements will be affected. When individual payer policies conflict with official coding rules and guidelines, these policies should be obtained in writing whenever possible. Reasonable efforts should be made to educate the payer on proper coding practices in order to influence a change in the payer's policy.

7. Coding professionals, as members of the healthcare team, should assist and educate physicians and other clinicians by advocating proper documentation practices, further specificity, resequencing or inclusion of diagnoses or procedures when needed to more accurately reflect the acuity, severity and the occurrence of events.

8. Coding professionals should participate in the development of institutional coding policies and should ensure that coding policies complement, not conflict with, official coding rules and guidelines.

9. Coding professionals should maintain and continually enhance their coding skills, as they have a professional responsibility to stay abreast of changes in codes, coding guidelines, and regulations.

10. Coding professionals should strive for the optimal payment to which the facility is legally entitled, remembering that it is unethical and illegal to maximize payment by means that contradict regulatory guidelines.

---

Revised December 1999.

# Appendix F
# Additional Resources

The following are not all-inclusive lists of resources. Numerous vendors, as well as additional organizations, offer compliance-related, benchmarking, and profiling products and services. Use of an Internet search engine is an effective means of finding information on available products and services. Many companies also advertise in healthcare and professional trade publications. Many states have been mandated to collect hospital-level data. Depending on the state, these data may or may not be available to the public. State hospital associations can provide information concerning the availability of comparative data.

Publication of the names of specific vendors does not constitute an endorsement by the AHIMA of any particular product or service.

The Web sites listed in this appendix were current and valid as of the date of publication. However, Web page addresses and the information on them may change or disappear at any time and for any number of reasons. Users are encouraged to perform their own general Web searches to locate any site addresses listed here that are no longer valid.

## Organizations

America's Health Insurance Plans
(202) 778-3200
www.ahip.org

American Health Information Management
Association
(312) 233-1100
www.ahima.org

American Health Lawyers Association
(202) 833-1100
www.healthlawyers.org

American Hospital Association
(312) 422-3000
www.aha.org

American Medical Association
(800) 621-8335
www.ama-assn.org

American Medical Group Association
(703) 838-0033
www.amga.org

Association of American Medical Colleges
(202) 828-0400
www.aamc.org

Association of Healthcare Internal
Auditors
(800) ASK AHIA
www.ahia.org

BlueCross/BlueShield Association
www.bcbs.com

Coalition Against Insurance Fraud
(202) 393-7330
www.insurancefraud.org

Health Care Compliance Association
(888) 580-8373
(952) 988-0141
www.hcca-info.org

Healthcare Billing and Management
Association
(877) 640-HBMA (4262) x203
www.hbma.com

Healthcare Financial Management
Association
(800) 252-HFMA (4362)
(708) 531-0032
www.hfma.org

Medical Group Management
Association
(303) 799-1111
(877) ASK-MGMA (275-6462)
www.mgma.com

National Health Care Anti-Fraud
Association
(202) 659-5955
www.nhcaa.org

Professional Association of Health Care
Office Management
(800) 451-9311
www.pahcom.com

Taxpayers Against Fraud
(202) 296-4826
(800) USFALSE (800)873-2573
www.taf.org

## Other Resources

Central Office on ICD-9-CM
(312) 422-3366
www.ahacentraloffice.org

National Correct Coding Initiative
United States Department of Commerce
National Technical Information Service
(703) 605-6000
www.ntis.gov

To subscribe to the American Medical Association's CPT Information Services
for answers to CPT coding questions:
(800) 621-8335

# Government Web Sites

Centers for Medicare and Medicaid Services: www.cms.gov

CMS' MDS home page: www.cms.hhs.gov/quality/mds30/

CMS' OASIS home page: www.oig.hhs.gov/

HHS Office of Inspector General: www.hhs.gov/oig

Home health PPS: www.cms.hhs.gov/providers/hhapps/

Long-term care hospital PPS: www.cms.hhs.gov/providers/longterm/

Long Term Care Resident Assessment Instrument User's Manual for the Minimum Data Set (MDS): www.cms.hhs.gov/medicaid/mds20/man-form.asp

Medicare manuals: www.cms.hhs.gov/manuals/SaleManuals.asp

Medlearn: www.cms.hhs.gov/medlearn/

National and local Medicare coverage determinations (NCDs and LCDs): www.cms.hhs.gov/mcd

Outpatient PPS: www.cms.hhs.gov/providers/hopps/

Rehabilitation PPS: www.cms.hhs.gov/providers/irfpps/

Skilled nursing facility PPS: www.cms.hhs.gov/providers/snfpps/

# Additional Internet Resources

CART (CMS Abstraction and Reporting Tool): www.qnetexchange.org

HHS Office of Inspector General's RATSTATS program: www.oig.hhs.gov/organization/oas/ratstats/ratstat.pdf

HIPAA rules and other resources: aspe.os.dhhs.gov/admnsimp/

Medicare Hospital Manual: www.cms.hhs.gov/manuals/10_hospital/ho00.asp

National Practitioner Data Bank and Health Care Integrity and Protection Data Bank: www.npdb-hipdb.com

Texas Medical Foundation Health Quality Institute (Hospital Payment Monitoring Program): www.tmf.org

OIG document titled *The Audit Process* oig.hhs.gov/organization/OAS/OIGAuditProcess.pdf

# Listservs

American Health Lawyers Association Compliance listserv: To subscribe, go to www.healthlawyers.org/listserves/manager/ and check off "Compliance."

Fraud-l: To subscribe, go to http://www.compliancealert.net and click on "Join the Fraud and Abuse Listserv."

## Sources of Comparative Data

Comparative data are necessary to establish internal coding data monitors. Data may be obtained from a variety of sources, usually for a charge. Many private companies offer access to giant databases, often in a user-friendly electronic format. Many states, through state data organizations or hospital associations, release claims data for all payers. Peer review organizations often provide comparative data reports. The most notable comparative data are Medicare MedPar data, which can be obtained from CMS at www.cms.hhs.gov/statistics/medpar/default.asp.

The PEPPER reports, which provide short-term, acute care hospitals with summary statistics of administrative claims on CMS target areas, are available from your QIO.

CMS also provides some public-use files free of charge. These can be accessed from CMS' home page at www.cms.hhs.gov/providers/pufdownload/default.asp#carrpuf. CMS' interim resource-based practice expense data files, CPT Procedure Code Utilization by Specialty, can be accessed at www.cms.hhs.gov/physicians/pfs/resource.asp.

Other sources of health data include:

- American Hospital Directory (www.ahd.com)
  *Analysis of facility-specific financial and DRG data*

- Data Advantage (www.data-advantage.com)
  *Comparative healthcare information products*

- Solucient (www.solucient.com) (800) 366-7526
  *Hospital benchmarking and profiling products*

- The MEDSTAT Group (www.medstat.com/) (734) 913-3000
  *Hospital benchmarking and profiling products*

- Iameter Inc. (www.iameter.com/) (650) 349-9100/(770) 279-8767
  *Hospital benchmarking and profiling products*

- National Center for Health Statistics (www.cdc.gov/nchs)
  *Data warehouse*

- National Health Information Resource Center (www.nhirc.org)
  *Links to sixty health data sites*

- QuadraMed Corporation (www.quadramed.com/) QUADRAMED (800) 393-0278
  *Hospital benchmarking*

In addition, the National Association of Health Data Organizations (www.nahdo.org) has published two books with information on health data sources: *State Health Data Resource Manual: Hospital Discharge Data Systems* and *A Guide to State-level Ambulatory Care Data Collection Activities.*

# Books and Journal Articles

The following list contains all references cited in the chapters of this book, resources used in developing the text, and additional items of interest.

Abraham, P.R. 2001 (May). Trends to watch in home health compliance. *Journal of American Health Information Management Association* 72(5):47.

Abraham, P.R. 2001. *Documentation and Reimbursement for Home Care and Hospice Programs.* Chicago: AHIMA.

Abraham, P.R., and R. Gottschalk. 2004. *ICD-9-CM Diagnostic Coding for Long-Term Care and Home Care.* Chicago: AHIMA.

AHIMA e-HIM Work Group on Computer-Assisted Coding. 2004 (November–December). Practice brief: Delving into computer-assisted coding. *Journal of American Health Information Management Association* (76)10:48A–H (with web extras).

AHIMA e-HIM Work Group on Maintaining the Legal EHR. 2005 (November-December). Update: Maintaining a legally sound health record—Paper and electronic. *Journal of American Health Information Management Association* 76(10):64A–L.

AHIMA Workgroup on Electronic Health Records Management. 2004 (October). The strategic importance of electronic health records management. Appendix A: Issues in electronic health records management. *Journal of American Health Information Management Association* 75(9):web extra.

AHIMA's Coding Policy and Strategy Committee. 2001. Payer's Guide to Healthcare Diagnostic and Procedural Data Quality. Available online from ahima.org.

Amatayakul, M., M. Brandt, and M. Dougherty. 2003 (October). Cut, copy, paste: EHR guidelines. *Journal of American Health Information Management Association* 72(9):72, 74.

American Health Information Management Association. 2001 (February). AHIMA position statement: Privacy official. Available online from www.ahima.org.

American Health Information Management Association. 2004. Code of Ethics. Available online from ahima.org.

American Health Information Management Association. 2004. Lifelong Learning Resolution. Available online from http://campus.ahima.org/.

American Health Information Management Association. 2006 (May 30). AHIMA's Coding Program Curriculum Guide. Available online from http://www.ahima.org/academics/documents/CEPAManualMay2006.doc.

American Health Information Management Association. Help wanted: Privacy officer. 2001 (June). *Journal of American Health Information Management Association* 72(6):37–39.

American Health Information Management Association. n.d. AHIMA's Internet-based Coding Assessment and Training Solutions. Distance education course catalog available online from http://campus.ahima.org/campus/catalog/catalog_all.htm.

American Health Information Management Association. n.d. Approved coding education programs. Available online from http://www.ahima.org/careers/college_search/search.asp.

American Health Information Management Association. n.d. Certification standards. Available online from http://www.ahima.org/certification/.

American Medical Association. 2006. *Current Procedural Terminology.* Chicago: AMA

American Medical Association. 2006. *International Classification of Diseases.* Chicago: American Medical Association.

American Psychiatric Association. 2000. *Diagnostic and Statistical Manual of Mental Disorders, Fourth Edition, Text Revision*. Arlington, VA: American Psychiatric Publishing.

Becker, J. 2002. GA Modifier. Document posted to AHIMA LCDs/LMRPs Community of Practice, Community Resources (proprietary content). Available online from https://www.ahimanet.org/COP/LocalCoverageDecisionsLMRPs?CFID=5466476&CFTOKEN=70106793.

Becker, J. 2002. GZ Modifier. Document posted to AHIMA LCDs/LMRPs Community of Practice, Community Resources (proprietary content). Available online from https://www.ahimanet.org/COP/LocalCoverageDecisionsLMRPs?CFID=5466476&CFTOKEN=70106793.

Cahaba GBA. 2006 (August). Coverage guidelines for home health agencies: Medicare fiscal intermediary. Available online from https://www.cahabagba.com/part_a/education_and_outreach/educational_materials/hh_coverage.pdf.

Cahaba GBA. 2006 (March 28). What happened to the HHABN?!? Created under contract for Centers for Medicare and Medicaid Services.

Campbell, J. 2002 (Oct.). Key compliance strategies for the physician practice. *Proceedings from the AHIMA 2002 National Convention, San Francisco*. Chicago: AHIMA.

Centers for Medicare and Medicaid Services. 2006. IPF PPS Overview. Available online from http://www.cms.hhs.gov/InpatientPsychFacilPPS/.

Centers for Medicare and Medicaid Services. 2006 (Jan. 23). Medicare Program: Inpatient Psychiatric Facilities Prospective Payment System Payment Update for Rate Year Beginning July 1, 2006 (RY 2007), Proposed Rule. 42 CFR Parts 412 and 424. *Federal Register* 71(14):3616–3752. Available online from http://a257.g.akamaitech.net/7/257/2422/01jan20061800/edocket.access.gpo.gov/2006/pdf/06-488.pdf.

Centers for Medicare and Medicaid Services. 2006 (Jan. 13). Teaching physician services. Pub 100-04: Medicare claims processing, transmittal 811. Available online from http://www.cms.hhs.gov/transmittals/downloads/R811CP.pdf.

Centers for Medicare and Medicaid Services. 2006 (Jan. 4). Prospective payment systems: General information. HIPPS codes. Available online from http://www.cms.hhs.gov/ProspMedicareFeeSvcPmtGen/02_HIPPSCodes.asp.

Centers for Medicare and Medicaid Services. 2005. OASIS user's manual. Available online from http://www.cms.hhs.gov/OASIS/.

Centers for Medicare and Medicaid Services. 2005 (Dec. 14). Elements of LTCH PPS. Available online from http://www.cms.hhs.gov.

Centers for Medicare and Medicaid Services. 2005 (Nov. 10). Medicare program; changes to the hospital outpatient prospective payment system and calendar year 2006 payment rates; final rule. *Federal Register*. 70(217):68515–9040. Available online from http://a257.g.akamaitech.net/7/257/2422/01jan20051800/edocket.access.gpo.gov/2005/pdf/05-22136.pdf.

Centers for Medicare and Medicaid Services. 2005 (Sept. 7). *Medicare Coverage Issues Manual*. Publication no. 06. Available online from http://www.cms.hhs.gov/Manuals/PBM/list.asp.

Centers for Medicare and Medicaid Services. 2005 (Aug. 26). *Medicare Program Integrity Manual*. Publication no. 100-08 Available online from http://www.cms.hhs.gov/Manuals/IOM/list.asp.

Centers for Medicare and Medicaid Services. 2005 (Aug. 12). Medicare benefit policy manual, Pub. 100-2, revision 27. Chapter 7: Home health services, item 30.1: Confined to the home. Available online from http://www.cms.hhs.gov/Manuals/.

Centers for Medicare and Medicaid Services. 2005 (Aug. 11). Medicare benefit policy manual, home health services. CMS Pub. 100-02, Ch 7 30.1. Available online from www.cms.hhs.gov/Manuals/iom/list.asp.

Centers for Medicare and Medicaid Services. 2004 (Dec. 17). CMS Manual System, Pub 100-04 Medicare Claims Processing, Transmittal 407, Change Request 3633. Available online from cms.hhs.gov/transmittals/downloads/R407CP.pdf.

Centers for Medicare and Medicaid Services. 2004 (Nov. 15). Medicare Program: Prospective Payment System for Inpatient Psychiatric Facilities, Final Rule. 42 CFR Parts 412 and 413. *Federal Register* 69(219):66922–67015. Available online from http://a257.g.akamaitech.net/7/257/2422/15nov20040800/edocket.access.gpo.gov/2004/pdf/04-24787.pdf.

Centers for Medicare and Medicaid Services. 2004 (Oct. 29). CMS Manual System, Pub 100-04 Medicare Claims Processing, Transmittal 347, Change Request 3503. Available online from cms.hhs.gov/transmittals/downloads/R347CP.pdf

Centers for Medicare and Medicaid Services. 2004 (June 25). CMS Manual System, Pub 100-04 Medicare Claims Processing, Transmittal 221, Change Request 3503. Available online from cms.hhs.gov/transmittals/downloads/R347CP.pdf

Centers for Medicare and Medicaid Services. 2004 (June). Long-term care hospital interrupted stay fact sheet. Available online from http://www.cms.hhs.gov/LongTermCareHospitalPPS/Downloads/interrupted_stay_fs.pdf.

Centers for Medicare and Medicaid Services. 2003 (Nov. 7). Medicare Program: Review of national coverage determinations and local coverage determinations, Final Rule. 42 CFR Parts 400, 405, and 426. *Federal Register* 68(216): 63692–731. Available online from www.access.gpo.gov/su_docs/fedreg/a031107c.html.

Centers for Medicare and Medicaid Services. 2003 (March 13). Program Memorandum—Carriers. Transmittal B-03-021, change request 2619. Provider education regarding home health consolidated billing (HH CB) and provider liability, Pub. 60B. Available online from http://www.cms.hhs.gov/transmittals/Downloads/b03021.pdf.

Centers for Medicare and Medicaid Services. 2002 (Nov. 22). Carriers Manual, Part 3—Claims Process, Transmittal 1780. Available online from cms.hhs.gov/Transmittals/Downloads/R1780B3.pdf.

Centers for Medicare and Medicaid Services. 2002 (November). LTCH PPS training guide. Available online from http://www.cms.hhs.gov.

Centers for Medicare and Medicaid Services. 2002. (Aug. 30). Medicare program: Prospective payment system for long-term care hospitals, final rule. 42 CFR, Parts 412, 413, and 476. *Federal Register* 67(169):55954–56001. Available online from http://www.cms.hhs.gov/LongTermCareHospitalPPS/downloads/55954-56002.pdf.

Centers for Medicare and Medicaid Services. 2001 (Sept. 26). Program memorandum, intermediaries/carriers: ICD-9-CM coding for diagnostic tests. Transmittal AB-01-144. Available online from http://www.cms.hhs.gov/Transmittals/downloads/AB01144.pdf.

Centers for Medicare and Medicaid Services. n.d. GA and GZ Modifiers. Available online from cms.hhs.gov.

Centers for Medicare and Medicaid Services. n.d. Medicare Provider Analysis and Review (MEDPAR) File. Available online from http://www.cms.hhs.gov/IdentifiableDataFiles/05_MedicareProviderAnalysisandReviewFile.asp.

Centers for Medicare and Medicaid Services. n.d. Medlearn. Available online from http://www.cms.hhs.gov/MLNGenInfo/.

Civil Monetary Penalties Law, 42 USC § 1320a-7a.

Drach, M., A. Davis, and C. Sagrati. 2001 (January). Ten steps to successful chargemaster reviews. *Journal of American Health Information Management Association* 72(1):42–48.

Dunn, R.T. 2003 (Nov. 14). ABNs: Always been neglected. AHIMA Community of Practice resource. Available online from www.ahima.org.

Equal Employment Opportunity Commission. n.d. Federal equal employment opportunity (EEO) laws. Available online from http://www.eeoc.gov/abouteeo/overview_laws.html.

Estrella, R. 2003 (July-August). What happened to PEPP? QIOs plan for hospital payment monitoring program. *Journal of American Health Information Management Association* 74(7):43-48.

Foundation of Research and Education of AHIMA. 2005 (July 11). Automated coding software: Development and use to enhance anti-fraud activities. HHS contract no. HHSP23320054100EC. Chicago: AHIMA.

Foundation of Research and Education of AHIMA. 2005 (Sept. 30). Use of health information technology to enhance and expand health care anti-fraud activities. HHS contract number: HHSP23320054100EC. Chicago: AHIMA.

Garvin, J.H., S. Moeini, and V. Watzlaf. 2006 (March). Fighting fraud, automatically: How coding automation can prevent healthcare fraud. *Journal of American Health Information Management Association* 77(3):32–36.

Government Accountability Office. 2005 (Dec. 15). Information on false claims act litigation: Briefing for Congressional requesters. Document no. GAO-06-320R. Available online from http://www.gao.gov/new.items/d06320r.pdf.

Government Accountability Office. 2001 (June 27). Health care: Consultants' billing advice may lead to improperly paid insurance claims. GAO-01-818. Available online from www.gao.gov/new.items/d01818.pdf.

Government Accountability Office. 1999 (April). Medicare: Early evidence of compliance effectiveness is inconclusive. GAO/HEHS-99-59. Available online from www.gao.gov/archive/1999/he99059.pdf.

Glondys, B. 2003 (May). Practice Brief: Ensuring legibility of patient records. *Journal of American Health Information Management Association* 74(5):64A–D.

Green-Shook, S. 2004 (October). *IFHRO Congress and AHIMA Convention Proceedings,* Washington, D.C.

Hammen, C. 2001 (October). Choosing consultants without compromising compliance. *Journal of American Health Information Management Association* 72(9):26, 28, 30.

Hanna, J. 2002 (July-August). Constructing a coding compliance plan. *Journal of American Health Information Management Association* 73(7):48–56.

Hanson, S.P., and B.S. Cassidy. 2006 (March). Fraud control: New tools, new potential. *Journal of American Health Information Management Association* 77(3):24–27, 30.

Health Care Compliance Association. 2003 (April 4). Evaluating and improving a compliance program: A resource for health care board members, health care executives, and compliance officers. Available online from http://www.hcca-info.org/Content/NavigationMenu/ComplianceResources/EvaluationImprovement/Eval-Improve03.pdf.

Health Care Financing Administration. 2000 (July 3). Medicare program; prospective payment system for home health agencies; final rule. 42 CFR 409, 410, 411, 413, 424, and 484. Federal Register 65(128):41127–214.

Hornung Garvin, J., S. Moeini, and V. Watzlaf. 2006 (March). Fighting fraud, automatically: How coding automation can prevent healthcare fraud. *Journal of American Health Information Management Association* 77(3):32–36.

Hull, S. 2003 (June). Long-term care hospital PPS creates opportunity for coders: Proposed rule addresses related coding issues. *Journal of American Health Information Management Association* 74(6):58–60.

Iowa Foundation for Medical Care. 1999–2001. MDS download. Available online from https://www.qtso.com/mdsdownload.html.

Jones, L. 2005. *Coding and Reimbursement for Hospital Outpatient Services.* Chicago: AHIMA.

Kaldal, K. 1998 (November-December). Benchmarks as the signposts on the fraud case trail. *Journal of American Health Information Management Association* 69(10):44–45.

King, E. 1998 (January). Playing a part: The FBI's role in healthcare fraud investigations. *Journal of American Health Information Management Association* 69(1):43.

Kuehn, L. 2001 (Oct.). Unlock the information secrets in your billing database. Proceedings from the AHIMA 2001 National Convention, Miami.

Kuehn, L. 2006. *CPT/HCPCS Coding and Reimbursement for Physician Services.* Chicago: AHIMA.

LeBlanc, M.M. 2006. Work design and performance improvement. Chapter 23 in LaTour, K., and S. Eichenwald *Health Information Management: Concepts, Principles, and Practice,* 2nd ed. Chicago: AHIMA.

*Lutwin v. Thompson,* 361 F.3d. 136(2d.Cir 2004).

Medical Group Management Association. n.d. Education/events. Available online from http://www.mgma.com/education/index.cfm.

Medicare Payment Advisory Commission. 2006 (March). Report to Congress: Medicare payment policy. Section 4D: Inpatient rehabilitation facility services. Available online from medpac.gov.

Micheletti, J.A., Shlala, T.J. 2006 (February). Documentation Rx: Strategies for Improving Physician Contribution to Hospital Records. *Journal of American Health Information Management Association* 77(2): 66–68.

Neville, D., and F. Katz. 2001 (May). Six steps to compliance for small practices. *Journal of American Health Information Management Association* 72(5):40–44.

Office of the Deputy Attorney General. 1998 (June 3). Memo: Guidance on the use of the false claims act in civil health matters. Available online from http://www.usdoj.gov/dag/readingroom/chcm.htm.

Office of Inspector General. 2006. Work Plan, fiscal year 2007. Available online from http://www.oig.hhs.gov/publications/docs/workplan/2007/Work%20Plan%202007.pdf.

Office of Inspector General. 2006 (March). Consultations in Medicare: Coding and reimbursement. Document no. OEI-09-02-00030. Available online from http://oig.hhs.gov/oei/reports/oei-09-02-00030.pdf.

Office of Inspector General. 2006 (January). Review of billing under the home health prospective payment system for therapy services. Document no. A-07-04-01010. Available online from http://www.oig.hhs.gov/oas/reports/region7/70401010.pdf.

Office of Inspector General. 2006 (January). Effect of the home health prospective payment system on the quality of home health care. Document no. OEI-01-04-00160. Available online from http://oig.hhs.gov/oei/reports/oei-09-02-00030.pdf.

Office of Inspector General. 2006. Work plan, fiscal year 2006. Available online from http://oig.hhs.gov/publications/docs/workplan/2007/Work%20Plan%202007.pdf.

Office of Inspector General. 2005 (Jan. 31). OIG supplemental compliance program guidance for hospitals. *Federal Register* 70(19): 4858–76. Available online from http://a257.g.akamaitech.net/7/257/2422/01jan20051800/edocket.access.gpo.gov/2005/pdf/05-1620.pdf.

Office of Inspector General. 2001 (June). Special Advisory Bulletin: Practices of business consultants. Available at http://oig.hhs.gov/fraud/docs/alertsandbulletins/consultants.pdf.

Office of Inspector General. 2000 (Oct. 5). OIG Compliance Program Guidance for Individual and Small Group Physician Practices. *Federal Register* 65(194):59434-52. Available online from http://oig.hhs.gov/authorities/docs/physician.pdf.

Office of Inspector General. 1998 (Feb. 23). OIG Compliance Program Guidance for Hospitals. *Federal Register* 63(35):8987–98. Available online from http://oig.hhs.gov/authorities/docs/cpghosp.pdf.

Office of Inspector General. 2006 (February). A review of nursing facility resource utilization groups. Report no. OEI-02-02-00830. Available online from http://www.oig.hhs.gov/oei/reports/oei-02-02-00830.pdf.

Office of Inspector General. n.d. Background on Civil Monetary Penalties. Available online from http://oig.hhs.gov/fraud/enforcement/administrative/cmp/cmp.html.

Office of Inspector General. n.d. Office of Audit Services, RAT-STATS program. Available online from http://www.oig.hhs.gov/organization/OAS/ratstat.html.

Office of Inspector General. 1998 (Aug. 24). OIG compliance program guidance for clinical laboratories. *Federal Register* 63(163):45076–87. Available online from oig.hhs.gov/authorities/docs/cpglab.pdf.

Office of Inspector General. 1998 (Dec. 18). OIG compliance program guidance for third party medical billing companies. *Federal Register* 63(243):70138-52. Available online from oig.hhs.gov/fraud/docs/complianceguidance/thirdparty.pdf.

Office of Inspector General. 2000 (Oct. 5). OIG compliance program for individual and small group physician practices. *Federal Register* 65(194): 59434–52. Available online from oig.hhs.gov/authorities/docs/physician.pdf.

Ortquist, S., and S. Vacca. 2004 (January). Evaluating compliance program effectiveness. *Journal of American Health Information Management Association* 75(1):74–75.

Prophet, S. 2001 (October). Practice brief: Developing a physician query process. *Journal of American Health Information Management Association* 72(9):88I–M.

Prophet, S. 2001 (October). Practice brief: Developing a physician query process. *Journal of American Health Information Management Association* 72(9):88I–M.

Prophet-Bowman, S. 2003 (March). Observation services present compliance challenges: Know these complex, changing requirements to avoid risk. *Journal of American Health Information Management Association* 74(3):60–65.

Rollins, G. 2006 (March). Following the digital trail: Weak auditing functions spell trouble for an electronic record. *Journal of American Health Information Management Association* 77(3):38–41.

Russo, R. 1998. *Seven Steps to HIM Compliance.* Marblehead, MA: Opus Communications.

Scichilone, R. 2004 (June 7). AHIMA home health services coding and reporting. Handouts from Continuing Education online course, Reimbursement Methods, Lesson 3.

Scichilone, R. 2002 (February). Best practices for medical necessity validation. *Journal of American Health Information Management Association* 73(2):48, 50.

Skurka, M.A. 2001 (July-August). Navigating the physician services maze. *Journal of American Health Information Management Association* 72(7):51–58.

Stanfill, M. 2003 (October). Strategies for effective auditing of physician evaluation and management services. *Proceedings of the AHIMA 2003 National Convention, San Francisco.*

Stewart, M.M. 2001. *Coding and Reimbursement under the Outpatient Prospective Payment System.* Chicago: AHIMA.

Tegan, A., et al. 2005 (May). The EHR's impact on HIM functions. *Journal of American Health Information Management Association* 76(5):56C–H.

TMF Health Quality Institute. 2005 (December). Hospital payment monitoring program compliance workbook. Available online from http://www.tmf.org/hpmp/tools/workbook/.

Williams, A. 2006 (February). Design for better data: How software and users interact onscreen matters to data quality. *Journal of American Health Information Management Association* 77(2):56–60.

# Index

Clinical Laboratory Improvement Amendments
(CLIA) certification levels, 128
CMS-1500 forms for repeat visits by same
patient, comparisons of, 142
Code assignments, 41–42
assessing accuracy of, 117. *See also* Coding
accuracy
Code changes, requests for, 29
Code jamming, 43, 193–94
Code of conduct, HIM, 11
Codes
assigned based on physician documentation,
30
crosswalk of diagnostic to reimbursement
behavioral care, 233–38
crosswalk of services to behavioral care,
238–39
maximization versus optimization of, 11
triggers for compliance review from illogical
patterns or changes in use of, 16
Coding accuracy
comparing code assignments with criteria and
documentation to assess, 117
factors to consider in monitoring, 86
reviews of, 71–72, 80–81
scope of, 71
standards for, 28
Coding advice, clarification of, 28
Coding and billing procedures and tools,
compliance issues for, 129
Coding assessment
compliance with EEOC guidelines for, 63
internal or external conduct of, 81
Coding certificate programs, 62
AHIMA-approved, 63
*Coding Clinic for ICD-9-CM*
interactive discussions of, 68
quarterly publication of, 201
situations appropriate for physician queries
listed in, 31
support of ICD-9-CM codes using advice and
directions from, 201
Coding compliance committee, 12
Coding policies and procedures
internal, 18
payment policies affecting code assignment
incorporated in, 34
Coding positions
in HIM compliance program, 8
qualifications for, 61–64
Coding practices, internal, 24–37
evaluation of, 73
Coding process
education on, 68
policies and procedures for, 26–28

Coding resources, 25–26, 129
Coding skills
assessing job candidate's, 63
insufficient, 70
Coding software, automating, 101–5
Comorbidities, 164, 167, 253
mental health DRG adjustment factors for,
234, 236
Compliance
areas of vulnerability for, 82
as element of performance review, 58
evidence of, 6
impact of EHRs on HIM, 95–111
Compliance considerations
in behavioral health facilities, 231–57
for computer-assisted coding technology, 103,
121
for physician practices, 125–44
Compliance guidance for all healthcare settings,
1–111
supplemental, 113–259
Compliance officer, involvement in design of
educational programs by, 68
Compliance program effectiveness, auditing,
88–93
Compliance program, HIM
addressing EHR issues in, 95–101
AHIMA development of model, 3
benefits of, 79
benefits of LTCH, 226
clarification of policies and procedures in, 13
coding and documentation in, 8
communication of violations of, 12–14
communication, productivity, and efficiency
in, 8
components of, 64, 103–4, 228–29
education in, 8, 66, 104
elements of, 9–20
enforcement of, 14–15
ethical practices in, 8–9
internal controls improved by, 7
interrupted stay processes in, 227
model, 4–5
oversight of, 11–12
overview of, 7–20
problem resolution and corrective action for,
15–20
reimbursement regulations and policies in,
3–4
training of newly hired coding professionals
in, 64
Compliance programs
assessing effectiveness of, 89–91
challenges for physicians in implementing, 143
*(continued on next page)*

management, 156–57
scheduled, 157
Mission statement, HIM, 10–11
Modifiers
    25, 122–23, 130, 135, 136
    59, 122–23, 130, 172
    CA, 120
    GA, 131
    GZ, 131, 132
Monitoring for improvement, 140–41

National Correct Coding Initiative (NCCI) edits
    CMS use for OPPS claims of, 116, 120
    modifiers used to inappropriately bypass, 123, 130
National coverage determinations (NCDs)
    publication of, 41
    resources for, 22
National Uniform Billing Committee, 25
National Uniform Claims Committee, 25
Nationwide Health Information Network (NHIN), 95
Natural language processing (NLP), 102
    combining automated coding with, 102
Noncompliance, reporting violations to government authorities for, 19
Notice of Medicare Provider Noncoverage, 197–200
Nursing home deficiencies related to MDS assessments and care planning, 150

Observation reporting, 121–22
Office of Audit Services Statistical Sampling Software, 75
Office of Inspector General (OIG) (HHS), 15
    audit recommendations by, 136, 139
    Compliance Program Guidance for Clinical Laboratories, 126, 129
    Compliance Program Guidance for Hospitals of, 38, 88
    Compliance Program Guidance for Individual and Small Group Physician Practices of, 125–26
    Compliance Program Guidance for Third-Party Medical Billing Companies of, 126
    compliance risks of IT noted by, 106
    "Effect of the Home Health PPS on the Quality of Home Health Care" study of, 183–84
    error rate in outpatient mental health services studied by, 233, 239
    guidance for physicians of, 125–26
    operating components of, 183
    physician office studies by, 140–41
    RAT-STATS of, 75
    resources identifying high-risk areas by, 22

"Review of Nursing Facility Resource Utilization Groups, A" report by, 147–48
    studies of error, code misuse, and fraud by, 130, 140
    subpoenas by, 191
    Supplemental Compliance Program Guidance (SCPG) of, 4, 26, 106, 119–21
    target areas for compliance of, 87, 242
    work plan of, 140, 148–50, 167, 183–84, 225, 242–43
Office of the National Coordinator for Health Information Technology (ONC) of HHS, reports of, 106–11
Official coding guidelines (Cooperating Parties), ICD-9-CM, 24
    facility-specific coding guidelines compatible with, 27
    HIPAA requirements for adherence to, 35, 45, 59
Outcome and assessment information set (OASIS), 175–79
    data elements of, 176
    documentation requirements of, 175
    as patient assessment instrument for home health agencies, 25
    purposes of, 175
Outcome and assessment information set (OASIS) assessments
    follow-up and transfer, 179
    locked, 192
Outpatient prospective payment system (OPPS), hospital
    actions to ensure compliance with requirements of, 116–18
    claims processing for, 116
    Final Rule for each year of, 120, 121
    implementation of, 115
Outpatient rehab providers, consolidated billing for, 190
Outpatient rehabilitation, 170–72
    certification and recertification of therapy for, 171
    documentation to support claim for, 172
    units billed for, 171–72
    written treatment plan required for reimbursement of, 170–71
Outpatient services, hospital, 115–24
Outsourced coding staff, 58
Overcoding, identifying, 143
Overpayments, 23
    audit results identifying problem with, 80
    refunding identified, 19

Paraprofessionals in service delivery, 241–43
Partial hospitalization program, billing under, 121